Phytotherapy in the Management of Diabetes and Hypertension

(Volume 3)

Edited by

Mohamed Eddouks

Faculty of Sciences and Techniques Errachidia
Moulay Ismail University of Meknes
Errachidia
Morocco

Phytotherapy in the Management of Diabetes and Hypertension

Volume # 3

Editor: Mohamed Eddouks

ISSN (Online): 2452-3232

ISSN (Print): 2452-3224

ISBN (Online): 978-981-14-5913-9

ISBN (Print): 978-981-14-5911-5

ISBN (Paperback): 978-981-14-5912-2

need for a court order if at any point you breach any terms of this License Agreement. In no event will any delay or failure by Bentham Science Publishers in enforcing your compliance with this License Agreement constitute a waiver of any of its rights.

3. You acknowledge that you have read this License Agreement, and agree to be bound by its terms and conditions. To the extent that any other terms and conditions presented on any website of Bentham Science Publishers conflict with, or are inconsistent with, the terms and conditions set out in this License Agreement, you acknowledge that the terms and conditions set out in this License Agreement shall prevail.

Bentham Science Publishers Pte. Ltd.
80 Robinson Road #02-00
Singapore 068898
Singapore
Email: subscriptions@benthamscience.net

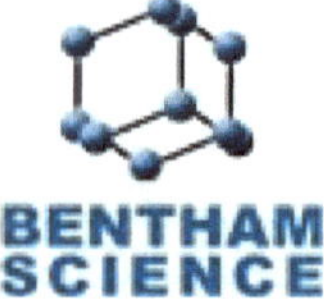

CONTENTS

PREFACE

The volume 1 of the present ebook series "Phytotherapy in the Management of Diabetes and Hypertension" has emphasized the basic Biochemistry of diabetes mellitus and hypertension, and described many aspects of these lifestyle diseases and its control or remediation through a cost effective, safe, easy-going, easy-adaptable method through the age-old practice validated by scientific research. In response to requests from WHO in providing safe and effective herbal medicines for use in national health-care systems and to prepare monographs of used medicinal plants around the world, the volume 2 of this e-book series has been published in 2016 and contained monographs related to antihypertensive and antidiabetic plants. The present volume 3 is dedicated to different aspects including the evaluation of the efficacy and safety of medicinal plants and their derivatives on diabetes and hypertension. The study of the mechanisms of action of medicinal plants is deeply discussed. This volume includes 7 complementary chapters that describe different aspects including the biochemistry of type 2 diabetes, the pathophysiology of diabetes and hypertension, the role of essential oils extracted from medicinal plants in the management of diabetes and hypertension, the mechanistic perspectives of the treatment of diabetes and hypertension, some important phytochemicals with beneficial action on diabetes and hypertension, and detailed monographs concerning some potential medicinal plants used in the treatment of diabetes and hypertension. This volume will be useful to the students, teachers, researchers, scientists, clinicians, herbalists, and even the common people interested to know about the subject.

ACKNOWLEDGMENTS AND GRANTS

The Editor would like to express his thanks to all the authors, the reviewers, and Miss Salma Sarfraz for their special effort during the preparation of this book. This work was supported by the Ministry of National Education, Vocational Training, Higher Education and the Scientific Research (Morocco) and the National Center for Scientific and Technical Research (CNRST) (Morocco) under grant N° PPR/2015/35.

Mohamed Eddouks
Faculty of Sciences and Techniques Errachidia
Moulay Ismail University of Meknes
Errachidia
Morocco

List of Contributors

Adki Kaveri M.
Shobhaben Pratapbhai Patel School of Pharmacy & Technology Management, SVKM's NMIMS, V.L. Mehta Road, Vile Parle (West), Mumbai-400056, India

Agrawal Ojaskumar D.
Shobhaben Pratapbhai Patel School of Pharmacy & Technology Management, SVKM's NMIMS, V.L Mehta Road, Vile Parle (W), Mumbai – 400 056, India
Vivekanand Education Society's College of Pharmacy, University of Mumbai, Chembur (E), Mumbai 400074, India

Cerón-Romero L.
Laboratorio de Farmacología, Facultad de Química, Universidad autónoma de Yucatán, Calle 43 No. 613 x Calle 90 Col. Inalámbrica. C.P. 97069, Mérida, Yucatán, Mexico

Choudhury Manabendra Dutta
Department of Life Science and Bioinformatics, Assam University, Silchar, India

Das Subrata
Department of Life Science and Bioinformatics, Assam University, Silchar, India

Ekambaram Sanmuga Priya
Department of Pharmaceutical Technology, University College of Engineering, BIT Campus, Anna University, Tiruchirappalli – 620 024, Tamil Nadu, India

El Zerey-Belaskri Asma
Laboratoire de recherche Biodiversité végétale: conservation et valorisation, Faculté des Sciences de la nature et de la Vie, Université de Sidi Bel Abbes, Algérie

Erusappan Thamizharasi
Department of Pharmaceutical Technology, University College of Engineering, BIT Campus, Anna University, Tiruchirappalli – 620 024, Tamil Nadu, India

Gaikwad Anil Bhanudas
Department of Pharmacy, Birla Institute of Technology and Science, Pilani, Pilani Campus Pilani- 333031, Rajasthan, India

Hanif Muhammad Asif
Nano and Biomaterials Lab, Department of Chemistry, University of Agriculture, Faisalabad-38040, Pakistan

Kulkarni Yogesh A.
Shobhaben Pratapbhai Patel School of Pharmacy & Technology Management, SVKM's NMIMS, V.L Mehta Road, Vile Parle (W), Mumbai – 400 056, India

Laddha Ankit P.
Shobhaben Pratapbhai Patel School of Pharmacy & Technology Management, SVKM's NMIMS, V.L. Mehta Road, Vile Parle (West), Mumbai-400056, India

Majeed Muhammad Irfan
Department of Chemistry, University of Agriculture, Faisalabad-38040, Pakistan

Nadeem Farwa
Nano and Biomaterials Lab, Department of Chemistry, University of Agriculture, Faisalabad-38040, Pakistan

Nawaz Haq
Nano and Biomaterials Lab, Department of Chemistry, University of Agriculture, Faisalabad-38040, Pakistan

Ningthoujam Sanjoy Singh
Department of Botany, Ghanapriya Women's College, Dhanamanjuri University, Imphal, India

Ortiz-Andrade R.
Laboratorio de Farmacología, Facultad de Química, Universidad autónoma de Yucatán, Calle 43 No. 613 x Calle 90 Col. Inalámbrica. C.P. 97069, Mérida, Yucatán, Mexico

Oza Manisha J.
Shobhaben Pratapbhai Patel School of Pharmacy & Technology Management, SVKM's NMIMS, V.L. Mehta Road, Vile Parle (West), Mumbai-400056, India
SVKM's Dr. Bhanuben Nanavati College of Pharmacy, V.L. Mehta Road, Vile Parle (West), Mumbai-400056, India

Perumal Senthamil Selvan
Department of Pharmaceutical Technology, University College of Engineering, BIT Campus, Anna University, Tiruchirappalli – 620 024, Tamil Nadu, India

Sánchez-Recillas A.
Laboratorio de Farmacología, Facultad de Química, Universidad Autónoma de Yucatán, Calle 43 No. 613 x Calle 90 Col. Inalámbrica. C.P. 97069, Mérida, Yucatán, Mexico

Sarfraz Maliha
Institute of Pharmacy, Physiology and Pharmacology, Department of Physiology and Pharmacology, University of Agriculture, Faisalabad, Pakistan

Talukdar Anupam Das
Department of Life Science and Bioinformatics, Assam University, Silchar, India

CHAPTER 1

Biochemistry of Type 2 Diabetes Mellitus

Ekambaram Sanmuga Priya[*], **Perumal Senthamil Selvan** and **Erusappan Thamizharasi**

Department of Pharmaceutical Technology, University College of Engineering, BIT Campus, Anna University, Tiruchirappalli, India

Abstract: Diabetes mellitus, a metabolic disorder, characterized by chronic hyperglycemia results from defects in insulin secretion, insulin action, or both. Insulin is an anabolic peptide hormone that possesses pleiotropic activity. It can hinder with multiple physiological processes by either upregulating or downregulating various metabolic intracellular pathways. The complex insulin signaling system makes it vital in a variety of biological responses. This chapter describes the biochemistry of type 2 diabetes mellitus, as well as the features underlying its pathophysiology.

Keywords: Diabetes, Glucose Uptake, Insulin, Insulin Receptor, Insulin Resistance, Metabolic Disorder.

INTRODUCTION

Diabetes mellitus (DM), a metabolic disorder, characterized by chronic hyperglycemia results from defects in insulin secretion, insulin action, or both. Diabetes mellitus is classically characterized into two types *viz.*Type 1 diabetes mellitus (T1DM) and Type 2 diabetes mellitus (T2DM). T1DM, which is also known as insulin dependent diabetes mellitus (IDDM), is caused due to deficiency of insulin secretion from β cells of the pancreas. T2DM, which is also known as non-insulin dependent diabetes mellitus (NIDDM), is associated with diminished sensitivity of insulin in target tissues. This reduced sensitivity to insulin is a characteristic of insulin resistance. The reduced insulin levels or the resistance to insulin reduced the uptake of glucose by most of the tissues of the body except the brain [1]. This leads to an increase in blood glucose concentration along with a decrease in utilization of glucose by cells which results in an increase in the utilization of fats and proteins. The clinical features of patients with T1DM and T2DM are shown in Table **1**.

[*] **Corresponding author Ekambaram Sanmuga Priya:** Department of Pharmaceutical Technology, University College of Engineering, BIT Campus, Anna University, Tiruchirappalli, India; E-mail: sanmug77@gmail.com

M. Eddouks (Ed.)

Table 1. Clinical features of patients with T1DM and T2DM [1].

Features	T1DM	T2DM
Age of onset	Usually less than 20 years	Usually greater than 30 years
Body mass	Low (wasted) to normal	Obese
Plasma insulin	Low or absent	Normal to high initially
Plasma glucagon	High, can be suppressed	High, resistant to suppression
Plasma glucose	Increased	Increased
Insulin sensitivity	Normal	Reduced
Therapy	Insulin	Weight loss, thiazolidinediones, metformin, sulfonylureas, insulin, DPP4 inhibitors, PPAR-γ agonists, incretins, SGLT2 inhibitors (canagliflozin, dapagliflozin, empagliflozin, and ertugliflozin)

EPIDEMIOLOGY OF T2DM

The number of people with T2DM is progressively increasing. According to the World Health Organisation (WHO), there were 422 million adults with diabetes worldwide in 2014. The prevalence in adults increased from 4.7% in 1980 to 8.5% in 2014, with a higher increase in low and middle-income countries compared to high-income ones [2]. Further, the International Diabetes Federation (IDF) estimates to have 374 million people at an increased risk of developing T2DM. Without any intervention to slow down this rise in T2DM, there will be at least 700 million people with diabetes by 2045. The demographics of T2DM and the percentage of the population by geographical location are illustrated in Fig. (1). The lower rate of diagnosis of diabetes and the difficult access to diabetes care in low- and middle-income countries lead to 90% of all diabetes-related premature deaths and, 87% of all diabetes-related deaths [3]. Consequently, high blood glucose causes almost 4 million deaths each year [2]. The demographic and geographic outline of diabetes worldwide is shown in Fig. (1).

ETIOLOGY OF T2DM

T2DM, the more prevalent form of diabetes, is a heterogeneous disorder triggered by a multitude of genetic factors related to diminished insulin secretion, insulin resistance and related factors, such as obesity, overeating, sedentary lifestyle, stress and aging [4]. This multifactorial disease involves numerous genes as well as environmental factors [5]. There is an acute need for insulin by the body in T2DM to avoid the ketoacidosis. Predominately it is not an autoimmune disorder. Also, there is no identification of the susceptible genes that may account for a predisposition to T2DM in most patients. This can be accounted to the heterogeneity of the genes accountable for the susceptibility to T2DM.

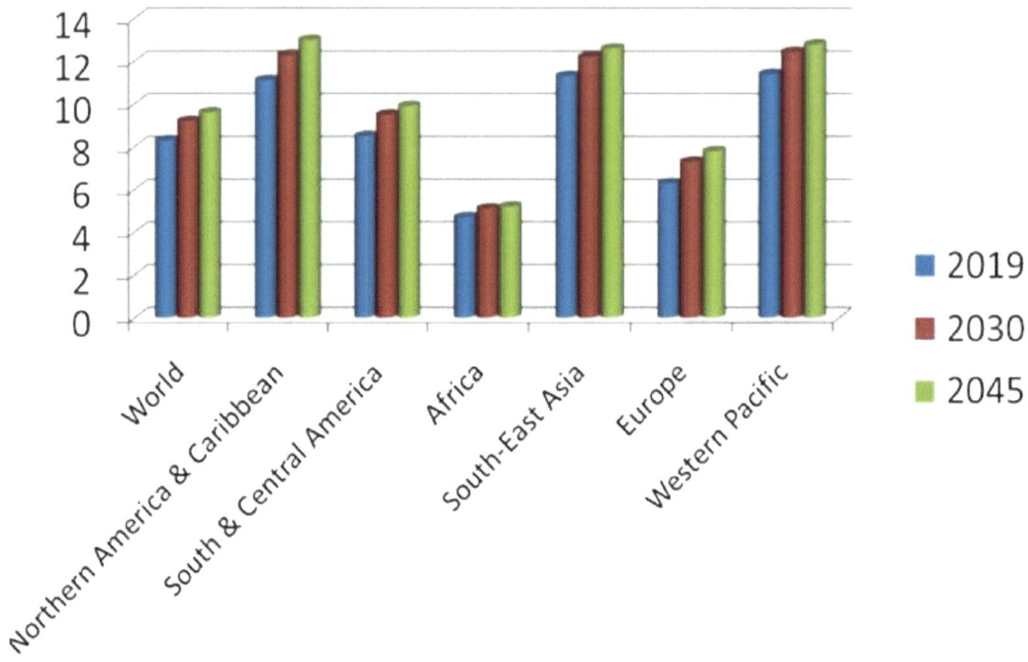

Fig. (1). Demographic and geographic outline of diabetes.

SOME MAJOR CAUSES OF DEVELOPING INSULIN RESISTANCE INCLUDE

1. Obesity, especially accumulation of adipose tissue surrounding the viscera.
2. Mutations in insulin receptor genes.
3. Mutations of the peroxisome proliferator activator receptor-γ (PPAR-γ) genes.
4. Mutations that cause genetic obesity, *e.g.*, melanocortin receptor mutations.
5. Higher glucocorticoids, *e.g.*, Cushing's syndrome or steroid therapy.
6. Higher growth hormone (acromegaly).
7. Pregnancy leading to gestational diabetes.
8. Polycystic ovary disease (PCOD).
9. Hypertension, *i.e.* (≥140/90 mmHg)
10. HDL cholesterol level(<35 mg/dL (0.90 mmol/L) or triglyceride level >250 mg/dL (2.82 mmol/L) or both).
11. Acquired or genetic lipodystrophy associated with accumulation of lipids in liver.
12. Hemochromatosis.

13. Female delivering a baby weighing >9 lb or prior diagnosis of Gestational Diabetes Mellitus [1, 6].

PATHOPHYSIOLOGY OF T2DM

T2DM is characterized by chronic hyperglycemia, which results from a multifactorial interaction between genetic predisposition and environmental factors [7, 8]. T2DM is the more common form of diabetes that accounts for at least 90% of all cases of diabetes mellitus [9]. The rise in prevalence is projected to be much greater in developing (69%) than in developed countries (20%) [10]. Several important pathophysiological studies have highlighted a clear understanding of insulin secretion and resistance in the course of disease onset and progression.

In T2DM, the first step is impaired insulin-stimulated glucose transport in skeletal muscles. The pancreatic β-cells increase the secretion of insulin to compensate for this impaired glucose transport which results into hyperinsulinemia. Thus, peripheral insulin resistance, along with the impaired insulin secretion in late-stage T2DM leads to hyperglycemia Fig. (**2**). At the end stage of T2DM, the inability to inhibit hepatic gluconeogenesis with endogenous insulin is accompanied by a decline of pancreatic β-cell function. The progression towards the severity of T2DM results when the over-secretion of insulin by the β-cell fails to compensate for insulin resistance. The obese euglycemic people have 30% reduced insulin sensitivity compared to lean euglycemic subjects therefore obese euglycemic people show increased insulin secretion to maintain the normal glucose tolerance. This phenomenon is known as "euglycemic hyperinsulinemia". Over the course of time, the obese euglycemic people develop further reduction in insulin sensitivity, which is no longer associated with compensatory hyperinsulinemia. This results in an increased blood glucose concentration termed as "hyperglycemic hyperinsulinemia" [11].

Two different hypotheses are proposed for adipose tissue dysfunction [12]:

1. **The Lipid Burden Hypothesis** PPAR-γ expression, that determines the ability to store triacylglycerol (TAG) is reduced in the adipose tissue of obese individuals. At the same time, the levels of PPAR- γ are elevated in their liver and muscles, which is ectopic. simultaneously, all the tissues like adipose, liver, and muscle tissues becomes less insulin sensitive.
2. **The Role Of Inflammation (The Inflammatory Hypothesis)** In obese individuals, the adipocytes release monocyte chemoattractant protein-1 (MCP-1) due to the overloading of TAG. This MCP-1 attracts macrophages which in-turn release TNF-α and other cytokines, hampering with the insulin signaling.

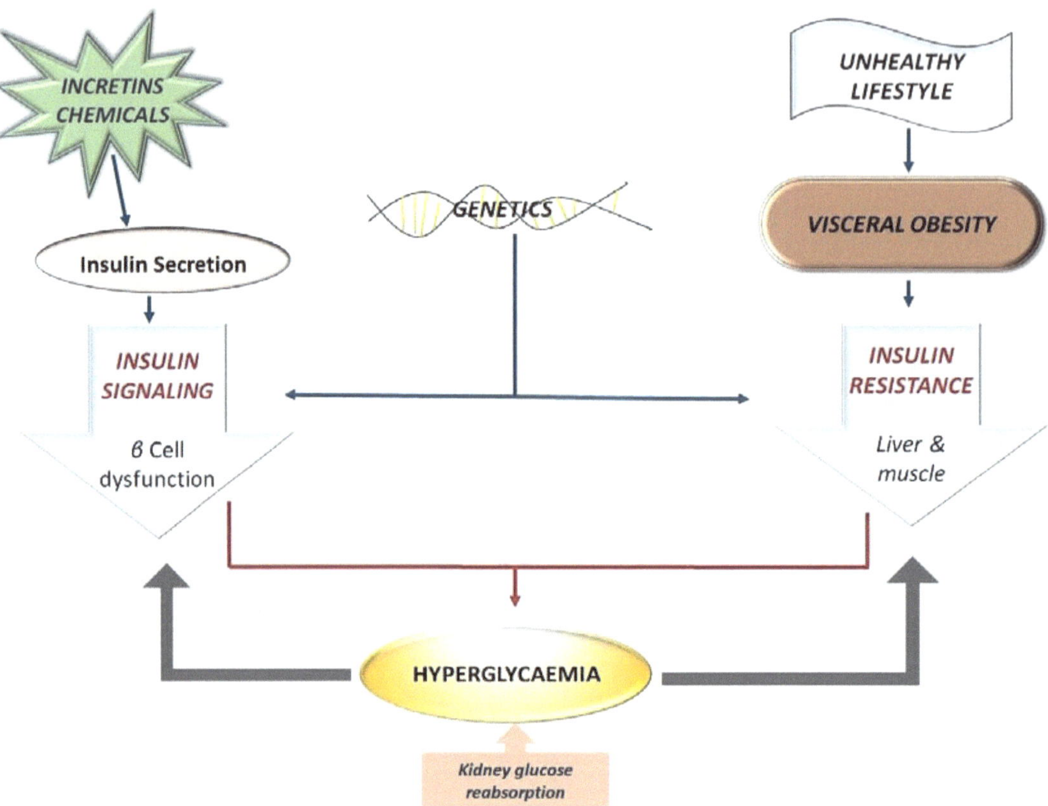

Fig. (2). Pathophysiology of T2DM.

The mechanism of insulin resistance in muscles and liver revolves around the role of the mitochondria. Dysfunction of adipose tissue causes fatty acid accumulation in the liver. In addition, excessive nutrition causes increase in malonyl-CoA in the liver, that inhibits carnitine palmitoyl transferase 1 (CPT1). This, in turn, inhibits fatty acid oxidation. Ultimately, the storage of triglycerides (TRIGs) increases in the lack of fatty acid oxidation. Due to CPT1 inhibition, the fatty acid metabolism also leads to the production of diacylglycerol (DAG) and ceramide. DAG triggers stress-induced kinases, and results in reduced insulin signaling. In the muscles, fatty acid accumulation causes an increase in beta oxidation and decreases the rate of citric acid cycle. The products of incomplete fat oxidation (acylcarnitines and reactive oxygen species) stimulate stress-induced kinases and reduce the insulin signaling [12].

Various studies on subjects with T2DM point to an increased gluconeogenesis, that occurs in spite hyperinsulinaemia, signifying hepatic insulin resistance as the main cause of fasting hyperglycemia [13]. The visceral obesity causes accumulation of fat in liver and muscles which leads to impaired insulin-mediated glucose uptake due to intracellular damage to insulin signaling [14].

The biochemistry of these adipose, muscle, and liver tissue dysfunction will be discussed in depth in this chapter.

GENETIC FACTORS ASSOCIATED WITH T2DM

A sedentary lifestyle coupled with a high calorie consumption is a major causative factor in the development of T2DM. However, a genetic predisposition also plays a contributing role in the development. Using the genome-wide linkage methods, various genes have been identified for polymorphisms correlated to T2DM [15].

1. **CAPN10** CAPN10 which codes for the cysteine protease calpain 10, was considered to be the first T2DM susceptibility gene that was identified through a genome-wide scan and positional cloning. The CAPN10 gene is situated on chromosome 2q37.3 and distances 1 kb, composed of 15 exons encoding a 672 amino acid protein. The genetic variants in CAPN10 may modify insulin secretion or insulin action and the production of glucose by the liver. The significant role of CAPN10 in the survival of pancreatic β-cells was revealed in the recent studies.
2. **Hepatocyte Nuclear Factor 4-A (HNF-4A)** HNF4A is a gene that acts as a switch to turn on and off other genes in the body. Variations in the HNF4A gene could lead to T2DM by reducing the amount of insulin secreted by the pancreas. The HNF4A gene is present on chromosome 20, a region that is related to T2DM. The HNF4A gene, located at 20q12–q13.1, is encoded in 12 exons. Single nucleotide polymorphisms (SNPs) in the HNF4A gene impact pancreatic β-cell function that leads to changes in the insulin secretion and also results in the progression of maturity onset diabetes of the young 1 (MODY1).
3. **PPAR-gamma** It is a transcription factor which binds to another transcription factor known as retinoid X receptor (RXR) on activation. These two transcription factors were found to interact and bind with specific PPAR response elements available in the target genes and regulate their expression. PPAR-γ is a key regulator of adipocyte differentiation and it stimulates the differentiation of fibroblasts as well as other undifferentiated cells into mature fat cells. Increasing evidence suggests that the mutations of PPAR-γ gene are linked to insulin resistance.
4. **(TCF7L2)** The transcription factor 7 like-2, is a T-cell specific HMG-box and also one of the four TCF proteins that are involved in the signaling pathways originating from the Wnt family of secreted growth factors. TCF7L2 gene contains the SNPs for two highly linked polymorphisms with T2DM.

B CELL DYSFUNCTION AND INSULIN RESISTANCE

The dynamics of β cell dysfunction and insulin resistance are illustrated in Fig. (**3**) [16]. The failure of pancreatic β-cells to function efficiently is the main cause for the manifestation of hyperglycemia in T2DM [16]. In genetically predisposed individuals, the augmented demand between insulin synthesis and secretion ultimately results in β-cell dysfunction [17, 18]. Studies suggest that the 'stressed' β-cells may kindle local inflammation and alter the balance between α- and β- cell mass and function within the Islets of Langerhans. Insulin tends to exert negative paracrine action on α-cells and limits the secretion of glucagon [19]. Consequently, the lack of insulin results in higher levels of glucagon, which cause a rise in the blood glucose concentration *via* hepatic gluconeogenesis.

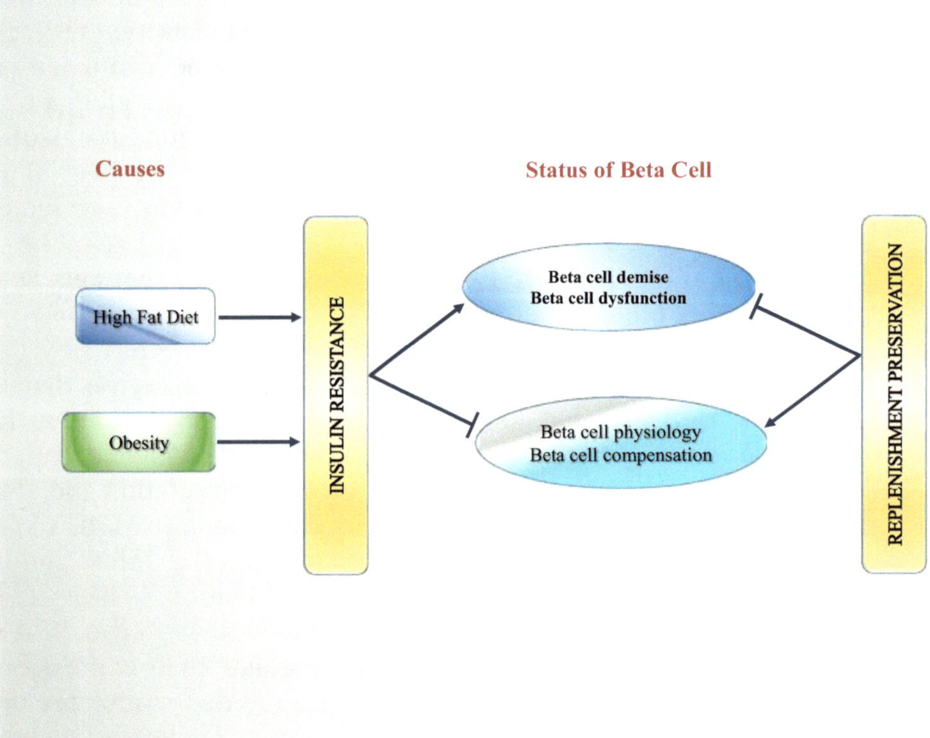

Fig. (3). Dynamics of βcell dysfunction and insulin resistance in T2DM: The relationship between βcell dysfunction and insulin resistance largely depends on metabolic state and it is dynamic. Insulin resistance could be triggered by high fat diet and obesity independently. Both βcell physiology and compensation has been impaired through insulin resistance, thereby it induces b cell demise and dysfunction. The use of novel therapeutic treatments both βcell physiology and compensation can be preserved. Thus, to avoid βcell dysfunction, βcell physiology must be maintained through βcell preservation.

Insulin resistance is compounded by β-cell dysfunction, which characterizes T2DM. β-cell dysfunction and insulin resistance can be activated by the onset of hyperglycemia which leads to the progression of T2DM. Further, β-cell failure is caused by proinflammatory-mediated cytokines, ER stress, oxidative stress, obesity, inflammation, and free fatty acids (FFA) [16].

ROLE OF INCRETINS

The central role of gut hormones or incretins which are involved in regulation of insulin secretion has been characterized in the past two to three decades. Two incretins, *i.e.* glucagon-like peptide-1 (GLP-1) and gastric inhibitory polypeptide (GIP), influence the secretion of insulin. GLP-1 secreted by L cells which are located in the ileum and colon. GIP is secreted by enteroendocrine K cells located in the duodenum and proximal jejunum [20]. These polypeptides are secreted after food ingestion and/or caloric liquid and assist in increasing insulin secretion as well as reduce glucagon secretion. Decreased secretion of GLP-1 is associated with T2DM [21], insulin resistance [22] and obesity [23].

INSULIN RESISTANCE MECHANISMS

The term "insulin resistance" is characterized by a poor biological response to either administered or secreted insulin. Insulin resistance is indicative of T2DM, which is a condition where the cells become irresponsive to insulin. Insulin resistance occurs mainly in insulin-sensitive tissues such as liver, muscles, and fat cells. The causes of insulin resistance are multifactorial and include genetic causes, lipotoxicity, inflammation, negative regulation by hyperglycemia, serine threonine phosphorylation, defects in glucose transport system, mitochondrial dysfunction and ROS generation, ER stress *etc.*

Various causes of insulin resistance, their molecular mechanism and biochemical effects are discussed below:

Obesity Intra-abdominal adiposity is mainly associated with insulin resistance and to different metabolic variables that include plasma glucose levels, insulin, total plasma cholesterol, triglyceride levels, and decreased plasma HDL cholesterol [24 - 26]. Although the link between intra-abdominal fat and abnormal metabolism is not well understood, several hypotheses have been derived. The accumulation of abdominal adipose tissue is resistant to the antilipolytic effects of insulin [27] which include changes in lipoprotein lipase activity. Further, it also causes an increased lipase activity and movement of fatty acids to the circulation where the portal circulation receives the highest fatty acid load. Additionally, the high levels of 11β-hydroxysteroid dehydrogenase type 1 (HSD11B1) present in the mesenteric fat leads to a higher conversion rate of inactive cortisone to active cortisol which causes increased local production of cortisol. This could trigger adipocytes to cause increased lipolysis and to modify the production of adipokines, that may directly control glucose metabolism.

Adipocyte Secretions Adipocytes control the uptake and release of FFAs. They not only take part in the glycerol FFA cycle and release leptin and other hormones responsible for energy status of the body but also release different cytokines containing hormonal, paracrine and autocrine actions [28]. The adipocyte can also be negatively affected by intake of excess nutrients, that leads to adverse events in the body. Due to an increase in the surface area of the adipocytes in obesity, there is an altered expression of leptin, IL-8, IL-6, MCP-1, and granulocyte colony-stimulating factor (GM-CSF). Cytokines attract proinflammatory macrophages (M1 type), that release TNF- α which has local and systemic inflammatory effects.

Mammalian Target Of Rapamycin (mTOR) mTOR is a part of the serine/threonine protein kinase complex, TORC. It integrates signaling from insulin and other growth factor receptors thereby regulating various cell processes including growth, autophagy, apoptosis, transcription and translation. Activation of TORC1 propagates anabolic signals through several downstream targets including inhibition of 4E-BP and S6K. This results in the stimulation of ribosomal translation, initiation of lipogenesis *via* the stimulation of sterol regulatory element–binding protein 1 (SREBP1), and upsurge in nucleotide synthesis by promoting flux through the pentose phosphate pathway [29]. S6K can also phosphorylate IRS1 at serine and prevent its activity resulting in downregulation of insulin signaling [30].

The association between obesity, adipocyte secretions, and mTOR signaling is explained in Fig. (**4a**).

Endoplasmic Reticulum (ER) Stress The major functions of ER is post-translational modification of proteins which includes protein folding, maturation, quality control and their transfer to other cellular compartments. When excess levels of unfolded or misfolded proteins accumulate in ER, the overall protein synthesis slows down, whereas the synthesis of chaperones and other proteins increases. This in turn increases the fidelity of protein processing. The ER membrane–associated proteins complexed to the ER protein BiP/GRP78 include eukaryotic initiation factor 2α (eIF2α), a kinase, known as PKR-like endoplasmic reticulum kinase (PERK), RNA-dependent protein kinase like PKR, the inositol-requiring enzyme 1 (IRE1) and the activating transcription factor 6 (ATF6). An Increase in unfolded proteins leads to dissociation of these proteins from BiP/GRP78. eIF2α gets phosphorylated by PERK resulting in inhibition of most of the protein synthesis and reduction in load on ER. IRE1 is also phosphorylated which triggers the cleavage of X-box binding protein 1 (XBP1), leading to the formation of a mRNA which gets translated into active transcription factor. In combination with ATF6α, XBP1 causes activation of transcription corresponding to the production of chaperones and other proteins involved in ER biogenesis, phospholipid synthesis, ER-associated protein degradation (ERAD) and secretion [31].

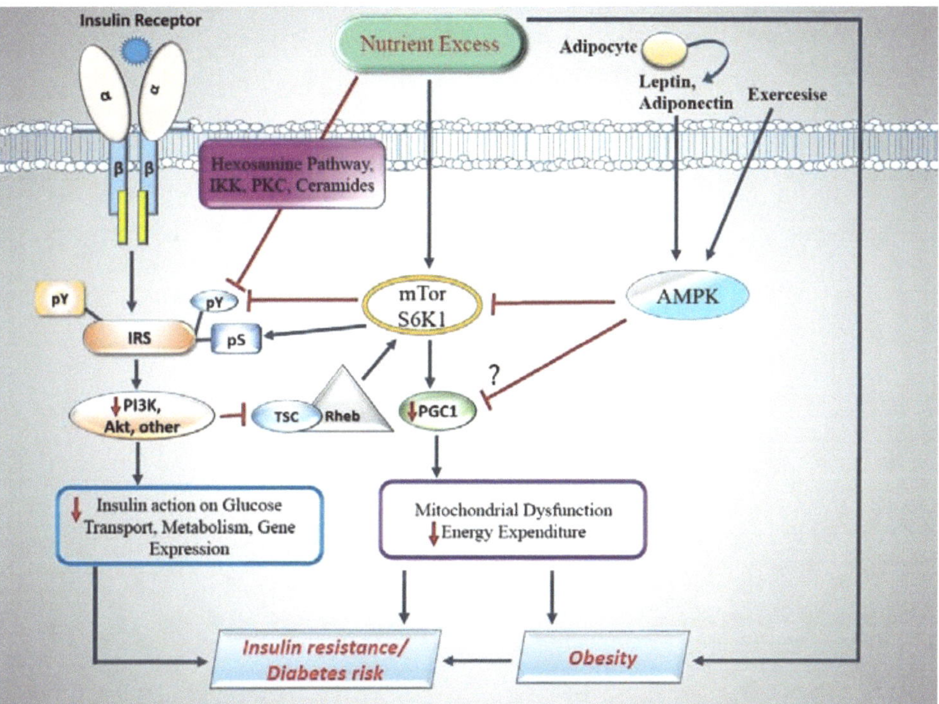

Fig. (4a). Association between mTOR, S6 kinase 1, excess nutrient with both obesity and insulin resistance. Nutrient based stimulation of mTOR and S6K decreases IRS tyrosine phosphorylation (pY) and upsurges serine phosphorylation (pS), thereby hindering downstream insulin signalling along with metabolic and transcriptional effects of insulin. On the other hand, AMP kinase–dependent pathways, triggered by exercise, leptin and adiponectin, may counteract the effect of nutrient excess at the level of mTOR and S6K. TSC (tuberous sclerosis complex). Rheb, RAS homolog enriched in brain. Pathways hindering and enabling insulin action are shown in red and blue, respectively.

Excessive food consumption and obesity activate the Unfolded Protein Response (UPR) which can be observed in adipose tissue, liver, muscles, pancreatic β-cells and other tissues Fig. (**4b**). The activation of UPR on excessive food consumption has several effects including activation of Janus kinase (Jak) and nuclear factor-κB (NF-κB)/inhibitor of κB kinase (IKK) pathways which causes a decrease in IRS1 activity, increase in the levels of endogenous inflammatory mediators, changes in SREBP1-mediated transcription, decrease in hepatic gluconeogenesis, cellular dysfunction and apoptosis [32].

Skeletal Muscles The skeletal muscles are the primary site of glucose clearance after food intake. In case of obesity, insulin resistance in skeletal muscles is manifests prior to irregularities in adipose tissue and liver which can be attributed to the limited nutrient storage capacity of skeletal muscles. An abnormal increase in FFAs points towards the progression of condition from impaired glucose tolerance (IGT) to diabetes [33].It is important to highlight that the FFAs might not be distinctly elevated in the periphery, due to an efficient uptake by the liver and skeletal muscles.

All these facts make it important to bring to notice that a minimal elevation in FFAs are not a true indicator of FFAs present in the peripheral tissues. Hence, an altered FFA movement into skeletal muscles, which is observed in increased visceral lipolysis, has been implicated in the inhibition of glucose uptake by muscles.

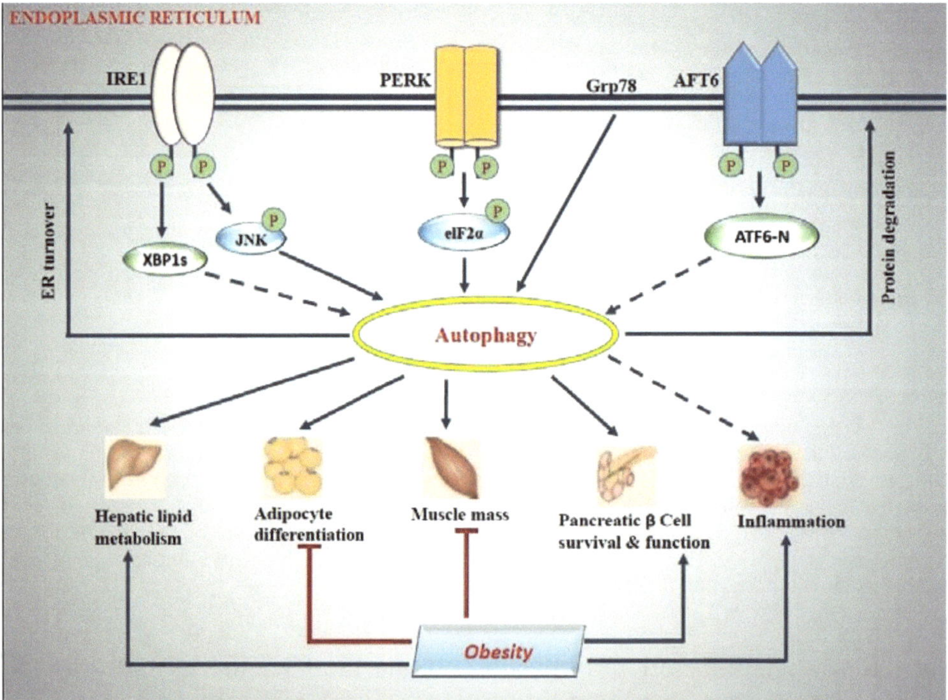

Fig. (4b). Association of ER stress, Autophagy, Obesity, Inflammation and Metabolism UPR has been implicated in ER stress-induced autophagy, thus connecting autophagy in ER homeostasis. On stress recovery, the actions of autophagy include degradation of misfolded proteins and the elevation of ER turnover. Autophagy is also known to involve in lipid droplet formation in the liver, survival and function of β cell, adipocyte differentiation, muscle mass control and inflammatory responses, all of which are known to be disturbed in obesity.

Various other causes of insulin resistance and their mechanisms are mentioned in the Table **2**.

Table 2. Other causes, molecular mechanisms and biochemical effects of insulin resistance.

Causes	Molecular Mechanism	Biochemical Effects	Reference
Genetic mutations	- Mutations in IR signaling molecules	- Increased insulin resistance and CV risk - Impaired insulin action and hyperglycemia - Increased risk of T2DM	[34-38]
Lipotoxicity – elevated free fatty acids (FFA)	- Hyperactivation of PP2A	- reactive oxygen and nitrogen species regulate effect on PP2A through post-translational methylation and nitration of resulting in metabolic dysregulation and cellular demise	[39]
Inflammation – cytokine mediated insulin resistance	- Cytokine-stimulated SOCS3 activation - Cytokine-stimulated reduction in gene expression - Cytokine stimulated activation of serine/threonine kinase, declining IRS-1, GLUT4, and PPAR-γ expression	- Blocking degradation of IRS- and -2 - Inhibition or IR tyrosine kinase phosphorylation - Competing IRS binding to IR - Increased IRS degradation - Reduced expression of insulin signaling molecules - Insulin resistance	[40-44] [43-46]
Hyperglycemia	- Glycation of insulin signaling molecules - Hyperactivation of PP2A	- Reduced affinity for IR - Decreased DNA-binding capacities of transcription factors - Reduced phosphorylation of IR and insulin signaling Molecules	[47-49] [39]
Hyperinsulinemia	- Hyperactivation of PHLPP1 and Grb14	- Reduced AKT Ser473 phosphorylation - Competing IRS binding to IR	[50-52]
Mitochondrial dysfunction through ROS generation	- Augmented metabolite flux into mitochondria, changes in mitochondrial proteins and diminished expression of antioxidant enzymes	- Increased ROS levels - Stimulation of stress kinases that activate insulin resistance by serine phosphorylation of IRS proteins	[53-55] [55]
Tumour necrosis factor –α	- Increased serine phosphorylation	- In 3T3-L1 adipocytes, decreased kinase activity in IR	[56-58]

Glucocorticoids	- Downregulation of IRS-1 - Profound inhibition of insulin and growth factor signaling	- Increasing hepatic glucose production *via* activation of gluconeogenesis - Insulin resistance in skeletal muscle	[59]

PLEIOTROPIC ACTION OF INSULIN

Insulin, an anabolic peptide hormone released by the β-cells of the pancreas, acts through insulin receptors (IRs) and enhances glucose conversion into glycogen and reduces glucose output. It also stimulates glucose uptake in skeletal muscles and fat tissues through translocation of GLUT4 (Fig. **5**). IRs are located in the membranes of the cells in target tissues, mainly in the liver and muscles.. Insulin also acts on other cells by pleiotropic effects. Insulin plays a critical role in human metabolism [60]. Although traditional role of insulin is considered as a glucose homeostasis regulating hormone, recent studies suggest that it has a much wider pleiotropic role.

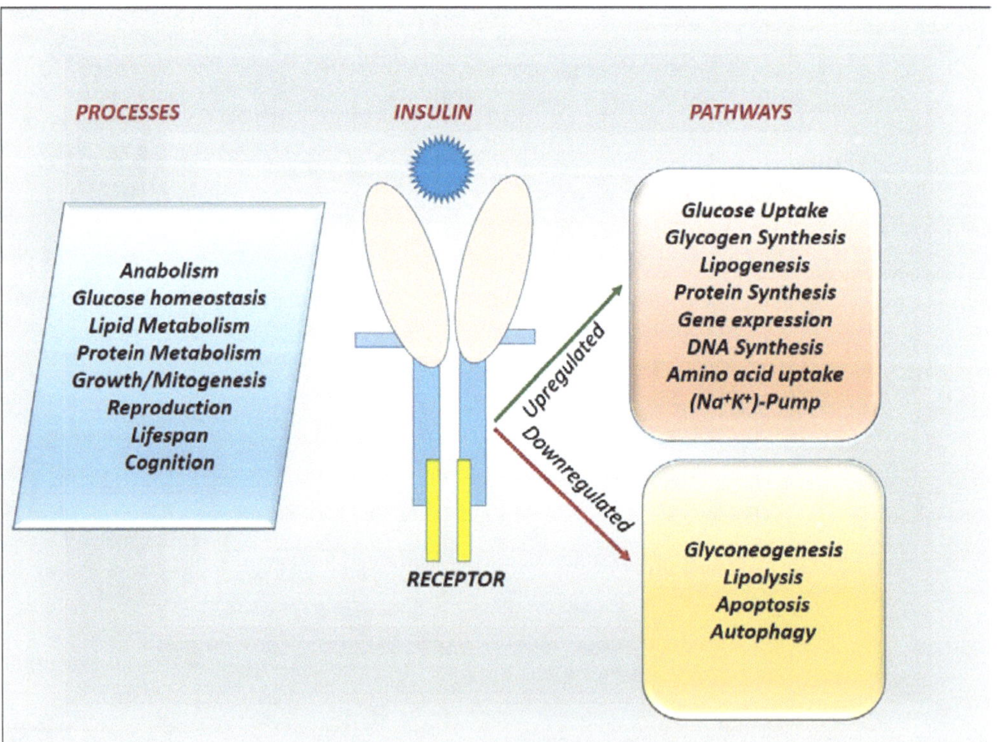

Fig. (5). Pleiotropic action of insulin. Insulin signaling of the IR influence numerous physiological processes in the organism by up regulating or down regulating many intracellular metabolic pathways.

The well characterized metabolic effects of insulin signaling through the IR can be categorized into three metabolic areas which are carbohydrate metabolism, lipid metabolism and, protein metabolism [61].

ROLE OF INSULIN IN CARBOHYDRATE METABOLISM

- Upregulates the glucose transport rate across the cell membrane as well as increases glycolysis in adipose tissue and muscles.
- Stimulates the glycogen synthesis rate in adipose tissue, muscles and liver.
- Decreases the rate of glycogen breakdown in muscles and liver.
- Inhibits the rate of glycogenolysis and gluconeogenesis in the liver.

ROLE OF INSULIN IN LIPID METABOLISM

- Stimulates the synthesis of FFAs and triacylglycerol in tissues to a certain extent.
- Increases the rate of formation of very-low-density lipoprotein (VLDL) as well as cholesterol in the liver.
- Increases the uptake of triglycerides in adipose tissue with a concomitant reduction in the rate of lipolysis thereby lowering plasma FFA levels.
- Decreases the rate of fatty acid oxidation in muscle and liver.

ROLE OF INSULIN IN PROTEIN METABOLISM

- Increases the rate of amino acid transport rate of protein synthesis in adipose tissues, muscles, liver, and other tissues.
- Decreases the rate of protein degradation in muscles and thereby the rate of formation of urea.

BIOCHEMISTRY OF GLUCOSE UPTAKE

In a normal individual, the normal plasma glucose ranges from 4 to 7 mM. These values represent the balance between: (a) transport of glucose into the circulation after its absorption from the intestine or by the conversion of stored glycogen to glucose in the liver and (b) utilization and metabolism of blood glucose by peripheral tissues [61, 62].

Glucose transport into the cells is facilitated by the specialized proteins called glucose transporters (GLUTs).The entry of glucose into the cells is restricted by the number of GLUTs as well as their affinity towards glucose. The basal glucose transporters, GLUT1 and GLUT3, have a higher affinity towards glucose and they are located nearly in all cells. Their K_m value for glucose is around 2-5 mM. As this value is less than the average blood glucose concentration (5-7 mM), the glucose uptake remains constant in most of the tissues, irrespective of the amount present in the blood.Muscle and fat cells possess a high-affinity insulin-responsive, third type of glucose transporter called GLUT4, with a K_m value of around 5 mM. Insulin is measured as the primary regulator of blood glucose levels as it reduces blood glucose levels by: (a) enhancing the uptake of glucose in the muscles and fat tissues *via* translocation of intracellular GLUT4 to the plasma membrane; (b) utilizing the fat and glycogen in the muscles, liver and adipose tissues *via* increased glycogenesis, lipogenesis and protein synthesis and (c) lowering the glucose production and its release by the liver *via* inhibition glycogenolysis. Insulin signaling also reduces the breakdown of fat (lipolysis) and protein.

INTRODUCTION TO THE INSULIN RECEPTOR (IR)

The IR belongs to the tyrosine kinase receptor super family which forms a heterotetramer of two α-subunits and two β-subunits. IR is similar to insulin-like growth factor-1 receptor (IGF-1R) and the insulin-related receptor. In basal conditions, the α-subunit acts as an allosteric inhibitor of the β-subunit. Stimulation by insulin inhibits the suppression of the β-subunit, followed by tyrosine kinase activity *via* a conformational change leading to transphosphorylation of tyrosine residues on specific β-subunit [63]. β-subunit has three tyrosine residues, Tyr-1158, -1162 and -1163, based on IR-isoform-B, and these residues are considered important in facilitating insulin signaling, Fig. (**6**). Among these, Tyr-1158 is the most critical residue as the mutation of Tyr-1158 causes ~80% reduction in tyrosine autophosphorylation and failure in detection of endogenous substrates [64]. Some evidences suggest that insulin, IGF-1, and insulin related receptors can form functional hybrids among each other and an inhibitory mutation that occurs in one of the receptor monomer can inhibit the activity of the other [65]. The tyrosine kinase activity of substrate proteins increases insulin signaling *via* tyrosine phosphorylation of substrate proteins that form a scaffold for multiple signaling events. The IR stimulates a complex intracellular signaling network *via* insulin receptor substrate (IRS) proteins and the canonical PI3K and ERK cascades. Insulin signaling in the β-cells and livers is emerging as a crucial determinant in preventing T2DM, through the consolidative role of molecules IRS2 and FOXO (Forkhead family of transcription factors) by preventing β-cell differentiation [66].

INSULIN SIGNALING

With the identification of IR, various substrate proteins of the receptor were also identified in which the first and best characterized substrate was IRS-1. It is 160 kDa docking/effector protein [67, 68]. Currently, there are nine insulin receptor substrate proteins which include IRS1-4, Dok, Gab-1, Cbl, APS, and isoforms of

Shc Fig. (**6**). With respect to insulin response, the IRS proteins on activation, employ other proteins such as PI3K, Nck, Grb2, and CrkII. These together and form a multifunctional signaling center which helps initiate the insulin action. Most of the SH2 proteins such as the p85 subunit of PI3K and Grb2 that bind to IRSs serve as the adapter molecules whereas other kinds of proteins carry out enzymatic functions themselves, *e.g.*, SHP2, a tyrosine phosphatase.

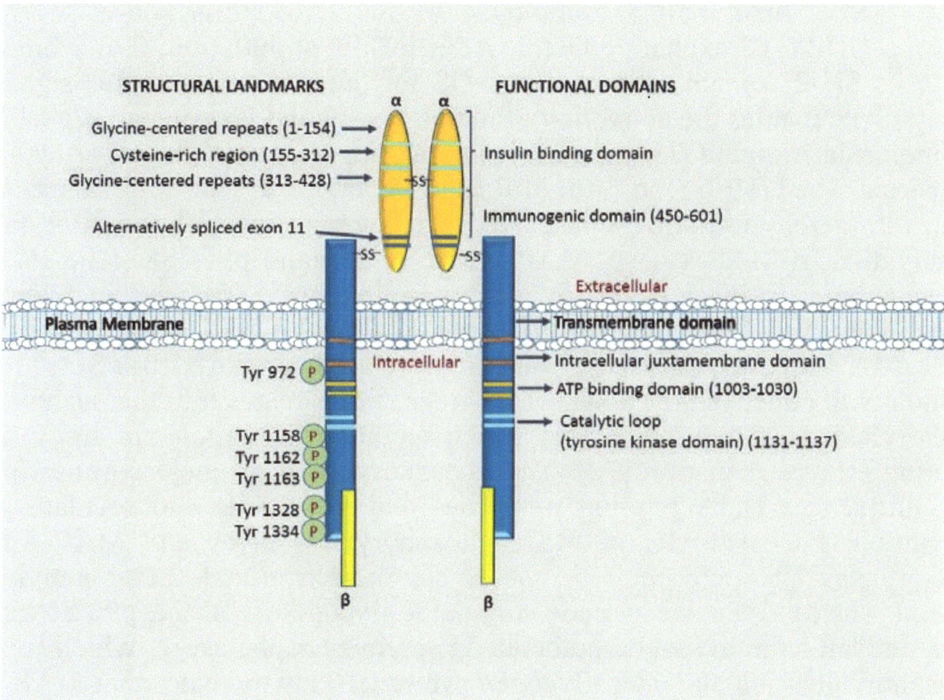

Fig. (6). Schematic diagram of IR indicating the structural landmarks and functional domains.

SH2-containing proteins bind to phosphotyrosine motifs and further dock with insulin receptor substrate proteins as well as enzymatic proteins such as PI3K, Fyn (tyrosine kinase), Csk (tyrosine kinase), SH2 domain-containing inositol 5-phosphatases-2 (SHIP-2; phosphotyrosine phosphatase) and other adapter proteins like Grb-2, Crk, APS, and Nck [69]. The adapter proteins also contain SH3 domains along with SH2 domains and bind to proline-rich sequences in other proteins containing consensus sequence PXXP. The adapter proteins interact with receptor substrates *via* their SH2 domains and employ other proteins that are bound to their SH3 domains. The SH3-bound proteins majorly constitute downstream signaling molecules and catalytic subunits, that contribute in the transduction of the insulin signal. Thus, insulin receptor substrates act as the fork in the insulin signal transduction pathways leading into the mitogenic (Ras/MAP kinase) and metabolic (PI3K) pathways.

MITOGENIC PATHWAY (RAS/MAP KINASE)

Grb-2 is a small SH2 domain containing cytosolic adapter protein which docks with IRSs Fig. (**7**). Grb-2 also contains an SH3 binding domain that binds with proteins through its interaction with proline-rich sequences, and one of such protein is SOS (mammalian homologue of the Drosophila son-of-sevenless protein), a GDP/GTP exchange factor. After insulin stimulation, Grb-2 binds to IRS *via* its SH-2 domain, and recruits SOS for the activation of Ras signaling pathway. SOS enables the activation of membrane-bound Ras, which is a 21 kDa small molecular weight GTPase, and it plays an important role in cell growth and oncogenesis. The GTP-bound form of Ras gets complexed with Raf-1 kinase and activates it, thereby initiating a cascade that leads to sequential phosphorylation and activation of MAP kinase, MAP kinase kinase and p90RSK. The IR also facilitates the activation of Ras/MAP kinase pathway *via* another substrate docking molecule called SHC [40]. In response to insulin, SHC also activates Ras and the MAP kinase pathway by making a complex with Grb-2/SOS. After activation with either IRS or SHC, MAP kinase translocates into the nucleus and phosphorylates transcription factors which facilitate the mitogenic and growth promoting effects of insulin [70]. The phosphorylation of nuclear transcription factors influences DNA binding properties and their ability to regulate gene transcription. For example, p90RSK phosphorylates c-fos and MAP kinase phosphorylates Elk-1and in both cases, the transcriptional factor activity is increased. The MAP kinase cascade stimulates glycogen synthase, p90 S6 kinase in turn activates the glycogen-associated protein phosphatase-1, which in turn dephosphorylates and activates glycogen synthase. This indicates that MAP kinase pathway is highly significant and possesses the potential to interact with various metabolic signaling pathways. However, MAP kinase pathway is not essential for the stimulation of glucose transport and thus is considered as being critically associated to the mitogenic effects of insulin. In adipocytes, inhibition of the MAP kinase pathway by dominant negative forms of Ras [71] or inhibitors of MAPKK [72] block the transcriptional effects but do not restrict the insulin stimulation of glucose transport or glycogen synthesis.

METABOLIC PATHWAY (PI3K/AKT)

The phosphorylation of IRS-1 or IRS-2 offers docking sites for the SH2 domains of the regulatory subunit p85 of PI3K that is bound to the catalytic subunit p110 as a heterodimer. The lipid products of PI3K include phosphatidylinositol bisphosphate (PIP2) and phosphatidylinositol triphosphate (PIP3) [73 - 75]. These lipid products induce the activation of protein serine kinase cascades through co-recruitment to the membranes *via* the PH domains of phosphoinositide-dependent kinase-1 (PDK1), its substrate kinases Akt/PKB and atypical protein kinase Cs (aPKCs). PDK1 is supposed to be constitutively active and it avoids membrane lipid binding for the effective phosphorylation of the substrates in the cytosol, whereas the binding to PIP2 and PIP3 is essential for the activation of few substrates like Akt, that need a proper orientation of the kinase and PH domains of PDK1 and Akt at the membrane. PDK1 partially stimulates the serine kinases Akt/PKB and aPKC by phosphorylation of a conserved threonine residue (Thr308 in Akt) in the kinase regulatory loop, whereas the full activation of Akt/PKB happens after the phosphorylation of a C-terminal hydrophobic motif that contains Ser473 which is catalyzed by a distinct enzyme mTORC2. The time-period and the intensity of Akt signaling are measured by the phosphatase PHLPP which acts on the hydrophobic phosphorylation motif [75].

Based on the cell type, the activated Akt/PKB phosphorylates various substrates and controls a variety of downstream processes. The well-established Akt/PKB substrates are GSK-3 that regulate glycogen synthesis, FOXO transcription factors that mobilize from the nucleus to the cytoplasm on phosphorylation and inhibit FOXO-dependent transcription of gluconeogenic and other genes, the Rheb GTPase activating complex TSC1/2 that regulates mTOR and protein synthesis, and the Rab GTPase activating protein AS160/TBC1D4 that regulatesthe glucose transport [75].

REGULATION OF GLUT 4 TRANSLOCATION

GLUT4 is one of 13 human glucose transporter (GLUT) isoform comprising of 12 membrane-spanning domains that are highly expressed in the adipose tissue and skeletal muscles. GLUTs catalyse hexose transport across the cell membranes *via* ATP-independent facilitative diffusion. In an unstimulated state, GLUT4 exists as intracellular disposition in the storage vesicles that are called as GLUT4 storage vesicles (GSVs). These GSVs are intensely redistributed in the plasma membrane [76]. With respect to insulin stimulation, GLUT4 gets translocated to the plasma membrane, through targeted exocytosis and endocytosis at the same time [77]. Thus, the concentration of GLUT4 at the cell surface and the its duration at the site determine the rate of glucose transport into muscles and fat cells.

GLUT4 exists in specialized vesicles that are sequestered within the cell, although the accurate intracellular location and the trafficking pathways of the vesicles are not clear. After GLUT-4 gets internalized, it localizes into the tubulovesicular and vesicular structures which are biochemically distinct but potentially interact with the recycling endosomal network [78]. Further, the microtubule network and actin cytoskeleton also play a significant role in the trafficking of GLUT4 either by connecting signaling components or by leading the movement of vesicles from the perinuclear region to the plasma membrane, in response to insulin. Cortical actin, a cytoskeletal protein is also considered essential for the translocation of GLUT4 in response to insulin into the plasma membrane [79], that is regulated by TC10.

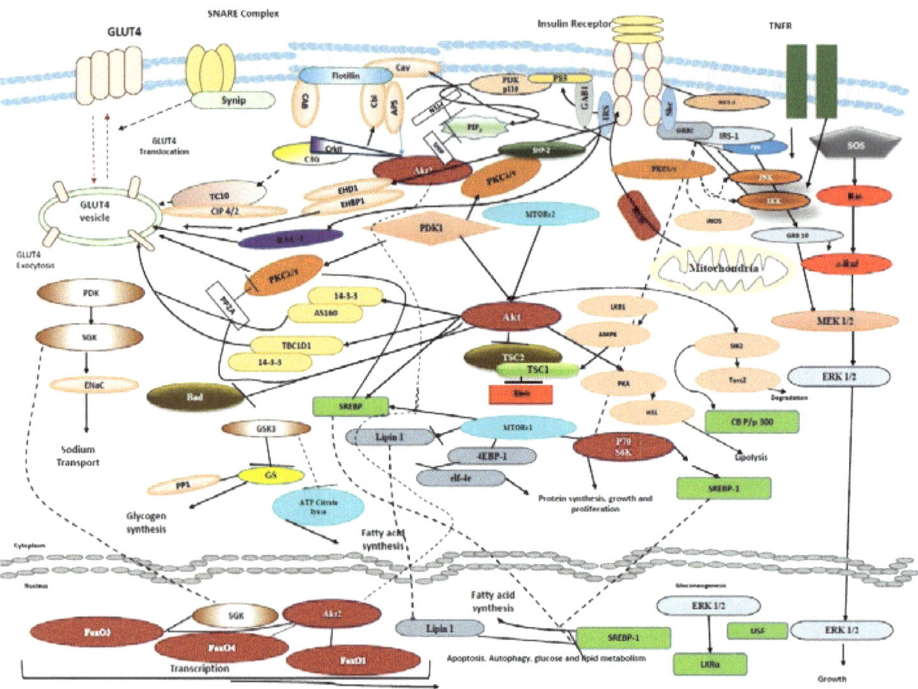

Fig. (7). Insulin signaling pathways (Metabolic and Mitogenic pathways). Insulin activates the insulin receptor tyrosine kinase (IR), which phosphorylates and recruits different substrate adaptors such as the IRS family of proteins. Tyrosine phosphorylated IRS then displays binding sites for numerous signaling partners. Among them, PI3K has a major role in insulin function, mainly *via* the activation of the Akt/PKB and the PKCζ cascades. Activated Akt induces glycogen synthesis through inhibition of GSK-3; protein synthesis *via* mTOR and downstream elements; and cell survival through inhibition of several pro-apoptotic agents (Bad, FoxO transcription factors, GSK-3, and MST1). Akt phosphorylates and directly inhibits FoxO transcription factors, which also regulate metabolism and autophagy. Inversely, AMPK is known to directly regulate FoxO3 and activate transcriptional activity. Insulin signaling also has growth and mitogenic effects, which are mostly mediated by the Akt cascade as well as by activation of the Ras/MAPK pathway. The insulin signaling pathway inhibits autophagy *via* the ULK1 kinase, which is inhibited by Akt and mTORC1, and activated by AMPK. Insulin stimulates glucose uptake in muscle and adipocytes *via* translocation of GLUT4 vesicles to the plasma membrane. GLUT4 translocation involves the PI3K/Akt pathway and IR-mediated phosphorylation of CAP, and formation of the CAP:CBL:CRKII complex. In addition, insulin signaling inhibits gluconeogenesis in the liver, through disruption of CREB/CBP/mTORC2 binding. Insulin signaling induces fatty acid and cholesterol synthesis *via* the regulation of SREBP transcription factors. Insulin signaling also promotes fatty acid synthesis through activation of USF1 and LXR. A negative feedback signal emanating from Akt/PKB, PKCζ, p70 S6K, and the MAPK cascades results in serine phosphorylation and inactivation of IRS signaling.

Thus, it is possible that the molecular motors initiate the movement of GLUT4 vesicles which is facilitated by microtubules and actin cytoskeletons. This may lead to dynamic remodeling in response to insulin. SNARE proteins act as the key mediators of GLUT4, movement in the insulin-sensitive cells. These proteins are involved in regulating the delivery of GLUT4 to the cell surface in response to insulin and control GLUT4 intracellular trafficking [80].

GSVs translocation involves PI3K/PDK1/AKT2 pathway as the major insulin signalling pathway, *via* phosphorylation of AS160 substrate Fig. (7). AS160 is a GTPase-activating protein which on phosphorylation activates small G proteins called RAB that are involved in membrane trafficking by blocking the exchange of GTP and GDP. Atypical Protein kinases C (aPKCs) isoforms are also involved in the downstream processing of PDK1 but not through AKT pathway [66]. Apart from insulin, exercise also stimulates glucose transport and GLUT4 translocation *via* an insulin-independent but AMK-dependent mechanism [76].

PROTEIN KINASE C

The isoforms of PKC are the mediators and modifiers of the metabolic action of insulin. With the three major classes of PKC, the atypical PKCs (aPKCs), PKC ζ and PKC λ/ι, are stimulated *via* PDK-1phosphorylation. aPKCs are considered important for the insulin-stimulated glucose transport and regulation of lipid synthesis. In obese and diabetic humans, the expression and/or activation of aPKCs is found to be decreased in the muscles. Both PKC-λ and PKC-ζ can act interchangeably in mediating the insulin-stimulated glucose transport [81]. In mice model, deletion of a muscle-specific PKC-λ leads to impairment in insulin resistance and insulin-stimulated glucose uptake. Similarly, deletion of liver-specific PKC-λ in a mice model showed decreased insulin-induced expression of SREBP1c and triglyceride content in the liver, which leads to increased insulin sensitivity [82].

INSULIN SIGNALING: NEGATIVE REGULATORS

Insulin and IGF-1 signaling are strongly regulated since the uncontrolled activity of the downstream pathways can cause severe disturbances in the metabolism and tumorigenesis.

Phosphoprotein Phosphatases PTP1B, the cytoplasmic protein tyrosine phosphatase, leukocyte antigen-related tyrosine kinase (LAR) and transmembrane phosphatase have been shown to cause dephosphorylation of the tyrosine residues on activated IR, IGF-1R and IRS proteins thereby diminishing their activity [83]. Protein phosphatase 1 (PP1), a serine/threonine phosphatase, is involved in the regulation of the metabolism of glucose and lipids including glycogen synthase, hormone-sensitive lipase, or acetyl CoA carboxylase [84]. Protein phosphatase 2A (PP2A), controls the activities of protein kinases like Akt, PKC, S6K, ERK, cyclin dependent kinases and IKK which are involved in insulin action [85]. Apart from these protein kinases, various other serine/threonine phosphatases involved in insulin action are protein phosphatases 2B (PP2B), otherwise known as calcineurin, and PH domain leucine-rich repeat protein phosphatases PHLPP-1 and -2, which dephosphorylate both Akt and PKCs [86].

Lipid Phosphatases Lipid phosphatases control insulin signaling by changing the PIP3 levels. PTEN dephosphorylates PIP3, and thus antagonizes the PI3K signaling in the cells [87]. It was identified that the regulatory subunit of PI3K, p85a binds directly and improves PTEN activity, thereby maintaining a balance between the generation and degradation of PIP3 [88]. PIP3 is also dephosphorylated by SHIP-1 and -2 [89].

Other negative modulators include the cytoplasmic adaptor proteins Grb10 and Grb14, that reduces the activity of IR and IGF-1R and prevent the access of substrates to the activated receptors [90]. The Suppressor of cytokine signaling (SOCS) proteins SOCS1 and SOCS3, negatively regulate insulin signaling by linking the cytokine signaling with insulin resistance [91]. The expression of Trb3, an adaptor protein of pseudo-kinase family is stimulated in the liver in the fasting as well as diabetic states. It disrupts insulin signaling *via* binding to Akt and hindering its activation [92]. In another study insulin and IGF-1 upregulated the IP7 levels, that cause inhibition of Akt translocation to the plasma membrane and following activation, creates a potential feedback mechanism that reduces insulin signaling [93].

Inhibitory Serine and Threonine Phosphorylation Altered inhibition of Ser/Thr phosphorylation of the proteins IR, IRS-1 and 2 takes place in response to cytokines, fatty acids, hyperglycemia, mitochondrial dysfunction, ER stress and insulin itself through the activation of multiple kinases [94]. Through the metabolic product DAG, the lipids can trigger classical PKC (α, β, γ) and novel PKC members (δ, θ, ε). These weaken the insulin signaling by stimulating multiple serine phosphorylation of IR and other IRS proteins [95]. mTORC1 is also considered to be an important module of the negative feedback loops in insulin signaling. Insulin signaling is inhibited by the activation of mTOR and S6K1 by cumulative serine phosphorylation and by decreasing IRS tyrosine phosphorylation [96].

INSULIN SIGNALING: ABNORMALITIES

The defects in the insulin signalling as well as glucose transport system have been well recognised in insulin resistant humans. Various studies have confirmed that the reduction in insulin-stimulated tyrosine phosphorylation of both IR and IRS-1decreased the association of PI3K with IRS-1, insulin-stimulated Akt phosphorylation [97 - 99] and serine phosphorylation of IRS-1 by ER [100].

Altered Glucose Transport System The multicompartmental nature of GLUT4 cellular trafficking involves a series of regulatory proteins that indicates the possibility of many potential target sites for defects that could impair GLUT4 translocation. In obesity and T2DM individuals, the cellular reduction of GLUT4 transporters in adipocytes is the primary reason behind insulin resistance [101], whereas GLUT4 expression is relatively normal in skeletal muscles [102]. In response to insulin in muscles and fat cells, GLUT4 gets accumulated or redistributed to a solid membrane compartment under basal conditions and causes impaired GLUT4 translocation [103, 104]. These data are indicative of a trafficking or directing abnormality that impairs GLUT4 translocation in tissues derived from insulin-resistant subjects.

Serine/Threonine Phosphorylation of the IR and IRS Serine-threonine phosphorylation of IR and IRS is considered to be the main mechanism of negative modulation of insulin signal transduction Fig. (**8**). Serine phosphorylation of IR reduces its tyrosine kinase activity [105], whereas the serine phosphorylation of IRS-1 and other IRSs diminishes the receptor-IRS coupling by hindering insulin-mediated receptor phosphorylation, tyrosine phosphorylation of IRS-1, binding and activation of PI3K and stimulation of glucose transport [106, 107]. IRS-1 is susceptible to a wide variety of serine-threonine kinases including PKC, Akt/PKB, PKA, MAP kinase, GSK3, Cdc2 kinase, casein kinase II, and JKN. These kinases have been shown to function as physiological modulators that cause desensitization of insulin signalling pathways [108].

Protein kinase C Serine-threonine phosphorylation of IRS results in the impairment of its ability to associate with IR and PI3K, leading to desensitization of the PI3K pathway. Hyperinsulinemia, hyperglycaemia, and elevated circulating FFAs cause an increment in the intracellular DAG that activates the conventional and novel PKC isoforms predominantly *via* their recruitment to the plasma membrane.

IMPAIRED INSULIN SIGNALING AND METABOLIC EFFECTS: The impaired insulin signaling in all the major insulin responsive tissues like liver, skeletal muscles, and adipose tissue leads to an increased rate of adipose tissue lipolysis resulting in an increased FFA delivery to liver and increased hepatic esterification of FFA into triglycerides Fig. (**9**). In hepatocytes, this process is controlled by a substrate push mechanism and it is independent of insulin signaling. In contrast to this, hepatic *de novo* lipogenesis, which is dependent on hepatic insulin signaling is significantly reduced [109].

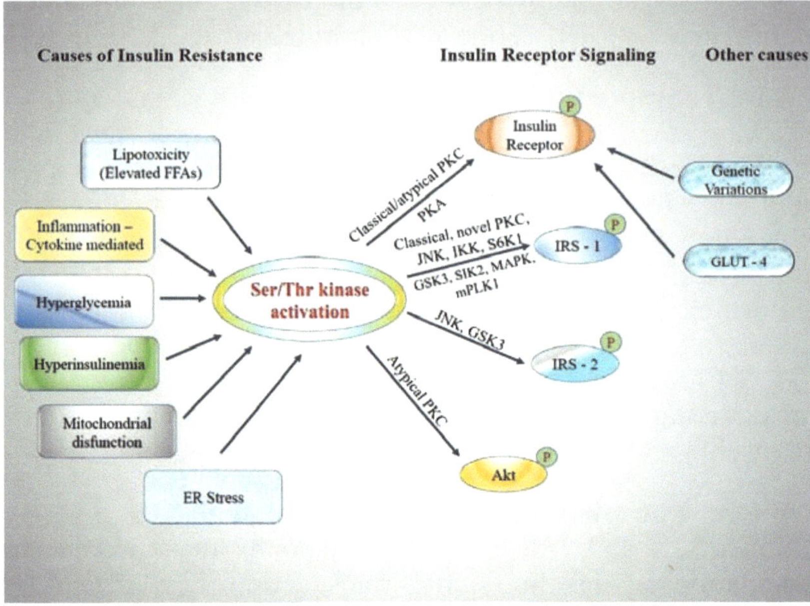

Fig. (8). Various causes of insulin resistance activate serine/threonine kinases that lead to inhibitory phosphorylation of IR and other signaling molecules. Causes of insulin resistance include lipotoxicity, cytokine mediated inflammatory activation, hyperglycemia, hyperinsulinemia, mitochondrial dysfunction and ER stress activates Ser/Thr kinases, inducing inhibitory Ser/Thr phosphorylation of IR, IRS proteins, and Akt on multiple residues causing insulin resistance. Genetic mutations of IR and other insulin signaling molecules and defects in GLUT-4 translocation system are other important causes of insulin resistance.

INDEPENDENT PATHWAYS FOR GLUCOSE TRANSPORT (CAP/CBL/TC10)

In addition to previously mentioned growth factors, other growth factor receptors like the platelet-derived growth factor receptor, cytokine receptors like IL-4, and few integrins that activate PI3K to the same level as like IR with the formation of PI(3,4,5)P3 are also widely present. These growth factors do not stimulate glucose transport [110]. Wortmannin, a PI3K inhibitor can block the stimulation of glucose transport. There is some evidence that other similar signaling pathways, that can act as a parallel complementary pathway for insulin-stimulated glucose transport are also present [111]. Evidence suggests that the CAP/Cbl/TC10 pathway is the complementary pathway for insulin stimulated glucose transport [62]. The pathway deviates from the PI3K pathway at the stage of the insulin receptor kinase, that facilitates tyrosine phosphorylation of Cbl proto-oncogene *via* a process which does not require IRSs. Various studies highlight the important role of CAP/Cbl/TC10 pathway as a complementary pathway for the stimulation of glucose transport [112 - 114].

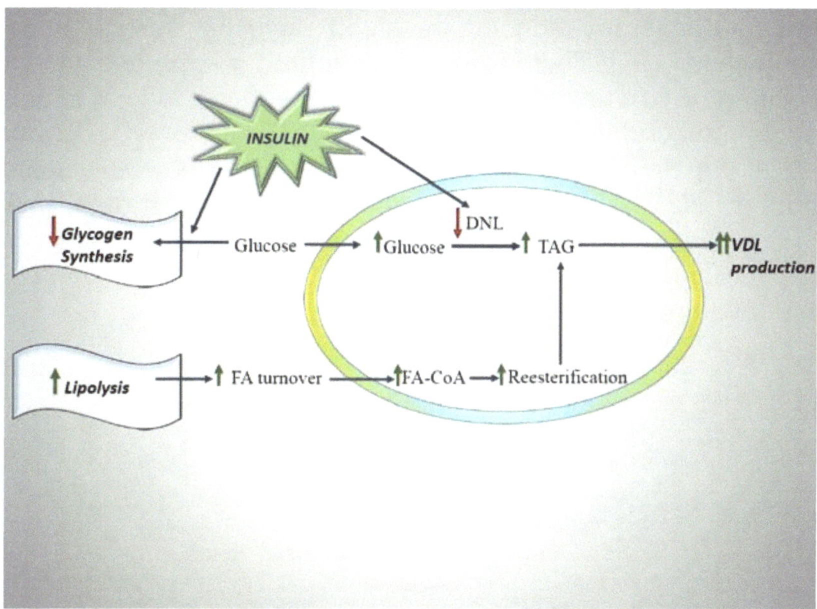

Fig. (9). Impaired insulin signaling and metabolic effects.

THERAPEUTICS OF T2DM

Therapeutic drugs used for the treatment of T2DM include metformin, sulfonylureas, insulin, dipeptidyl peptidase 4 (DPP4) inhibitors, PPAR-γ agonists, incretins and SGLT2 inhibitors. Metformin is the preferred and most widely used first-line pharmacotherapy to manage hyperglycaemia in T2DM. Metformin also reduces the HbA1c levels by hindering hepatic gluconeogenesis. Sulfonylureas and non-sulfonylureas are classified as insulin-secreting agents. These drugs elevate the secretion level of insulin by upregulating Ca^{2+} permeability through the voltage-gated ion channels. PPAR-γ agonists such as Thiazolidinediones increase the insulin sensitivity of muscles, liver, and adipose tissue through mechanisms that are not well understood. However, they do stimulate gene production that increases sensitivity of glucose in muscles and adipose tissue. Furthermore, thiazolidinediones preserve β–cell function which contributes to an improved glycaemic control [115]. Various biochemical changes and drug targets that are involved in T2DM are highlighted in Fig. (**10**).

SGLT2 inhibitors are the recent therapeutic agents which are used for T2DM. SGLT2 inhibitors exhibit a lower hypoglycemia risk, which has gained particular attention, and is used in combination with metformin and DPP4 inhibitors. SGLT2 is a highly efficient transporter gene, which facilitates reabsorption of glucose and sodium in the kidney. The SGLT2 inhibitors act by inhibiting SGLT2 in the proximal convoluted tubule to prevent reabsorption of glucose and facilitate its excretion in urine thereby reducing the blood glucose levels and improving the glycemic parameters [116]. There is a mild potential for hypoglycemia but no risk of overstimulation or fatigue to the β cells [117]. As their mode of action depends on normal renal glomerular-tubular function, the efficacy of SGLT2 inhibitors is reduced in renal impaired patients. Currently, FDA and EMA have approved four SGLT2 inhibitors *viz.* canagliflozin, dapagliflozin, empagliflozin, and, ertugliflozin for the management of T2DM. Pleiotropic effects of SGLT2 comprise of weight loss, persistent reduction in BP, alteration in lipid profile, natriuresis and reduction in intraglomerular pressure.

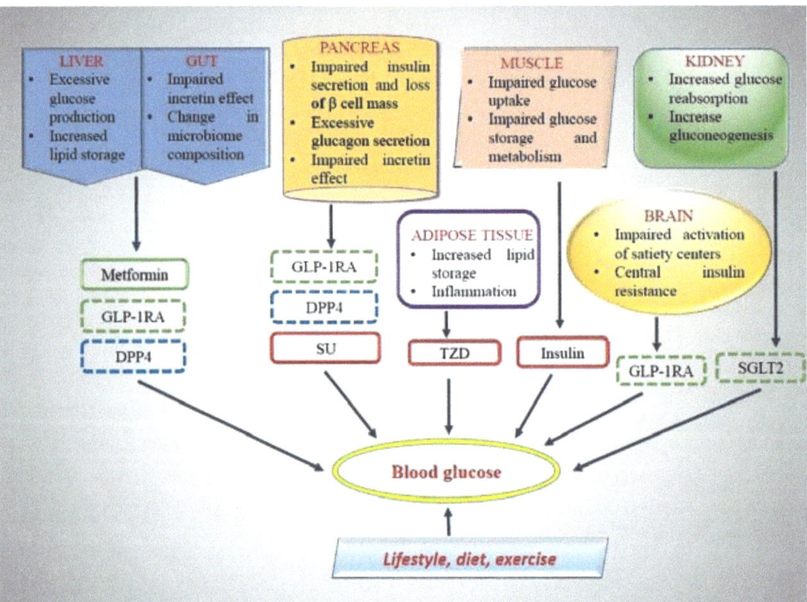

Fig. (10). Biochemical changes in vital organs and drug targets involved in T2DM: Insulin resistance of liver, adipose, and skeletal muscle tissue causes impaired insulin-induced reduction of hepatic glucose production (HGP), lipolysis, and impaired insulin-stimulated glucose uptake [120]. Hyperglycemia evolves when pancreatic β-cells are unable to secrete sufficient insulin to overcome insulin resistance. α-cell dysfunction, characterized by fasting and postprandial hyperglucagonemia also stimulates HGP, which further augments hyperglycemia. Further, the efficacy of gut-derived incretin hormones (GLP-1 and GIP) in facilitating meal-related insulin release and glucagon suppression is also impaired. The kidneys contribute to hyperglycemia by increasing tubular glucose reabsorption, presumably through upregulation of SGLT2 and increased renal gluconeogenesis [121]. Finally, in the development of T2D, impaired activation of satiety centers in the brain stimulates excessive food intake, and insulin resistance in the brain that may alter the control of metabolic homeostasis [122]. Pleiotropic drug effects are illustrated by the frame and color of the boxes. Green indicates body weight loss, blue indicates body weight neutrality, and red indicates body weight gain. A dotted frame indicates blood pressure reduction, and a solid frame indicates blood pressure neutrality. SU, sulfonylurea; TZD, thiazolidinedione.

Incretins are peptides that are gut-derived and are members of the glucagon superfamily. The major physiological incretins are glucagon-like peptide-1 (GLP-

1) and gastric inhibitory peptide (GIP), which are rapidly deactivated by DPP4 enzyme. Both glucagon-like peptide–1 receptor agonists and dipeptidyl peptidase–4 inhibitors are common therapies used in controlling the glycemic level. GLP-1 increases the insulin secretion but inhibits the secretion of glucagon in a glucose-dependent manner [118]. GLP-1 also increases the synthesis of insulin, increases glucose sensitivity to the resistant β-cells, stimulates the proliferation of β-cells, and inhibits β-cell apoptosis.

TCF7L2, a transcription factor activated by the Wnt/b-catenin pathway, plays a key role in the physiology of β-cells. The gene variations in TCF7L2 are considered as the strongest known genetic risk factors for the dysfunction of β-cells and T2DM. The stimulation of GLP-1R increases the phosphorylation and stabilization of β-catenin *via* a cAMP/PKA mechanism sensitive to AKT and ERK1/2 inhibition and improves β-catenin/TCF7L2-mediated transcription of cyclin D1 mRNA, that leads to altered β-cell proliferation [119].

Increase in incretin activity, using either GLP-1 agonists or DPP4 inhibitors represents a novel therapeutic concept by eliciting anti-hyperglycemic, as well as substantial pleiotropic effects (Fig. **10**). The DPP4 inhibitors and GLP-1 agonists extend its benefits to various organ system of the human body by providing cardiovascular stability, weight loss, neuronal-protection, skeletal health, hepatoprotection, and improvement in insulin resistance. Owing to their notable pleiotropic activities, incretin agonism and SGLT2 inhibition evidently represent the future of anti-diabetic therapies.

FUTURE AREAS OF RESEARCH

Genome wide association studies (GWAS) have identified at least 25 additional genes that are associated with T2DM and/or elevated fasting plasma glucose levels. These are enlisted in Table **3**.

Table 3. Additional Genes Associated with T2DM Susceptibility [15].

Name of the Gene/ Gene Symbol	Functions of the Gene	Mechanism of the Disease
Cyclin-dependent kinase-5 regulatory subunit associated protein 1-like 1/ CDKAL1	Inhibitor of cyclin-dependent kinase 5 (CDK5)	β-cell dysfunction, impaired insulin secretion
Haematopoietically expressed homeobox / HHEX	Transcriptional repressor in liver cells is a target of the Wnt signaling pathway	β-cell dysfunction, impaired insulin secretion

(Table 3) cont.....

Name of the Gene/ Gene Symbol	Functions of the Gene	Mechanism of the Disease
Melatonin receptor 1B / MTNR1B	High affinity G-protein coupled receptor, expressed primarily in pancreatic β-cells	β-cell dysfunction, impaired insulin secretion
Ca^{2+}/calmodulin-dependent protein kinase 1-δ / CAMK1D	Activation of extracellular signal-regulated protein kinase 1 (ERK1) activity	β-cell dysfunction
Cell division cycle 123 homolog / CDC123	CDC123 is in the same chromosomal region as the CAMK1D gene	β-cell dysfunction
Cyclin-dependent kinase inhibitor 2A / CDKN2A/B	CDKN2A gene produces 2 major proteins: p16(INK4), which is a cyclin-dependent kinase inhibitor, and p14(ARF), which binds the p53-stabilizing protein MDM2, p14 is also called CDKN2B	β-cell dysfunction
Insulin degrading enzyme / IDE	Extracellular thiol metalloprotease with preference for insulin, also degrades amyloid-β protein; the IDE gene resides within the same chromosomal locus as HHEX	β-cell dysfunction
Insulin-like growth factor-2 mRNA binding protein 2 / IGF2BP2	Binds to the IGF2 mRNA	β-cell dysfunction
Juxtaposed with another zinc-finger gene 1: TAK1(TGFβ-activated kinase-1)-interacting protein 27 / JAZF1 also called TIP27	Acts as a transcriptional repressor, exhibits antiapoptotic activity	β-cell dysfunction
Potassium in wardly-rectifying channel, subfamily J, member 11 / KCNJ11	Forms the core of the ATP-sensitive potassium (KATP) channel involved in insulin secretion	β-cell dysfunction
Potassium channel, voltage-gated, KQT-like subfamily, member 1 / KCNQ1	Pore-forming α-subunit of a cardiac delayed rectifier potassium channel; also referred to as KvLQT because the gene resides in a critical region for the cardiac long QT syndrome-1 disorder which is a region that is also in the imprinted locus associated with Beckwith-Weidemann syndrome.	β-cell dysfunction
Leucine-rich repeat containing G-protein coupled receptor 5 / LGR5	Gene is expressed exclusively in the cycling crypt base of the columnar cells of the gut and hair follicle, protein is a glycoprotein that associates with integrins, the gene is a marker for intestinal stem cells, expression is regulated by Wnt signaling	β-cell dysfunction
Solute carrier family 30 (zinc transporter), member 8 / SCL30A8	Allows cellular efflux of zinc	β-cell dysfunction
Tetraspanin 8 / TSPAN8	Tetraspanins are proteins that contain 4 transmembrane domains	β-cell dysfunction

(Table 3) cont.....

Name of the Gene/ Gene Symbol	Functions of the Gene	Mechanism of the Disease
Wolfram syndrome gene; also called diabetes insipidus, diabetes mellitus, optic atrophy, and deafness (DIDMOAD) / WFS1	Integral ER membrane glycoprotein, associates with the C-terminal domain of the ER-localized Na^+/K^+ATPase β-1 subunit (ATP1B1)	β-cell dysfunction
Fat mass- and obesity-associated gene / FTO	Catalyzes the iron- and 2-oxoglutarate-dependent demethylation of N6-methyladenosine in mRNA; expression upregulated in hypothalamus in response to food intake; increased expression in hypothalamus regulates energy intake.	Obesity
Melanocortin 4 receptor / MC4R	Single exon gene, mutations in this gene are the most frequent genetic cause of severe obesity, receptor binds α-melanocyte stimulating hormone (α-MSH)	Obesity
Thyroid adenoma-associated gene / THADA	Protein contains an ARM repeat (ARM = armadillo which is a fruit fly gene involved in segment polarity), the ARM repeat is involved in protein-protein interactions	Unknown
Notch homolog 2 / NOTCH2	One of three mammalian homologues of the Notch gene of fruit flies which regulates cellular differentiation	Unknown
Disintegrin-like and metalloproteinase (ADAM) with thrombospondin type 1 motif, 9 / ADAMTS9	Proteolytically cleave bovine versican and aggrecan	Unknown

CONCLUSION

Insulin, an anabolic peptide hormone, displays pleiotropic action by influencing multiple physiological processes as well as through upregulation and downregulation of various intracellular metabolic pathways. Insulin and IGF-1 act *via* specific tyrosine kinase receptors activating two pathways which include PI3K-PDK-1-Akt and Grb2-SOS-Ras-MAPK pathways that control the cellular growth and metabolism in organisms. The complexity of the insulin signaling system makes it highly essential to mediate the variety of biological responses. As a normal physiological process, actions of insulin are negatively regulated by phosphatases and certain inhibitory proteins, *e.g.*, SOCS3. The mechanisms of insulin resistance are multifactorial. The major causes of insulin resistance are identified as lipotoxicity (lipid burden), inflammation (cytokine-mediated), mitochondrial dysfunction, ER stress, and hyperglycemia which lead to impaired insulin signaling through serine/threonine kinase activation. Other causes include genetic mutation in IR and insulin signaling molecules, defective GLUT4 translocation system, TNF-α, and glucocorticoid mediated mechanisms. Future research on the contribution of additional genes involved in the pathophysiology of T2DM and focus on incretin agonism and SGLT2 inhibition as effective therapeutic aids can reduce the burden of T2DM and improve their quality of life.

CONSENT FOR PUBLICATION

Not applicable.

CONFLICT OF INTEREST

The author(s) confirms that there is no conflict of interest.

ACKNOWLEDGEMENTS

Declared none.

REFERENCES

[1]   Guyton AC, Hall JE. Unit XIV Endocrinology and reproduction. Textbook of medical physiology. 11th Edition New Delhi Elsevier Inc 2006; p. 972.

[2]   World Health Organization.. Global report on diabetesGeneva.

[3]   IDF diabetes atlas. International Diabetes Federation. 9[th]Edition 2019.Brussels

[4]   Kaku K. Pathophysiology of type 2 diabetes and its treatment policy. Japan Med Assoc J 2010; 53(1): 41-6.

[5]   Holt G I. Br J Psychol 2004; 184: s55-63.
        [http://dx.doi.org/10.1192/bjp.184.47.s55]

[6]   Grant RW, Kirkman MS. Trends in the evidence level for the American Diabetes Association's "Standards of Medical Care in Diabetes" from 2005 to 2014. Diabetes Care 2015; 38(1): 6-8.
        [http://dx.doi.org/10.2337/dc14-2142] [PMID: 25538309]

[7]   Tripathi BK, Srivastava AK. Diabetes mellitus: complications and therapeutics. Med Sci Monit 2006; 12(7): RA130-47.
        [PMID: 16810145]

[8]   Wu Y, Ding Y, Tanaka Y, Zhang W. Risk factors contributing to type 2 diabetes and recent advances in the treatment and prevention. Int J Med Sci 2014; 11(11): 1185-200.
        [http://dx.doi.org/10.7150/ijms.10001] [PMID: 25249787]

[9]   González EL, Johansson S, Wallander MA, Rodríguez LA. Trends in the prevalence and incidence of diabetes in the UK: 1996-2005. J Epidemiol Community Health 2009; 63(4): 332-6.
        [http://dx.doi.org/10.1136/jech.2008.080382] [PMID: 19240084]

[10]   Shaw JE, Sicree RA, Zimmet PZ. Global estimates of the prevalence of diabetes for 2010 and 2030. Diabetes Res Clin Pract 2010; 87(1): 4-14.
        [http://dx.doi.org/10.1016/j.diabres.2009.10.007] [PMID: 19896746]

[11]   Jallut D, Golay A, Munger R, *et al.* Impaired glucose tolerance and diabetes in obesity: a 6-year follow-up study of glucose metabolism. Metabolism 1990; 39(10): 1068-75.
        [http://dx.doi.org/10.1016/0026-0495(90)90168-C] [PMID: 2215253]

[12]   https://www.cureffi.org/2013/12/13/biochemistry-12-diabetes/

[13]   Ferrannini E, Gastaldelli A, Miyazaki Y, *et al.* Predominant role of reduced beta-cell sensitivity to glucose over insulin resistance in impaired glucose tolerance. Diabetologia 2003; 46(9): 1211-9.
[http://dx.doi.org/10.1007/s00125-003-1169-6] [PMID: 12879253]

[14]   DeFronzo RA. Pathogenesis of type 2 diabetes mellitus. Med Clin North Am 2004; 88(4): 787-835, ix.
[http://dx.doi.org/10.1016/j.mcna.2004.04.013] [PMID: 15308380]

[15]   King WM. Diabetes Mellitus 2020.https://themedicalbiochemistrypage.org/diabetes.php#niddm

[16]   Cerf ME. Beta cell dysfunction and insulin resistance. Front Endocrinol (Lausanne) 2013; 4: 37.
[http://dx.doi.org/10.3389/fendo.2013.00037] [PMID: 23542897]

[17]   Ahlqvist E, Ahluwalia TS, Groop L. Genetics of type 2 diabetes. Clin Chem 2011; 57(2): 241-54.
[http://dx.doi.org/10.1373/clinchem.2010.157016] [PMID: 21119033]

[18]   Halban PA, Polonsky KS, Bowden DW, *et al.* β-cell failure in type 2 diabetes: postulated mechanisms and prospects for prevention and treatment. Diabetes Care 2014; 37(6): 1751-8.
[http://dx.doi.org/10.2337/dc14-0396] [PMID: 24812433]

[19]   Xu E, Kumar M, Zhang Y, *et al.* Intra-islet insulin suppresses glucagon release *via* $GABA\text{-}GABA_A$ receptor system. Cell Metab 2006; 3(1): 47-58.
[http://dx.doi.org/10.1016/j.cmet.2005.11.015] [PMID: 16399504]

[20]   Reimann F. Molecular mechanisms underlying nutrient detection by incretin-secreting cells. Int Dairy J 2010; 20(4): 236-42.
[http://dx.doi.org/10.1016/j.idairyj.2009.11.014] [PMID: 20204054]

[21]   Holst JJ, Knop FK, Vilsbøll T, Krarup T, Madsbad S. Loss of incretin effect is a specific, important, and early characteristic of type 2 diabetes. Diabetes Care 2011; 34(2) (Suppl. 2): S251-7.
[http://dx.doi.org/10.2337/dc11-s227] [PMID: 21525464]

[22]   Rask E, Olsson T, Söderberg S, *et al.* Northern Sweden Monitoring of Trends and Determinants in Cardiovascular Disease (MONICA). Impaired incretin response after a mixed meal is associated with insulin resistance in nondiabetic men. Diabetes Care 2001; 24(9): 1640-5.
[http://dx.doi.org/10.2337/diacare.24.9.1640] [PMID: 11522713]

[23]   Muscelli E, Pereira JA, Lazarin MA, da Silva CA, Pareja JC, Saad MJ. Lack of insulin inhibition on insulin secretion in non-diabetic morbidly obese patients. Int J Obes Relat Metab Disord 2001; 25(6): 798-804.
[http://dx.doi.org/10.1038/sj.ijo.0801607] [PMID: 11439292]

[24]   Taniguchi A, Nakai Y, Sakai M, *et al.* Relationship of regional adiposity to insulin resistance and serum triglyceride levels in nonobese Japanese type 2 diabetic patients. Metabolism 2002; 51(5): 544-8.
[http://dx.doi.org/10.1053/meta.2002.31984] [PMID: 11979383]

[25]   von Eyben FE, Mouritsen E, Holm J, *et al.* Intra-abdominal obesity and metabolic risk factors: a study of young adults. Int J Obes Relat Metab Disord 2003; 27(8): 941-9.
[http://dx.doi.org/10.1038/sj.ijo.0802309] [PMID: 12861235]

[26]   Després JP, Lemieux I, Bergeron J, *et al.* Abdominal obesity and the metabolic syndrome: contribution to global cardiometabolic risk. Arterioscler Thromb Vasc Biol 2008; 28(6): 1039-49.
[http://dx.doi.org/10.1161/ATVBAHA.107.159228] [PMID: 18356555]

[27]   Mittelman SD, Van Citters GW, Kim SP, *et al.* Longitudinal compensation for fat-induced insulin resistance includes reduced insulin clearance and enhanced beta-cell response. Diabetes 2000; 49(12): 2116-25.
[http://dx.doi.org/10.2337/diabetes.49.12.2116] [PMID: 11118015]

[28]   Iyer A, Fairlie DP, Prins JB, Hammock BD, Brown L. Inflammatory lipid mediators in adipocyte function and obesity. Nat Rev Endocrinol 2010; 6(2): 71-82.
[http://dx.doi.org/10.1038/nrendo.2009.264] [PMID: 20098448]

[29]   Howell JJ, Ricoult SJ, Ben-Sahra I, Manning BD. A growing role for mTOR in promoting anabolic metabolism. Biochem Soc Trans 2013; 41(4): 906-12.
[http://dx.doi.org/10.1042/BST20130041] [PMID: 23863154]

[30]   Patti ME, Kahn BB. Nutrient sensor links obesity with diabetes risk. Nat Med 2004; 10(10): 1049-50.
[http://dx.doi.org/10.1038/nm1004-1049] [PMID: 15459705]

[31]   Ron D, Walter P. Signal integration in the endoplasmic reticulum unfolded protein response. Nat Rev Mol Cell Biol 2007; 8(7): 519-29.
[http://dx.doi.org/10.1038/nrm2199] [PMID: 17565364]

[32]   Hotamisligil GS. Endoplasmic reticulum stress and the inflammatory basis of metabolic disease. Cell 2010; 140(6): 900-17.
[http://dx.doi.org/10.1016/j.cell.2010.02.034] [PMID: 20303879]

[33]   Defronzo RA, Tripathy D, Schwenke DC, *et al.* ACT NOW Study. Prediction of diabetes based on baseline metabolic characteristics in individuals at high risk. Diabetes Care 2013; 36(11): 3607-12.
[http://dx.doi.org/10.2337/dc13-0520] [PMID: 24062330]

[34]   George S, Rochford JJ, Wolfrum C, *et al.* A family with severe insulin resistance and diabetes due to a mutation in AKT2. Science 2004; 304(5675): 1325-8.
[http://dx.doi.org/10.1126/science.1096706] [PMID: 15166380]

[35]   Prudente S, Hribal ML, Flex E, *et al.* The functional Q84R polymorphism of mammalian Tribbles homolog TRB3 is associated with insulin resistance and related cardiovascular risk in Caucasians from Italy. Diabetes 2005; 54(9): 2807-11.
[http://dx.doi.org/10.2337/diabetes.54.9.2807] [PMID: 16123373]

[36]   Hribal ML, Tornei F, Pujol A, *et al.* Transgenic mice overexpressing human G972R IRS-1 show impaired insulin action and insulin secretion. J Cell Mol Med 2008; 12(5B): 2096-106.
[http://dx.doi.org/10.1111/j.1582-4934.2008.00246.x] [PMID: 18208559]

[37]   Dash S, Sano H, Rochford JJ, *et al.* A truncation mutation in TBC1D4 in a family with acanthosis nigricans and postprandial hyperinsulinemia. Proc Natl Acad Sci USA 2009; 106(23): 9350-5.
[http://dx.doi.org/10.1073/pnas.0900909106] [PMID: 19470471]

[38]   Prudente S, Scarpelli D, Chandalia M, *et al.* The TRIB3 Q84R polymorphism and risk of early-onset type 2 diabetes. J Clin Endocrinol Metab 2009; 94(1): 190-6.
[http://dx.doi.org/10.1210/jc.2008-1365] [PMID: 18984671]

[39]   Kowluru A, Matti A. Hyperactivation of protein phosphatase 2A in models of glucolipotoxicity and diabetes: potential mechanisms and functional consequences. Biochem Pharmacol 2012; 84(5): 591-7.
[http://dx.doi.org/10.1016/j.bcp.2012.05.003] [PMID: 22583922]

[40]   Rui L, Yuan M, Frantz D, Shoelson S, White MF. SOCS-1 and SOCS-3 block insulin signaling by ubiquitin-mediated degradation of IRS1 and IRS2. J Biol Chem 2002; 277(44): 42394-8.
[http://dx.doi.org/10.1074/jbc.C200444200] [PMID: 12228220]

[41]   Ueki K, Kondo T, Kahn CR. Suppressor of cytokine signaling 1 (SOCS-1) and SOCS-3 cause insulin resistance through inhibition of tyrosine phosphorylation of insulin receptor substrate proteins by discrete mechanisms. Mol Cell Biol 2004; 24(12): 5434-46.
[http://dx.doi.org/10.1128/MCB.24.12.5434-5446.2004] [PMID: 15169905]

[42]   Ueki K, Kondo T, Tseng YH, Kahn CR. Central role of suppressors of cytokine signaling proteins in hepatic steatosis, insulin resistance, and the metabolic syndrome in the mouse. Proc Natl Acad Sci USA 2004; 101(28): 10422-7.
[http://dx.doi.org/10.1073/pnas.0402511101] [PMID: 15240880]

[43]   Rotter V, Nagaev I, Smith U. Interleukin-6 (IL-6) induces insulin resistance in 3T3-L1 adipocytes and is, like IL-8 and tumor necrosis factor-alpha, overexpressed in human fat cells from insulin-resistant subjects. J Biol Chem 2003; 278(46): 45777-84.
[http://dx.doi.org/10.1074/jbc.M301977200] [PMID: 12952969]

[44]   Jager J, Grémeaux T, Cormont M, Le Marchand-Brustel Y, Tanti JF. Interleukin-1beta-induced insulin resistance in adipocytes through down-regulation of insulin receptor substrate-1 expression. Endocrinology 2007; 148(1): 241-51.
[http://dx.doi.org/10.1210/en.2006-0692] [PMID: 17038556]

[45]   Zhang J, Gao Z, Yin J, Quon MJ, Ye J. S6K directly phosphorylates IRS-1 on Ser-270 to promote insulin resistance in response to TNF-(alpha) signaling through IKK2. J Biol Chem 2008; 283(51): 35375-82.
[http://dx.doi.org/10.1074/jbc.M806480200] [PMID: 18952604]

[46]   Fan Y, Yu Y, Shi Y, *et al.* Lysine 63-linked polyubiquitination of TAK1 at lysine 158 is required for tumor necrosis factor alpha- and interleukin-1beta-induced IKK/NF-kappaB and JNK/AP-1 activation. J Biol Chem 2010; 285(8): 5347-60.
[http://dx.doi.org/10.1074/jbc.M109.076976] [PMID: 20038579]

[47]   Federici M, Giaccari A, Hribal ML, *et al.* Evidence for glucose/hexosamine *In vivo* regulation of insulin/IGF-I hybrid receptor assembly. Diabetes 1999; 48(12): 2277-85.
[http://dx.doi.org/10.2337/diabetes.48.12.2277] [PMID: 10580414]

[48]   Riboulet-Chavey A, Pierron A, Durand I, Murdaca J, Giudicelli J, Van Obberghen E. Methylglyoxal impairs the insulin signaling pathways independently of the formation of intracellular reactive oxygen species. Diabetes 2006; 55(5): 1289-99.
[http://dx.doi.org/10.2337/db05-0857] [PMID: 16644685]

[49]   Housley MP, Rodgers JT, Udeshi ND, *et al.* O-GlcNAc regulates FoxO activation in response to glucose. J Biol Chem 2008; 283(24): 16283-92.
[http://dx.doi.org/10.1074/jbc.M802240200] [PMID: 18420577]

[50]   Cariou B, Capitaine N, Le Marcis V, *et al.* Increased adipose tissue expression of Grb14 in several models of insulin resistance. FASEB J 2004; 18(9): 965-7.
[http://dx.doi.org/10.1096/fj.03-0824fje] [PMID: 15059968]

[51]   Cozzone D, Fröjdö S, Disse E, *et al.* Isoform-specific defects of insulin stimulation of Akt/protein kinase B (PKB) in skeletal muscle cells from type 2 diabetic patients. Diabetologia 2008; 51(3): 512-21.
[http://dx.doi.org/10.1007/s00125-007-0913-8] [PMID: 18204829]

[52]   Andreozzi F, Procopio C, Greco A, *et al.* Increased levels of the Akt-specific phosphatase PH domain leucine-rich repeat protein phosphatase (PHLPP)-1 in obese participants are associated with insulin resistance. Diabetologia 2011; 54(7): 1879-87.
[http://dx.doi.org/10.1007/s00125-011-2116-6] [PMID: 21461637]

[53]   Fridlyand LE, Philipson LH. Reactive species and early manifestation of insulin resistance in type 2 diabetes. Diabetes Obes Metab 2006; 8(2): 136-45.
[http://dx.doi.org/10.1111/j.1463-1326.2005.00496.x] [PMID: 16448517]

[54]   Evans JL, Maddux BA, Goldfine ID. The molecular basis for oxidative stress-induced insulin resistance. Antioxid Redox Signal 2005; 7(7-8): 1040-52.
[http://dx.doi.org/10.1089/ars.2005.7.1040] [PMID: 15998259]

[55]   Dokken BB, Saengsirisuwan V, Kim JS, Teachey MK, Henriksen EJ. Oxidative stress-induced insulin resistance in rat skeletal muscle: role of glycogen synthase kinase-3. Am J Physiol Endocrinol Metab 2008; 294(3): E615-21.
[http://dx.doi.org/10.1152/ajpendo.00578.2007] [PMID: 18089761]

[56]   Hotamisligil GS, Peraldi P, Budavari A, Ellis R, White MF, Spiegelman BM. IRS-1-mediated inhibition of insulin receptor tyrosine kinase activity in TNF-α- and obesity-induced insulin resistance. Science 1996; 271(5249): 665-8.
[http://dx.doi.org/10.1126/science.271.5249.665] [PMID: 8571133]

[57]   Lorenzo M, Fernández-Veledo S, Vila-Bedmar R, Garcia-Guerra L, De Alvaro C, Nieto-Vazquez I.

Insulin resistance induced by tumor necrosis factor-alpha in myocytes and brown adipocytes. J Anim Sci 2008; 86(14) (Suppl.): E94-E104.
[http://dx.doi.org/10.2527/jas.2007-0462] [PMID: 17940160]

[58]	Nieto-Vazquez I, Fernández-Veledo S, Krämer DK, Vila-Bedmar R, Garcia-Guerra L, Lorenzo M. Insulin resistance associated to obesity: the link TNF-alpha. Arch Physiol Biochem 2008; 114(3): 183-94.
[http://dx.doi.org/10.1080/13813450802181047] [PMID: 18629684]

[59]	Rafacho A, Ortsäter H, Nadal A, Quesada I. Glucocorticoid treatment and endocrine pancreas function: implications for glucose homeostasis, insulin resistance and diabetes. J Endocrinol 2014; 223(3): R49-62.
[http://dx.doi.org/10.1530/JOE-14-0373] [PMID: 25271217]

[60]	White MF. Springer Science+Business Media. LLC. Springer 2012.Mechanisms of insulin action.4th Edition
[http://dx.doi.org/10.1007/978-1-4614-1028-7_2]

[61]	Newsholme EA, Dimitriadis G. Integration of biochemical and physiologic effects of insulin on glucose metabolism. Exp Clin Endocrinol Diabetes 2001; 109 (Suppl. 2): S122-34.
[http://dx.doi.org/10.1055/s-2001-18575] [PMID: 11460564]

[62]	Saltiel AR, Kahn CR. Insulin signalling and the regulation of glucose and lipid metabolism. Nature 2001; 414(6865): 799-806.
[http://dx.doi.org/10.1038/414799a] [PMID: 11742412]

[63]	Hubbard SR. The insulin receptor: both a prototypical and atypical receptor tyrosine kinase. Cold Spring Harb Perspect Biol 2013; 5(3)a008946
[http://dx.doi.org/10.1101/cshperspect.a008946] [PMID: 23457259]

[64]	Emkey R, Kahn CR. Molecular Aspects of Insulin Signaling.Supplement 21. Handbook of physiologyThe Endocrine System. The Endocrine Pancreas and Regulation of Metabolism 2011.
[http://dx.doi.org/10.1002/cphy.cp070212]

[65]	Butler AA, LeRoith D. Minireview: tissue-specific *versus* generalized gene targeting of the igf1 and igf1r genes and their roles in insulin-like growth factor physiology. Endocrinology 2001; 142(5): 1685-8.
[http://dx.doi.org/10.1210/endo.142.5.8148] [PMID: 11316729]

[66]	De Meyts P. The Insulin Receptor and Its Signal Transduction Network 2016.
https://www.ncbi.nlm.nih.gov/books/NBK378978/

[67]	Machado-Neto JA, Fenerich BA, Rodrigues Alves APN, *et al.* Insulin Substrate Receptor (IRS) proteins in normal and malignant hematopoiesis. Clinics (Sao Paulo) 2018; 73(suppl 1): 11.e566s

[68]	Mardilovich K, Pankratz SL, Shaw LM. Expression and function of the insulin receptor substrate proteins in cancer. Cell Commun Signal 2009; 7: 14.
[http://dx.doi.org/10.1186/1478-811X-7-14] [PMID: 19534786]

[69]	White MF. IRS proteins and the common path to diabetes. Am J Physiol Endocrinol Metab 2002; 283(3): E413-22.
[http://dx.doi.org/10.1152/ajpendo.00514.2001] [PMID: 12169433]

[70]	Cargnello M, Roux PP. Activation and function of the MAPKs and their substrates, the MAPK-activated protein kinases. Microbiol Mol Biol Rev 2011; 75(1): 50-83.
[http://dx.doi.org/10.1128/MMBR.00031-10] [PMID: 21372320]

[71]	Mor A, Aizman E, George J, Kloog Y. Ras inhibition induces insulin sensitivity and glucose uptake. PLoS One 2011; 6(6)e21712
[http://dx.doi.org/10.1371/journal.pone.0021712] [PMID: 21738773]

[72]	Lazar DF, Wiese RJ, Brady MJ, *et al.* Mitogen-activated protein kinase kinase inhibition does not block the stimulation of glucose utilization by insulin. J Biol Chem 1995; 270(35): 20801-7.

[http://dx.doi.org/10.1074/jbc.270.35.20801] [PMID: 7657664]

[73] Brognard J, Hunter T. Protein kinase signaling networks in cancer. Curr Opin Genet Dev 2011; 21(1): 4-11.
[http://dx.doi.org/10.1016/j.gde.2010.10.012] [PMID: 21123047]

[74] Hanks SK, Quinn AM. Protein kinase catalytic domain sequence database: identification of conserved features of primary structure and classification of family members. Methods Enzymol 1991; 200: 38-62.
[http://dx.doi.org/10.1016/0076-6879(91)00126-H] [PMID: 1956325]

[75] Siddle K. Signalling by insulin and IGF receptors: supporting acts and new players. J Mol Endocrinol 2011; 47(1): R1-R10.
[http://dx.doi.org/10.1530/JME-11-0022] [PMID: 21498522]

[76] Huang S, Czech MP. The GLUT4 glucose transporter. Cell Metab 2007; 5(4): 237-52.
[http://dx.doi.org/10.1016/j.cmet.2007.03.006] [PMID: 17403369]

[77] Chang L, Chiang SH, Saltiel AR. Insulin signaling and the regulation of glucose transport. Mol Med 2004; 10(7-12): 65-71.
[http://dx.doi.org/10.2119/2005-00029.Saltiel] [PMID: 16307172]

[78] Martin S, Millar CA, Lyttle CT, *et al.* Effects of insulin on intracellular GLUT4 vesicles in adipocytes: evidence for a secretory mode of regulation. J Cell Sci 2000; 113(Pt 19): 3427-38.
[PMID: 10984434]

[79] Brozinick JT Jr, Hawkins ED, Strawbridge AB, Elmendorf JS. Disruption of cortical actin in skeletal muscle demonstrates an essential role of the cytoskeleton in glucose transporter 4 translocation in insulin-sensitive tissues. J Biol Chem 2004; 279(39): 40699-706.
[http://dx.doi.org/10.1074/jbc.M402697200] [PMID: 15247264]

[80] Bryant NJ, Gould GW. SNARE proteins underpin insulin-regulated GLUT4 traffic. Traffic 2011; 12(6): 657-64.
[http://dx.doi.org/10.1111/j.1600-0854.2011.01163.x] [PMID: 21226814]

[81] Sajan MP, Rivas J, Li P, Standaert ML, Farese RV. Repletion of atypical protein kinase C following RNA interference-mediated depletion restores insulin-stimulated glucose transport. J Biol Chem 2006; 281(25): 17466-73.
[http://dx.doi.org/10.1074/jbc.M510803200] [PMID: 16644736]

[82] Matsumoto M, Ogawa W, Akimoto K, *et al.* PKClambda in liver mediates insulin-induced SREBP-1c expression and determines both hepatic lipid content and overall insulin sensitivity. J Clin Invest 2003; 112(6): 935-44.
[http://dx.doi.org/10.1172/JCI200318816] [PMID: 12975478]

[83] Galic S, Hauser C, Kahn BB, *et al.* Coordinated regulation of insulin signaling by the protein tyrosine phosphatases PTP1B and TCPTP. Mol Cell Biol 2005; 25(2): 819-29.
[http://dx.doi.org/10.1128/MCB.25.2.819-829.2005] [PMID: 15632081]

[84] Brady MJ, Saltiel AR. The role of protein phosphatase-1 in insulin action. Recent Prog Horm Res 2001; 56: 157-73.
[http://dx.doi.org/10.1210/rp.56.1.157] [PMID: 11237211]

[85] Ugi S, Imamura T, Maegawa H, *et al.* Protein phosphatase 2A negatively regulates insulin's metabolic signaling pathway by inhibiting Akt (protein kinase B) activity in 3T3-L1 adipocytes. Mol Cell Biol 2004; 24(19): 8778-89.
[http://dx.doi.org/10.1128/MCB.24.19.8778-8789.2004] [PMID: 15367694]

[86] Brognard J, Newton AC. PHLiPPing the switch on Akt and protein kinase C signaling. Trends Endocrinol Metab 2008; 19(6): 223-30.
[http://dx.doi.org/10.1016/j.tem.2008.04.001] [PMID: 18511290]

[87] Carracedo A, Pandolfi PP. The PTEN-PI3K pathway: of feedbacks and cross-talks. Oncogene 2008;

27(41): 5527-41.
[http://dx.doi.org/10.1038/onc.2008.247] [PMID: 18794886]

[88]	Chagpar RB, Links PH, Pastor MC, *et al.* Direct positive regulation of PTEN by the p85 subunit of phosphatidylinositol 3-kinase. Proc Natl Acad Sci USA 2010; 107(12): 5471-6.
[http://dx.doi.org/10.1073/pnas.0908899107] [PMID: 20212113]

[89]	Suwa A, Kurama T, Shimokawa T. SHIP2 and its involvement in various diseases. Expert Opin Ther Targets 2010; 14(7): 727-37.
[http://dx.doi.org/10.1517/14728222.2010.492780] [PMID: 20536411]

[90]	Holt LJ, Siddle K. Grb10 and Grb14: enigmatic regulators of insulin action--and more? Biochem J 2005; 388(Pt 2): 393-406.
[http://dx.doi.org/10.1042/BJ20050216] [PMID: 15901248]

[91]	Sachithanandan N, Fam BC, Fynch S, *et al.* Liver-specific suppressor of cytokine signaling-3 deletion in mice enhances hepatic insulin sensitivity and lipogenesis resulting in fatty liver and obesity. Hepatology 2010; 52(5): 1632-42.
[http://dx.doi.org/10.1002/hep.23861] [PMID: 20799351]

[92]	Koo SH, Satoh H, Herzig S, *et al.* PGC-1 promotes insulin resistance in liver through PPAR-alph--dependent induction of TRB-3. Nat Med 2004; 10(5): 530-4.
[http://dx.doi.org/10.1038/nm1044] [PMID: 15107844]

[93]	Chakraborty A, Koldobskiy MA, Bello NT, *et al.* Inositol pyrophosphates inhibit Akt signaling, thereby regulating insulin sensitivity and weight gain. Cell 2010; 143(6): 897-910.
[http://dx.doi.org/10.1016/j.cell.2010.11.032] [PMID: 21145457]

[94]	Boucher J, Kleinridders A, Kahn CR. Insulin receptor signaling in normal and insulin-resistant states. Cold Spring Harb Perspect Biol 2014; 6(1)a009191
[http://dx.doi.org/10.1101/cshperspect.a009191] [PMID: 24384568]

[95]	Turban S, Hajduch E. Protein kinase C isoforms: mediators of reactive lipid metabolites in the development of insulin resistance. FEBS Lett 2011; 585(2): 269-74.
[http://dx.doi.org/10.1016/j.febslet.2010.12.022] [PMID: 21176778]

[96]	Um SH, Frigerio F, Watanabe M, *et al.* Absence of S6K1 protects against age- and diet-induced obesity while enhancing insulin sensitivity. Nature 2004; 431(7005): 200-5.
[http://dx.doi.org/10.1038/nature02866] [PMID: 15306821]

[97]	Cusi K, Maezono K, Osman A, *et al.* Insulin resistance differentially affects the PI 3-kinase- and MAP kinase-mediated signaling in human muscle. J Clin Invest 2000; 105(3): 311-20.
[http://dx.doi.org/10.1172/JCI7535] [PMID: 10675357]

[98]	Li Y, Tian M, Yang M, *et al.* Central Sfrp5 regulates hepatic glucose flux and VLDL-triglyceride secretion. Metabolism 2020; 103154029
[http://dx.doi.org/10.1016/j.metabol.2019.154029] [PMID: 31770545]

[99]	Zierath JR, Krook A, Wallberg-Henriksson H. Insulin action and insulin resistance in human skeletal muscle. Diabetologia 2000; 43(7): 821-35.
[http://dx.doi.org/10.1007/s001250051457] [PMID: 10952453]

[100]	Aguirre V, Werner ED, Giraud J, Lee YH, Shoelson SE, White MF. Phosphorylation of Ser307 in insulin receptor substrate-1 blocks interactions with the insulin receptor and inhibits insulin action. J Biol Chem 2002; 277(2): 1531-7.
[http://dx.doi.org/10.1074/jbc.M101521200] [PMID: 11606564]

[101]	Govers R. Molecular mechanisms of GLUT4 regulation in adipocytes. Diabetes Metab 2014; 40(6): 400-10.
[http://dx.doi.org/10.1016/j.diabet.2014.01.005] [PMID: 24656589]

[102]	Richter EA, Hargreaves M. Exercise, GLUT4, and skeletal muscle glucose uptake. Physiol Rev 2013; 93(3): 993-1017.

[http://dx.doi.org/10.1152/physrev.00038.2012] [PMID: 23899560]

[103] Tremblay F, Lavigne C, Jacques H, Marette A. Defective insulin-induced GLUT4 translocation in skeletal muscle of high fat-fed rats is associated with alterations in both Akt/protein kinase B and atypical protein kinase C (ζ/λ) activities. Diabetes 2001; 50(8): 1901-10.
[http://dx.doi.org/10.2337/diabetes.50.8.1901] [PMID: 11473054]

[104] Maianu L, Keller SR, Garvey WT. Adipocytes exhibit abnormal subcellular distribution and translocation of vesicles containing glucose transporter 4 and insulin-regulated aminopeptidase in type 2 diabetes mellitus: implications regarding defects in vesicle trafficking. J Clin Endocrinol Metab 2001; 86(11): 5450-6.
[http://dx.doi.org/10.1210/jcem.86.11.8053] [PMID: 11701721]

[105] Draznin B. Molecular mechanisms of insulin resistance: serine phosphorylation of insulin receptor substrate-1 and increased expression of p85α: the two sides of a coin. Diabetes 2006; 55(8): 2392-7.
[http://dx.doi.org/10.2337/db06-0391] [PMID: 16873706]

[106] Tanti JF, Gual P, Grémeaux T, Gonzalez T, Barrès R, Le Marchand-Brustel Y. Alteration in insulin action: role of IRS-1 serine phosphorylation in the retroregulation of insulin signalling. Ann Endocrinol (Paris) 2004; 65(1): 43-8.
[http://dx.doi.org/10.1016/S0003-4266(04)95629-6] [PMID: 15122091]

[107] Paz K, Hemi R, LeRoith D, *et al.* A molecular basis for insulin resistance. Elevated serine/threonine phosphorylation of IRS-1 and IRS-2 inhibits their binding to the juxtamembrane region of the insulin receptor and impairs their ability to undergo insulin-induced tyrosine phosphorylation. J Biol Chem 1997; 272(47): 29911-8.
[http://dx.doi.org/10.1074/jbc.272.47.29911] [PMID: 9368067]

[108] Tanti JF, Jager J. Cellular mechanisms of insulin resistance: role of stress-regulated serine kinases and insulin receptor substrates (IRS) serine phosphorylation. Curr Opin Pharmacol 2009; 9(6): 753-62.
[http://dx.doi.org/10.1016/j.coph.2009.07.004] [PMID: 19683471]

[109] Samuel VT, Shulman GI. The pathogenesis of insulin resistance: integrating signaling pathways and substrate flux. J Clin Invest 2016; 126(1): 12-22.
[http://dx.doi.org/10.1172/JCI77812] [PMID: 26727229]

[110] Whiteman EL, Chen JJ, Birnbaum MJ. Platelet-derived growth factor (PDGF) stimulates glucose transport in 3T3-L1 adipocytes overexpressing PDGF receptor by a pathway independent of insulin receptor substrates. Endocrinology 2003; 144(9): 3811-20.
[http://dx.doi.org/10.1210/en.2003-0480] [PMID: 12933652]

[111] Watson RT, Pessin JE. Intracellular organization of insulin signaling and GLUT4 translocation. Recent Prog Horm Res 2001; 56: 175-93.
[http://dx.doi.org/10.1210/rp.56.1.175] [PMID: 11237212]

[112] Baumann CA, Ribon V, Kanzaki M, *et al.* CAP defines a second signalling pathway required for insulin-stimulated glucose transport. Nature 2000; 407(6801): 202-7.
[http://dx.doi.org/10.1038/35025089] [PMID: 11001060]

[113] Kimura A, Baumann CA, Chiang SH, Saltiel AR. The sorbin homology domain: a motif for the targeting of proteins to lipid rafts. Proc Natl Acad Sci USA 2001; 98(16): 9098-103.
[http://dx.doi.org/10.1073/pnas.151252898] [PMID: 11481476]

[114] Watson RT, Shigematsu S, Chiang SH, *et al.* Lipid raft microdomain compartmentalization of TC10 is required for insulin signaling and GLUT4 translocation. J Cell Biol 2001; 154(4): 829-40.
[http://dx.doi.org/10.1083/jcb.200102078] [PMID: 11502760]

[115] Bhowmick A, Banu S. Therapeutic targets of type 2 diabetes: an overview. MOJ Drug Des Develop Ther 2017; 1(3): 60-4.

[116] Hummel CS, Lu C, Loo DD, Hirayama BA, Voss AA, Wright EM. Glucose transport by human renal Na+/D-glucose cotransporters SGLT1 and SGLT2. Am J Physiol Cell Physiol 2011; 300(1): C14-21.

[http://dx.doi.org/10.1152/ajpcell.00388.2010] [PMID: 20980548]

[117] Nauck MA. Update on developments with SGLT2 inhibitors in the management of type 2 diabetes. Drug Des Devel Ther 2014; 8: 1335-80.
[http://dx.doi.org/10.2147/DDDT.S50773] [PMID: 25246775]

[118] Drucker DJ, Nauck MA. The incretin system: glucagon-like peptide-1 receptor agonists and dipeptidyl peptidase-4 inhibitors in type 2 diabetes. Lancet 2006; 368(9548): 1696-705.
[http://dx.doi.org/10.1016/S0140-6736(06)69705-5] [PMID: 17098089]

[119] Liu Z, Habener JF. Glucagon-like peptide-1 activation of TCF7L2-dependent Wnt signaling enhances pancreatic beta cell proliferation. J Biol Chem 2008; 283(13): 8723-35.
[http://dx.doi.org/10.1074/jbc.M706105200] [PMID: 18216022]

[120] Holst JJ, Vilsbøll T, Deacon CF. The incretin system and its role in type 2 diabetes mellitus. Mol Cell Endocrinol 2009; 297(1-2): 127-36.
[http://dx.doi.org/10.1016/j.mce.2008.08.012] [PMID: 18786605]

[121] Muskiet MHA, Tonneijck L, Smits MM, *et al.* GLP-1 and the kidney: from physiology to pharmacology and outcomes in diabetes. Nat Rev Nephrol 2017; 13(10): 605-28.
[http://dx.doi.org/10.1038/nrneph.2017.123] [PMID: 28869249]

[122] van Baar MJB, van Ruiten CC, Muskiet MHA, van Bloemendaal L, IJzerman RG, van Raalte DH. SGLT2 Inhibitors in Combination Therapy: From Mechanisms to Clinical Considerations in Type 2 Diabetes Management. Diabetes Care 2018; 41(8): 1543-56.
[http://dx.doi.org/10.2337/dc18-0588] [PMID: 30030256]

CHAPTER 2

Diabetes Mellitus and Protective Approaches of Medicinal Plants: Present Status and Future Prospects

Maliha Sarfraz[*]

Institute of Physiology and Pharmacology, University of Agriculture Faisalabad, Pakistan

Abstract: Diabetes mellitus is one of the major health problem worldwide, its incidence and mortality are increasing day by day. Conventional antidiabetic drugs are available with unavoidable side effects. On the other hand, medicinal plants act as an alternative source of antidiabetic agents. From ancient times, herbs and spices have been widely used in the food and for medicinal purposes. In culinary practices, these are used as colorant, preservatives, and flavor substitution. In medicine, oxidative stress and inflammation associated with noncommunicable diseases can be treated or managed through herbs and spices. Phytochemicals like carotenoids, phenolic compounds, sterols, terpenes, alkaloids, glucosinolates, and other sulfur-containing compounds may be responsible for their protective and therapeutic effects. In this modern era, it is necessary to inform consumers about the benefits of botanical compounds. Many herbal plants have potential health claims that are not significantly demonstrated. Since herbs and spices can be used to get better food value and human health, as functional food ingredients they are helpful to decrease the risk of chronic diseases. Much trial evidence for the use of herbal plants to treat diabetes mellitus has uniformly demonstrated safety. However, further studies are needed to explore the health beneficial effects of these herbal plants used for diabetes mellitus.

DIABETES MELLITUS

Diabetes includes a varied set of ailments categorized as the production of sufficient insulin or decreased sensitivity due to many reasons; chronically increased glucose concentration is one of the common characteristics. Due to this, several metabolic complications raised; in blood, increased ketone bodies due to stern insulin deficiency [1]. In the pathogenesis of diabetic complications, hyperglycemia plays a significant role and those people are at higher risk, who have poor glycemic control. Although in various studies it has been mentioned that the destruction of beta cells and insulin resistance are the major factors of

[*] **Corresponding author Maliha Sarfraz:** Institute of Physiology and Pharmacology, University of Agriculture Faisalabad, Pakistan; E-mail: maliha.sarfraz@yahoo.com

diabetes, several signaling pathways are also involved in diabetes as summarized in Fig. **(1)** [2].

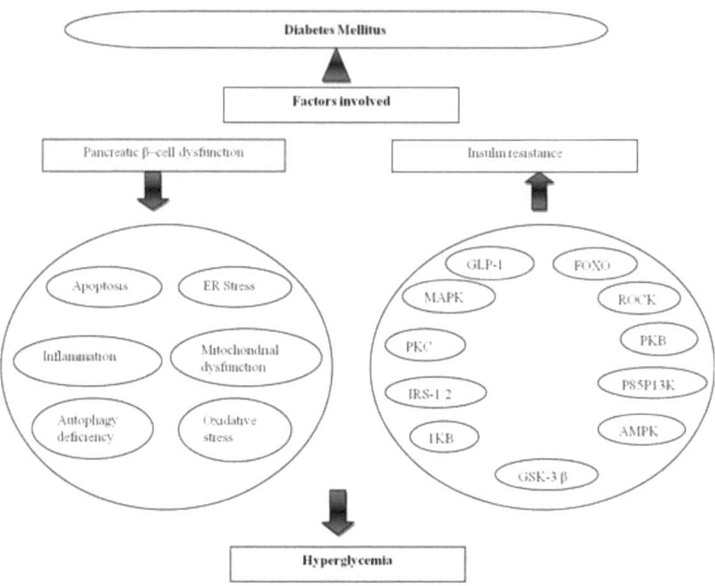

Fig. (1). Representative mechanism involved in the development of diabetes mellitus. Glucagon-like peptide 1 (GLP-1); insulin receptor substrate 1 and 2 (IRS-1/2); mitogen-activated protein kinases (MAPK); AMP-activated protein kinase (AMPK); IkB kinase (IkB); protein kinase C (PKC); Rho-associated coiled-coil containing protein kinase (ROCK); protein kinase B (PKB); forkhead box protein O (Foxo); PI3K subunit (p85); phosphatidylinositol 3-kinase (PI3K); Glycogen synthase kinase-3b (GSK-3b).

Pathophysiology and Complications

The specific acute metabolic complications of diabetes mellitus are diabetic ketoacidosis, lactic acidosis, hyperosmolar non-ketotic coma and hypoglycemia. In addition to acute complications, the long–lasting consequences of diabetes mellitus are the progressive development of some severe complications like retinopathy with prospective blindness, nephropathy that can cause kidney failure, neuropathy and diabetic foot, *etc.* Persistent hyperglycemia in diabetes may result in macroangiopathy and microangiopathy that are considered to be poly etiological disorders. Diabetic patients are generally more prone to coronary artery disease, diabetic cardiomyopathy, peripheral vascular and cerebrovascular disease [3].

Effects of Diabetes Mellitus on Biological Parameters

In diabetic animals, a strong relationship exists between hyperglycemia and reduced body weight. Weight decreased may be due to body's inability to utilize and storage of glucose which leads to malnourishment and weight loss [4]. Pancreatic beta cells produce insulin which helps glucose transportation across cell membrane. Insulin insufficiency disturb the transportation of glucose in blood as a result level increased in blood and urine [5]. Carbohydrate and fat metabolism is impaired during diabetes. In mammals, various sites of lipid metabolism are affected by insulin. In hyperglycemic state, lipid peroxidation alterations are very common which is related to free radicals. These radicals cause lipid disruption . They are also involved in diabetes complications. Antioxidants neutralize these radicals which prevent complications induced by diabetes in experimental animal models [6]. In hyperglycemic condition, increased lipid peroxidation and accumulation of its products is caused by oxidative stress. Adefegha and Ganiyu, reported that in alloxan-induced diabetic rats malondialdehyde levels increased as compared to normal rats. Imbalance between oxygen free radicals production and cell defense mechanism also cause destruction of liver and pancreatic tissues that leads to complications [7]. Ragavan and Krishnakumari, studied that in diabetic conditions liver sections revealed structural alterations (hepatocyte necrosis) due to insulin absence [8]. Moreover, Hashemnia described the degenerative changes in hepatocytes such as hepatic cord disorganization, congestion of central veins and infiltrated sinusoids in diabetic rats [9].

Diabetes Mellitus Management

Managing of a disease is very important. Several aspects, such as less physical activity, obesity, smoking and use of alcohol, effects the incidence of diabetes. Lifestyle modifications can reduce the risk of disease incidence. High fiberous and low total fats diet will prevent diabetes. WHO also recommended that improving factors of lifestyle like stay away from fatness lastly from hyperglycemia [10].

Conventional and Traditional Treatments for Diabetes

Diabetes is considered a global problem world widely. The purpose of its treatment to get better life and prevention from its complications. Most commonly for type 1 diabetes short and long acting insulin and for type 2 biguanides and sulfonylureas are used in allopathy. The sulfonylureas include tolbutamide, glibenclamide, chlorpropamide, glipizide, acetohexamide, gliclazide and tolazamide. Several factors have been involved in therapeutic effects of sulfonylureas for type II diabetic patients, including pancreatic and extrapancreatic. Sulfonylureas directly encourage release of insulin from the β-cells in the islets of Langerhans, and this effect does not require the existence of glucose or other secretagogues [11]. From since 1960s among biguanides, metformin and phenformin have been employed for oral diabetic therapy. In contrast to sulfonylureas, metformin has blood glucose reducing effect only in diabetes; and it does not produce hypoglycemia in normal subjects. Pancreas or isolated islets of nondiabetic animal model have no effect on release of basal insulin by use of metformin. Some new drugs which are used for diabetes type 2 include troglitazone and repaglinides. For the treatment of type 2 sitagliptin, saxagliptin and vildagliptin are effective [10].

DIABETES AND BOTANICAL MEDICINES

Before the advent of insulin for the management of diabetes plant remedies were used. The World Health Organization (WHO) advised scientists to observe whether old-style medications have any useful therapeutic efficacy. In plants, various numbers of biologically active compounds are present, and they may be serving as basis for synthetic equivalents and an interesting means that can be useful as improved type of biological mechanisms shown in Fig. (**2**). From last 20 years, scientific studies have evidenced the effectiveness of these preparations, few of them extremely effective. Different herbal plants with combinations were used for treatment [12]. Herbal remedies when used in combinations their constituents have synergic potential and less side effects. So, inspite of single herb usage, combinations are preferable [13, 14].

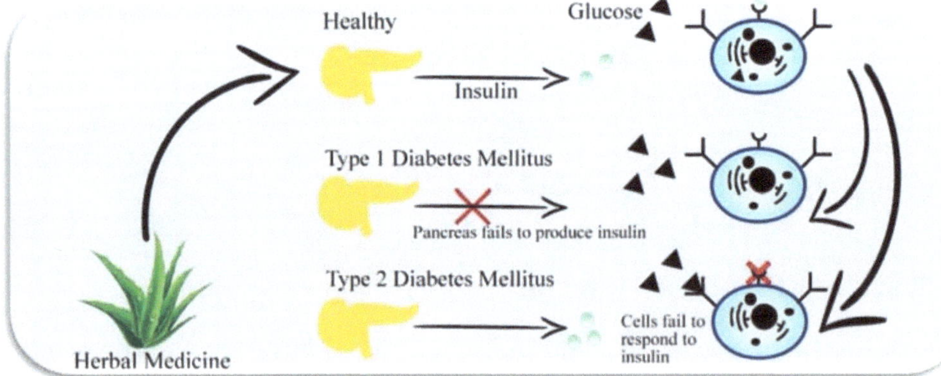

Fig. (2). Herbal medicine and diabetes mellitus.

Numerous bioactive compounds are identified by their hypoglycemic activity like flavonoids, alkaloids, polysaccharides and glycosides. For example, like mechanism of sulfonylureas, few plants increased insulin release and needs less number of β-cells to do function. Euphorbia prostrata, Momordica foetida,

Fumaria parviflora and Taraxacum officinale are one of these plants. Like metformin, few plants extracts *e.g.* Aloe, Momordica charantia, Cecropia obtusifolia, Coccinia indica and Hammada salicornia, act by altering the metabolism of glucose . Few of them affect on complication of diabetes like masoprocol, isolated from Larrea tridentata, effects on cholesterol free fatty acids and triglyceride in hyperglycemic rats [15].

NOMENCLATURE AND CHEMICAL CONSTITUENTS OF MEDICINAL PLANTS

Curcumin is the most active ingredient that has been the topic of many systematic research. There are forty tropical Asian specie of this genus is found. It is widely used as spice [16]. G. sylvestre is a woody plant found in tropical region of Africa and Australia. G. sylvestre roots and leaves in dried form have therapeutic properties. For the treatment of diabetes, respiratory diseases, kidney stones, stomach disorders it is used. *Piper nigrum* is generally used in medicine of ayurvedic system. It is cultivated overall in the world; also, known as natural spice; as a spice, its usage is documented. *Sesamum indicum* is also an ancient spice. Its seed is rich with oil and proteins. It is used as cooking oil world widely and belong to family Pedaliaceae [17]. For thousands of years in the Middle East dates fruit are used as essential part of the diet. It is commercially important crop of Saudi Arabia, Egypt and Emirates. Dates have high nutritional and therapeutics value, its products are commonly used for human and animal consumption, cosmetics, carpentry and pharmaceuticals [18]. Ajwa date is solitary cultivated in Saudia and has prominent role for disease treatment. It has defensive role in hepatic toxicity [19]. Fenugreek is very important in Ayuredic and Chinese medicine. It is one of the oldest medicinal plants. The leaves and seeds are used to prepare extracts or powders for medicinal use. In Egypt, Rome and Chinese medicine it is used as a tonic for various disease remedies [20, 21]. Nomenclature and different chemical constituents with their antidiabetic activity are shown in Tables **1** and **2**.

Table 1. Nomenclature and chemical constituents of medicinal plants.

Nomenclature	Curcuma longa	Gymnema sylvestre	Piper nigrum	Sesamum indicum	Phoenix dactylifera	Trigonella foenum-graecum
Kingdom **Division** **Class** **Order** **Family** **Genus** **Specie**	Plantae Tracheophyta Magnoliopsida Zingiberales Zingiberaceae Curcuma C. longa	Plantae Magnoliophyta Magnoliopsida Gentianales Asclepiadaceae Gymnema G. Sylvestre	Plantae Manoliophyta Magnoliopsida Piperales Piperaceae Piper P. nigrum	Plantae Tracheophyta Magnoliopsida Lamiales Pedaliaceae Sesamum S. Indicum	Plantae Magnoliophyta Liliopsida Arecales Arecaceae Phoenix P. dactylifera	Plantae Magnoliophyta Magnoliopsida Febales Febaceae Trigonella *T. foenum-graceum*
Chemical Constituents	Edgeworthin Curcumin Curcuminoids Curcumene [22]	Gymnemic acid Gymnemasin B, C, and D Gymnamine Gurmarin Gypenoside [23]	Piperine Alkaloids Steroid Terpenes Propenyphenols [24]	Sesamin, Sesame lignans Sesamol Episesamin, Sesamolin Fatty acids [25]	Phenolic Flavonoids Steroids Fatty acids Carotenoids [26]	Nicotinic acid Coumarin Alkaloid Trogonelline [27]

Table 2. Sources, structure, and target of potential antidiabetic phytochemicals.

Compound	Source	Structure	Target	Reference
Curcumin	Curcuma longa	Curcumin	Lowers blood glucose and glycosylated hemoglobin level	[28]
Gymnemic acid	Gymnema sylvestre	Gymnemic acid 1	It stimulates insulin secretion from the pancreas and delays glucose absorption	[29]
Piperine	*Piper nigrum*	Piperine	Lowers blood glucose level by the bio-enhancing the effect of piperine with metformin	[30]

(Table 2) cont.....

Compound	Source	Structure	Target	Reference
Sesame	Sesamum indicum	Sesamine	Blood glucose level reduced	[31]
Flavonoids (Quercetin)	Phoenix dactylifera	Quercetin	It activates Akt/cAMP response element-binding protein pathway	[32]
Edgeworthin	Trigonella foenum-graceum	Edgeworthin	α –glucosidase αamylase pathways stimulated to control blood glucose level	[33]

PROTECTIVE EFFECT OF MEDICINAL PLANTS

Curcumin biological activities have been reported in various studies. These involved reviews focusing on anti-carcinogenic and chemo preventive activities, mechanism of action, and role in management of ailment [34]. In different research works anti-oxidant potential of curcumin has been documented. Vitamin C a water-soluble antioxidant that can repair the resulting phenoxyl radicle [35] Free radicles like superoxide, hydroxyl radical and single oxygen can be scavenged directly by curcumin but also increased endogenous defense by exerting antioxidant activity against oxidative damage. It is reported that glutathione expression increased in cultured alveolar epithelial cells (A549) and its activity increased in kidneys of mice fed with dietary curcumin 2% when compared with normal rats [36]. Possible hypoglycemic activity of curcuma longa is shown in Fig. (3). In a variety of animals, antioxidant and scavenging of radical activities have been documented in different studies. Some of them are summarized here. Cadmium and lead caused lipid peroxidation in rat model, curcumin helps to protect brain homogenate. In rodents, hepatic oxidative damage decreased significantly if they were pretreated with curcumin. The rat forebrain oxidative injury can be protected with curcumin treatment [37].

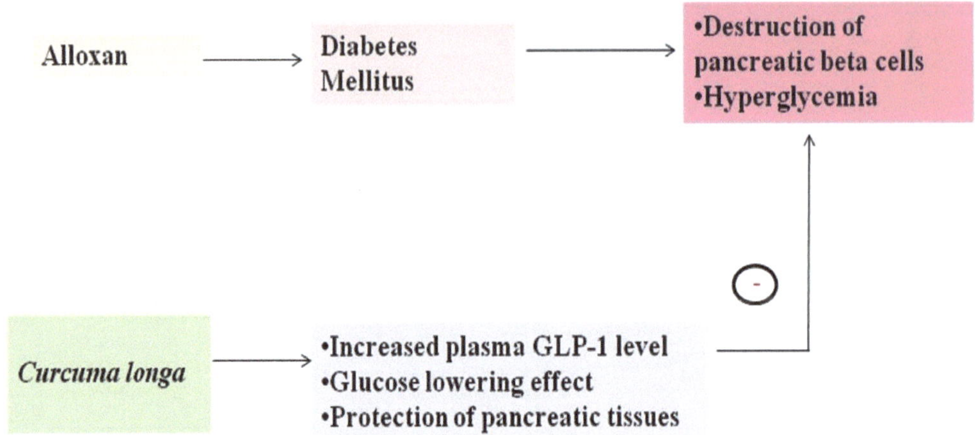

Fig. (3). Hypoglycemic activity of Curcuma longa.

A high fat atherogenic diet fed rabbit receiving 1.66 mg/kg hydroethanolic turmeric extract for four weeks significantly lowered oxidative damage [38]. The 1% turmeric extracts in diet for one week in mice decreased triglyceride level and erythrocyte phospholipid hydroperoxides as compared to control animals. While Kempaiah and Srinivasan reported that high fat diet fed rats for 8 weeks with 0.2% dietary curcumin significantly decreased lipid peroxidation and reduced intracellular antioxidants in erythrocyte [39]. In streptozotocin diabetic rats' lipid peroxidation level was reduced significantly when treated with 200mg/kg curcumin but superoxide dismutase and catalase level was not affected [40]. In another study, it was documented that same curcumin dose for 8 weeks significantly reduced AGE products that involved in oxidative stress [41]. In nicotine-induced lung toxicity antioxidant activity and lipid peroxidation status was significantly improved by curcumin treatment [42]. Dietary ethanol induced oxidative stress in rats caused increase level of lipid peroxidation and liver enzymes, curcumin helps to improve this effect, due to this reason it can be suggested as protective in liver disease [43]. Kumar reported in their study that low dietary curcumin dose helps to delay cataract formation in hyperglycemic rats [44]. In rodents, drug-induced oxidative organ damage curcumin helps to protect this damage. Curcumin helps to reduce bleomycin induced oxidative lung injury, adrinamycin induced cardiotoxicity and nephrotoxicity [45]. Renal oxidative damage caused by Gentamycin in rats' turmeric helps to improve it [46]. It also decreased clastogenesis by radicle scavenging activity formed due to cisplatin induced toxicity but did not show any significant effect at nephrotoxicity and lipid peroxidation level. It was also reported that under few circumstances curcumin promotes the production of reactive oxygen species [47].

In different studies anti-inflammatory activity of curcumin is studied. It is observed that activation of transcription factor NFκB was inhibited by curcumin. Inflammatory cytokines participate in NFκB activation and curcumin inhibit these cytokines. At 5µM concentration, curcumin inhibited lipopolysaccharide induced production of IL-1 and TNF by a cell line of human monocytic macrophage [48], while C- reactive protein IL-1β levels were reduced in rats with adjuvant inflammation [49]. During the inflammatory response, endothelial cells migrate to tissues through vascular system following leukocyte recruitment. TNF treated endothelial cells caused adherence of monocytes which results in endothelial leukocyte adhesion molecule-1 and vascular cell adhesion molecule-1; their bond completely blocked by curcumin pre-treatment [50]. Curcumin also inhibit protein expression in UVB-irradiated keratinocytes and COX-2 mRNA [51]. Along with that curcumin blocks phosphorylation and thus affects on arachidonic acid metabolism by PLA2 enzyme and also inhibit 5 LOX activity [52]. Endothelial tissue factors inhibited by curcumin which help in coagulation by (AP-1) and NFκB [53]. Nitric oxide an inflammatory mediator its derivative (nitrite and peroxynitrite) caused carcinogenicity its expression also inhibited by curcumin; its inhibition is observed in mouse peritoneal cells, while production of NO and iNOS expression inhibition was documented in microglial cells of rat [54]. Many signaling pathways like JNK, MAPK and NFκB are involved in curcumin inhibition. Mice injected with LPS reduced iNOS RNA hepatic expression about 50-70% when treated with curcumin 92ng/g body weight in *in-vivo* study [55]. It was observed that bioavailability of curcumin interfered when given after food and inhibition was seen only when given after fasting. Curcumin have important biological activity when given orally in low doses. It decreased the inflammatory response in glial cells of rodent brain by inhibiting the signaling of Janus kinase-STAT [56].

The anti-tumor activity of curcumin has been documented in many studies [57] but in human few studies are documented; those have been carried out are explorative in nature. At dose 3.6g curcumin for seven days in colorectal cancer patients' significantly reduced malignant tissues but COX-2 levels were unaffected [58]. In external cancer patients, curcumin mixed ointment and turmeric ethanolic extract provide relief. In several studies, it was reported that curcumin acts as an anticancer agent through different mechanisms at different stages [59]. A major mechanism seems to be the apoptosis induction by mitochondrial pathway because curcumin decrease membrane potential of mitochondria [60]. In human renal cancer cells curcumin-induced apoptosis was initiated with death receptor expression upregulation [61]. COX-2 plays an important role in carcinogenesis due to this reason in various malignant cells its expressions are elevated so it is considered as a molecular target for chemoprevention. In tumor, growth of COX-2 has been implicated [62].

Particularly COX-2 has prominent role in colon cancer. Along with that in many studies it was documented that in cancer cells curcumin down regulate COX-2 [63]. Curcumin has pharmacological activities like immunological effects, antihyperglycemic effects and hepatoprotective action. Curcumin and its derivatives reduce histamine release from leukemia cells. Endothelial dysfunction due to homocysteine improved by curcumin. In rats with glomerular disease curcumin had anti-fibrotic action and decreased a variety of inflammatory fragments [64]. Curcumin as a diet at 0.002% in rats protects cataract formation and had potent anti-ulcer effects by preventing glutathione depletion, protein oxidation and lipid peroxidation [65]. It enhanced healing of wound by gamma-irradiation and was also helpful in wound healing of diabetic rodents. In animal models of inflammatory bowel disease curcumin has positive results; this outcome is related to NFκB expression inhibition [66]. In another study patients with ulcerative proctitis have produced hopeful results [67]. Many studies reported that for treatment and prevention of Alzheimer's disease curcumin is helpful. For the treatment of cystic fibrosis curcumin was proposed as a beneficial agent [2].

Aqueous extract of G. sylvestre was administered to both normal and alloxan induced diabetic rats for thirty days and results showed that levels of glucose, creatinine, urea and uric acid were also turned to normal [68]. Along with that another study results showed that G. sylvestre aqueous leaf extract have turned fasting blood glucose, serum triglyceride and cholesterol turned to normal [69]. In one study hydrochloric extract of G. sylvestre was determined in hyperlipidemic rats. Hyperlipidemia was induced in rats by feeding high cholesterol diet. The results of the study demonstrated that significant reduction in serum cholesterol, triglyceride, LDL-C levels and improvement in HDL-C level was observed when compared with standard drug atorvastatin [70]. Hypoglycemic activity of Gymnema sylvestre shown in Fig. (**4**)

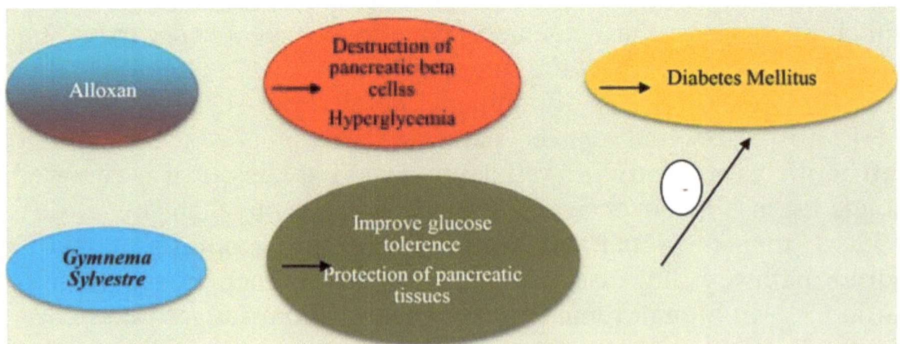

Fig. (4). Hypoglycemic activity of *Gymnema Sylvestre*.

Ethanol extract of G. sylvestre has hypoglycemic potential, for this purpose *in vitro* and *in vivo* trial were performed to check antioxidants potential in streptozotocin-induced diabetic rats. Extract was given for four weeks. Results showed that glucose, glutamate pyruvate transaminase and Glutathione peroxidase levels reduced to normal and they also have antioxidant potential activity [71]. A study was conducted in which hydrochloric extract G. sylvestre was administered to streptozotocin induced hyperglycemic rats for forty five days. Results of the study showed that serum glucose, insulin, cholesterol, triglyceride, ALT and AST levels were turned towards normal after treatment [72]. Shafey were also determined the antidiabetic effect of G. sylvestre extract in streptozotocin-induced diabetic rats. The results of the study demonstrated that plasma glucose, cholesterol, LDL, triglyceride and malondialdhyde level were reduced significantly whereas level of insulin, HDL and superoxide dismutase were increased significantly in diabetic control rats [73]. In another study interaction of gliclazide with G. sylvestre extract on pharmacodynamic response for 12 hours was observed in normal and alloxan-induced diabetic rats. G. sylvestre reduced blood glucose level at 3 hour at a dose of 100mg/kg body weight and gliclazide reduced blood glucose at 3 and 8 hour at a dose of 2mg/kg body weight. The results of the study showed that administration of G. sylvestre before administration of gliclazide significantly reduced blood glucose level [74]. Aantidiabetic activity of G. sylvestre leaf and Clerodendrum phlomidis leaf extract in alloxan- induced hyperglycemic rats were determined. Treatment showed significant decrease in blood glucose level, glycosylated haemoglobin and liver glycogen while serum cholesterol, triglyceride, LDL, HDL and VLDL levels were also reduced to normal in treated rats [75]. Another *in-vitro* study reported that ethanolic extract of this plant had strong antioxidant activity due to the presence of saponins, tannins, alkaloids, flavonoids and phenols [76].

Black pepper has diverse biological activities similar to analgesic, antipyretic, diuretic, digestive, alexiteric, CNS stimulant, carminative and antifeedant activities. It is also useful in asthma, cough, fever, arthritis, dyspepsia, dermopathy and hemorrhoids [77]. Several studies evaluated that oxidative stress related problems were resolved using antioxidants. Different piper species were documented for defense of renal, cardiac and hepatic antioxidant status in atherogenic hamsters. These also act against oxidative stress [78]. Agbor results also showed that oxidative stress and atherosclerosis caused due to increased lipid concentration in the blood and piper species have antioxidant and antiatherosclerosis activities in atherogenic diet fed hamsters [79]. They also reported that these piper species also have role in intoxication. Several medicinal plants have antioxidant activity and central nervous system effects. The food supplements have attracted more attention to cure cognitive function contrary to cognitive deficit condition including in Alzheimer's disease. Piperine was more effective in Alzheimer's disease for neurodegeneration and memory presentation in animal model [80]. *Piper nigrum* hypoglycemic action is summarized in Fig. (5).

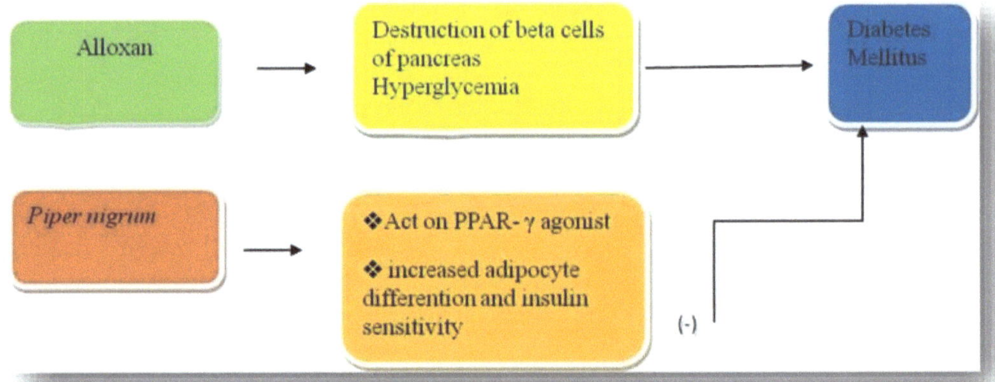

Fig. (5). Hypoglycemic activity of *Piper nigrum*.

It was reported that in mice during the preweaning period, safrole injection and tannic acid induced tumors in different organs, while d-limonene force feeding reversed carcinogenic activity caused due to these injections and piperine did not have any noteworthy outcome to reverse carcinogenic activity [81]. Bae reported in their study that phenolic component of black pepper; inhibit lipopolysaccharide induced inflammatory responses [82]. Chatterjee study showed that phenolic compounds in green pepper have antioxidant potential. They documented that lignin's from M. fragrans were assessed for capability to scavenge DPPH radical and plasmid DNA damage protection. Piperine effects glucose level in diabetic mice was also documented in acute and subacute models [83]. In acute study, they raised blood glucose level at high doses while in subacute study they documented that it has antihyperglycemic effect [84]. By the use of third-instar larvae of Aedes aegypti larvicidal activity of piper essential oil was tested. The oils have aryl-propanoids were more active [85]. By the use of wing Somatic Mutation and Recombination Test (SMART) in drosophila melanogaster modifying activity of black pepper and bell pepper with methyl methane sulfonate and ethyl carbamate was reported by Hamss [86]. They documented that the antimutagenic activity of spice may be due to suppression or interaction of metabolic activation with the mutagens of active groups.

The literature on S. indicum oil shows that they exhibit biological and antioxidant activities due to the presence of certain active phytochemical constituents [87]. In STZ induced diabetic rats 6% S. indicum oil were fed for forty two days and results of the study showed that blood glucose level reduced significantly as compared to diabetic control rats [88]. Another study showed that glucose level was reduced to 20% and 15% respectively when 35g of S. indicum oil per day in salad for two months and 36% decrease in glucose level was observed with combination therapy of S. indicum oil and glibenclamid. In Fig. (**6**) hypoglycemic activity of S. indicum is shown.

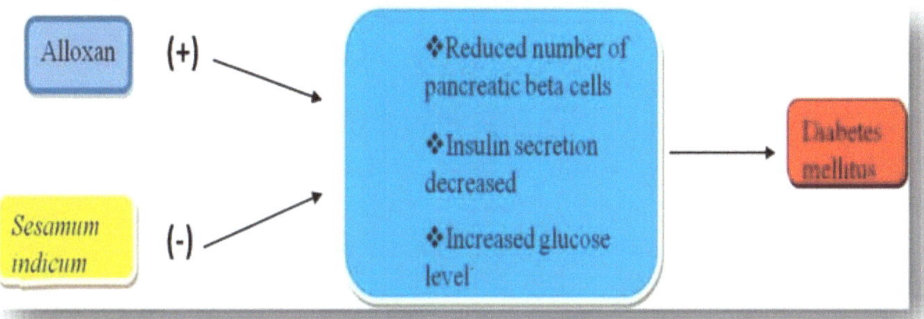

Fig. (6). Hypoglycemic activity of *Sesamum indicum*.

In another research study it was determined that steroids and terpenoids were present in very high concentration while flavonoids, phenols, alkaloids and saponins in moderately high concentration. Cardiac glycosides and phlabotannins were absent. Results showed that presence of phytocostitutes indicate its pharmacological activities [89]. Another study results showed that white sesame seed extract possesses better antioxidant activity as compared to black sesame seed extract [17]. A study results showed the effect of *S. indicum* seeds supplemented diet for five weeks significantly reduced blood glucose level in treated rats and triglyceride, total cholesterol and LDL levels were also turned towards normal as compared to diabetic control rats [90].

For a long time, date fruits are considered in Arab as a source of food. It is used in domestic preparation. It is useful to cure lead induced haemotoxicity. Date fruit, seed, bark and leaves have antimutagenic, antiulcerative, antihypertensive, anti-inflammatory, antidiarrheal, antifungal, antibacterial and antiviral potential [91]. Antioxidants neutralize the free radicals, but they do not cause damage. Free radicals action prevention is the first step for management of disease. Those plants have medicinal importance with antioxidant activity play important role to deactivate the free radicals [92]. *Phoenix dactylifera* exhibits effective antioxidative activity. Reduction of intrinsic defense system in fruit prevented by oxidative cell damage and contributes in reducing cell damage defense system [93]. Date fruit has capability to neutralize free radicals documented in earlier studies and its aqueous extract has potent anti-mutagenic, antioxidant and antimicrobial activity [94, 95]. Literature has shown that due to the presence of carotenoids and antioxidants constituents' 80400 μmol/100g and phenolic compounds with quantity 3942 mg/100g dates are a good source of antioxidants [96]. A study reported that when black pepper and ajwa seed aqueous extract used in combination they improved the liver enzyme activities and glucose level in alloxanized diabetic rats [97]. The antioxidant and hepatoprotective activity of date fruit depend upon the presence of phenolic and flavonoids contents. Those date varieties have high phenolic and flavonoids content have high potential to cure disease [98, 99]. Al-Shoaibi strongly suggest in their study the use of *Phoenix dactylifera* as dietary habit for better health due to their antioxidant potential [100]. In another study, hepatotoxicity induced rats, ajwa date was given as treatment is proved as hepatoprotective and may boost antioxidant enzymes [19]. Possible hypoglycemic activity of *Phoenix dactylifera* is shown in Fig. (**7**).

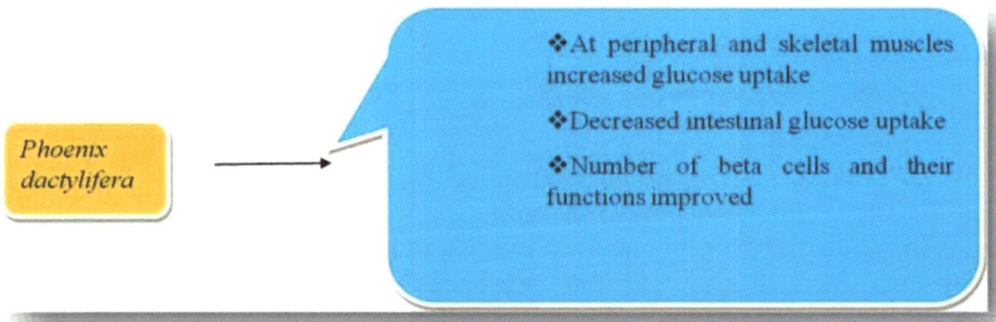

Fig. (7). Hypoglycemic activity of *Phoenix dactylifera*.

In biological defense mechanism inflammation plays important role. LOX and NF-kB transcriptional factors show prominent part in hyperglycemia and cancer. Transcriptional factor inhibitors played important role in prevention of transcription factors action. Unfortunately, the transcriptional inhibitors are expensive and have side effects. An important medication for NF-kB inhibition is natural product, which acts as anti-inflammatory agents. Phenolics and flavonoids are outstanding anti-inflammatory agents. Date fruit is also act as an excellent ant-inflammatory agent [101]. Elberry studied that date pollen has probable defensive action by varied cytokines expression [102]. It is also studied that date fruit methanolic extract have key part in declining the foot swelling and plasma fibrinogen [103]. Eddine, reported in their study that date leaves have good anti-oxidant and anti-inflammatory potential [104]. Vayalil, reported in his study that extract of *Phoenix dactylifera* pollen grains are effective in anticancer and antimutogenesis [105]. Its anticancer activity is also reported by Biglari *et al.*, its study showed the effect of *Phoenix dactylifera* fruits as anticancer for lymphoma

[106]. Al-Qawari *et al.*, reported in their study that date pulp and seed extracts are helpful in reduction of creatinine and urea concentration and perfected proximal tubular damage in gentamicin induced nephrotoxicity in rats [107].

In animals and small human trials fenugreek seeds have found to lower serum glucose level. Gupta *et al.* reported in their study that fenugreek has positive glycemic effects on glucose and insulin levels [108]. In another study Gaddam *et al.* reported the results of a randomized, controlled, crossover trial of fenugreek seeds and the results presented that in the fenugreek-treated patients, statistically significant mean improvements were reported for glucose tolerance and serum-clearance rates of glucose [109]. Goyal *et al.* conducted controlled studies in patients with type 2 diabetes and results demonstrated that significant mean improvements in fasting blood glucose levels and glucose-tolerance were observed in the fenugreek-treated patients [110]. Results from several additional case studies suggest that its seeds improve glycemic control in type 2 diabetes [111]. Hypoglycemic activity of T. foenum graceum is shown in Fig. (**8**).

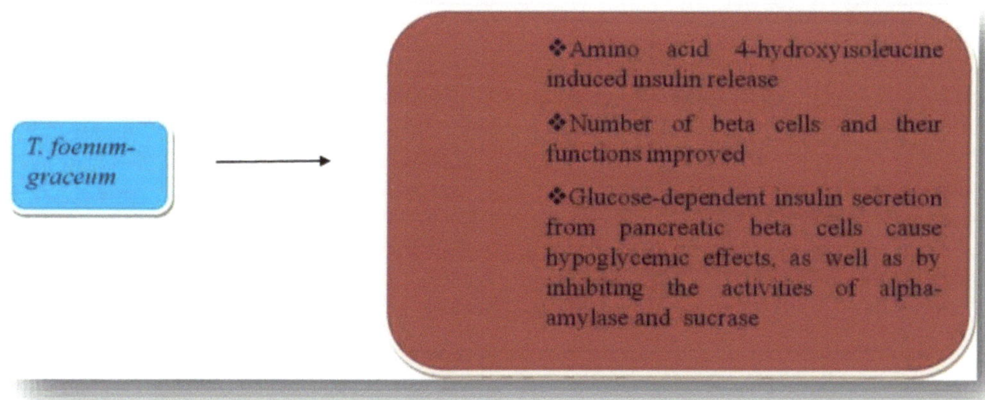

Fig. (8). Hypoglycemic activity of *T. foenum-graceum.*

FUTURE PROSPECTIVE

The evidence in relation to the hypoglycemic effect of phytochemicals is not very consistent; however, phytochemicals have the potential of improving the metabolic profile of patients with diabetes mellitus, mainly with regard to lipid levels, and reducing the associated complications. In addition, phytochemicals could have interesting interactions with conventional antidiabetic drugs that can positively affect diabetes treatment. Therefore, the use of phytochemicals as a coadjutant for diabetes mellitus therapy is a topic that merits to be considered. Finally, considering those clinical trials on phytochemicals antidiabetic properties are no conclusive and many issues regarding its bioavailability need to be resolved, some questions emerge: despite its pharmacokinetic issues, is phytochemicals able to produce pharmacological effects at tiny concentrations? Is there a point of convergence for diabetes mellitus and other diseases in which phytochemicals have been reported to exert a beneficial effect? And if this is true, is that point of convergence a target for phytochemicals?

CONSENT FOR PUBLICATION

Not applicable.

CONFLICT OF INTEREST

There is no conflict of interest declared.

ACKNOWLEDGEMENT

Declared none.

REFERENCES

[1]   Ramachandran S, Koikaramparambil RN, Baskaran R, Mohammad A, Aiyalu R. Antidiabetic, antihyperlipidemic and *in vivo* antioxidant potential of aqueous extract of Anogeissus latifolia bark in type 2 diabetic rats. Asian Pac J Trop Dis 2012; 15: S596-602.
[http://dx.doi.org/10.1016/S2222-1808(12)60229-1]

[2]   Susana RM, Trujillo J, Chaverri J P. The utility of curcumin for the treatment of diabetes mellitus: evidence from preclinical and clinical studies J Nut & Intermediatory metabolism 2018.

[3]   Pop-Busui R, Boulton AJM, Feldman EL, *et al*. Diabetic Neuropathy: A position statement by the American diabetes association. Diabetes Care 2017; 40(1): 136-54.
[http://dx.doi.org/10.2337/dc16-2042] [PMID: 27999003]

[4]   Zafar J, Bhatti F, Akhtar N, *et al*. Prevalence and risk factors for diabetes mellitus in a selected urban population of a city in Punjab. J Pak Med Assoc 2011; 61(1): 40-7.
[PMID: 22368901]

[5]   Tanaka H, Yoshida S, Oshima H, *et al*. Chronic treatment with novel GPR40 agonists improve whole-body glucose metabolism based on the glucose-dependent insulin secretion. J Pharmacol Exp Ther 2013; 346(3): 443-52.
[http://dx.doi.org/10.1124/jpet.113.206466] [PMID: 23853170]

[6]   Shahwar D, Muhammad AR, Afifa S, *et al*. Antioxidant potential of the extracts of Putranjiva roxburghii, Conyza bonariensis, Woodfordia fruticosa and Senecio chrysanthemoides. Afr J Biotechnol 2012; 18: 4288-95.

[7]   Adefegha SA, Ganiyu O. Phytochemistry and mode of action of some tropical spices in the management of type-2 diabetes and hypertension. Afr J Pharm Pharmacol 2013; 7: 332-46.
[http://dx.doi.org/10.5897/AJPPX12.014]

[8]   Ragavan B, Krishnakumari S. Effect of T. Arjuna stem bark extract on histopathology of liver, kidney and pancreas of alloxan-induced diabetic rats. Afr J Biomed Res 2006; 9: 189-97.

[9]   Hashemnia M, Ahmad O, Ahmad RH, Adel M. Blood glucose levels and pathology of organs in alloxan-induced diabetic rats treated with hydro-ethanol extracts of Allium sativum and Capparis spinosa. Afr J Pharm Pharmacol 2012; 21: 1559-64.

[10]   Wu Y, Ding Y, Tanaka Y, Zhang W. Risk factors contributing to type 2 diabetes and recent advances in the treatment and prevention. Int J Med Sci 2014; 11(11): 1185-200.
[http://dx.doi.org/10.7150/ijms.10001] [PMID: 25249787]

[11]   Wiwanitkit S, Wiwanitkit V. Therapeutic goal of diabetes mellitus. J Midlife Health 2011; 2(2): 94-5.
[PMID: 22408342]

[12]   Parveen A, Parveen R, Akhatar A, Parveen B, Siddiqui KM, Iqbal M. Concepts and Quality Considerations in Unani System of Medicine. J AOAC Int 2019.
[PMID: 31547901]

[13]   Afsheen N, Khalil R, Nazish J. Attenuation of Chemically Induced Diabetes in Rabbits with Herbal Mixture (Citrullus colocynthis and Cicer arietinum). Pak Vet J 2012; 1: 41-4.

[14]   Herrera TA. Iriondo-DeHond, J Uribarri, M D Castillo. Beneficial Herbs and Spices. Nutrition, Fitness, and Mindfulness 2020; pp. 65-85.

[15]   Veyrat-Durebex C, Bris C, Codron P, *et al.* Metabo-lipidomics of Fibroblasts and Mitochondrial-Endoplasmic Reticulum Extracts from ALS Patients Shows Alterations in Purine, Pyrimidine, Energetic, and Phospholipid Metabolisms. Mol Neurobiol 2019; 56(8): 5780-91.
[http://dx.doi.org/10.1007/s12035-019-1484-7] [PMID: 30680691]

[16]   Gupta A, Gupta R, Lal B. Effect of *Trigonella foenum-graecum* (fenugreek) seeds on glycaemic control and insulin resistance in type 2 diabetes mellitus: a double blind placebo controlled study. J Assoc Physicians India 2001; 49: 1057-61.
[PMID: 11868855]

[17]   Vishwanath HS, Anilakumar KR, Harsha SN, Khanum F, Bawa AS. *In vitro* antioxidant activity of *Sesamum indicum* seeds. Asian. J Pharm Clin Res 2012; 5: 56-60.

[18]   Robinson ML, Brown B, Williams CF. 2012.The date palm in southern Nevada http://www.unce.unr.edu/publications/files/ho/2002/sp0212.pdf

[19]   Abdu SB. The protective role of Ajwa date against the hepatotoxicity induced by Ochratoxin A. Egyp J Nat Tox 2011; 8: 1-15.

[20]   Ambachew Y, Kashy S, Tasfey R. Prevalence of diabetes mellitus among patients visiting the medical outpatient department of Ayder Referral Hospital, Mekelle, Ethiopia: A three years pooled data. Int J Pharm Sci Res 2015; 6: 215.

[21]   Oresanya IO, Sonibare MA, Gueye B, *et al.* Isolation of flavonoids from Musa acuminata Colla (Simili radjah, ABB) and the *in vitro* inhibitory effects of its leaf and fruit fractions on free radicals, acetylcholinesterase, 15-lipoxygenase, and carbohydrate hydrolyzing enzymes. J Food Biochem 2020; 44(3)e13137
[http://dx.doi.org/10.1111/jfbc.13137] [PMID: 31899556]

[22]   Evans WC. Trease and Evans Pharmacognosy. 15th ed., Edinburgh: WB Saunders 2002.

[23]   Leach MJ. Gymnema sylvestre for diabetes mellitus: a systematic review. J Altern Complement Med 2007; 13(9): 977-83.
[http://dx.doi.org/10.1089/acm.2006.6387] [PMID: 18047444]

[24]   Bano G, Raina RK, Zutshi U, Bedi KL, Johri RK, Sharma SC. Effect of piperine on bioavailability and pharmacokinetics of propranolol and theophylline in healthy volunteers. Eur J Clin Pharmacol 1991; 41(6): 615-7.
[http://dx.doi.org/10.1007/BF00314996] [PMID: 1815977]

[25]   Saleem MTS, Chetty MC, Kavimani S. Putative antioxidant property of sesame oil in an oxidative stress model of myocardial injury. J Cardiovasc Dis Res 2013; 4(3): 177-81.
[http://dx.doi.org/10.1016/j.jcdr.2013.07.001] [PMID: 24396257]

[26]   Vembu S, Sivanasan D, Prasanna G. Effect of *Phoenix dactylifera* on high-fat diet-induced obesity. J Chem Pharm Res 2012; 4(1): 348-52.

[27]   Singh AB, Tamarkar AK, Narender T, Srivastava AK. Antihyperglycaemic effect of an unusual amino acid (4-hydroxyisoleucine) in C57BL/KsJ-db/db mice. Nat Prod Res 2010; 24(3): 258-65.
[http://dx.doi.org/10.1080/14786410902836693] [PMID: 20140804]

[28]   Kunwar A, Priyadarsini KI, Gupta SC, Prasad S, Aggarwal BB. Curcumin and its role in chronic diseases.Advances in Experimental Medicine and Biology. Cham, Switzerland. Springer International Publishing 2016; 928: 1-26.

[29]   Atal S, Agrawal RP, Vyas S, Phadnis P, Rai N. Evaluation of the effect of piperine per se on blood glucose level in alloxan-induced diabetic mice. Acta Pol Pharm 2012; 69(5): 965-9.
[PMID: 23061294]

[30]   Tiwari P, Mishra BN, Sangwan NS. Phytochemical and pharmacological properties of *Gymnema sylvestre*: an important medicinal plant. BioMed Res Int 2014; 2014830285
[http://dx.doi.org/10.1155/2014/830285] [PMID: 24511547]

[31]   Thuy TD, Phan NN, Wang CY, *et al.* Novel therapeutic effects of sesamin on diabetes-induced cardiac dysfunction. Mol Med Rep 2017; 15(5): 2949-56.
[http://dx.doi.org/10.3892/mmr.2017.6420] [PMID: 28358428]

[32]   Li XH, Xin X, Wang Y, *et al.* Pentamethylquercetin protects against diabetes-related cognitive deficits in diabetic Goto-Kakizaki rats. J Alzheimers Dis 2013; 34(3): 755-67.
[http://dx.doi.org/10.3233/JAD-122017] [PMID: 23271319]

[33]   Pari L, *et al.* Antihyperlipidemic effect of coumarin in experimental type 2 diabetic rats. Biomedicine & Prev Nutr 2014; 2: 171-6.
[http://dx.doi.org/10.1016/j.bionut.2014.02.003]

[34]   Aggarwal BB, Harikumar KB. Potential therapeutic effects of curcumin, the anti-inflammatory agent, against neurodegenerative, cardiovascular, pulmonary, metabolic, autoimmune and neoplastic diseases. Int J Biochem Cell Biol 2009; 41(1): 40-59.
[http://dx.doi.org/10.1016/j.biocel.2008.06.010] [PMID: 18662800]

[35]   Jovanovic SV, Boone CW, Steenken S, Trinoga M, Kaskey RB. How curcumin works preferentially with water soluble antioxidants. J Am Chem Soc 2001; 123(13): 3064-8.
[http://dx.doi.org/10.1021/ja003823x] [PMID: 11457017]

[36]   Yu W, Wu J, Cai F, *et al.* Curcumin alleviates diabetic cardiomyopathy in experimental diabetic rats. PLoS One 2012; 7(12)e52013
[http://dx.doi.org/10.1371/journal.pone.0052013] [PMID: 23251674]

[37]   Daniel A. The benefits of curcumin in various diseases and the extension of its application through various technological approaches. Knowledge International Journal 2018; 28: 2.

[38]   Mesa MD, Aguilera CM, Ramírez-Tortosa CL, *et al.* Oral administration of a turmeric extract inhibits erythrocyte and liver microsome membrane oxidation in rabbits fed with an atherogenic diet. Nutrition 2003; 19(9): 800-4.
[http://dx.doi.org/10.1016/S0899-9007(03)00093-5] [PMID: 12921893]

[39]   Kempaiah RK, Srinivasan K. Influence of dietary curcumin, capsaicin and garlic on the antioxidant status of red blood cells and the liver in high-fat-fed rats. Ann Nutr Metab 2004; 48(5): 314-20.
[http://dx.doi.org/10.1159/000081198] [PMID: 15467281]

[40]   Anand P, Kunnumakkara AB, Newman RA, Aggarwal BB. Bioavailability of curcumin: problems and promises. Mol Pharm 2007; 4(6): 807-18.
[http://dx.doi.org/10.1021/mp700113r] [PMID: 17999464]

[41]   Na LX, Zhang YL, Li Y, *et al.* Curcumin improves insulin resistance in skeletal muscle of rats. Nutr Metab Cardiovasc Dis 2011; 21(7): 526-33.
[http://dx.doi.org/10.1016/j.numecd.2009.11.009] [PMID: 20227862]

[42]   Kalpana C, Menon VP. Inhibition of nicotine-induced toxicity by curcumin and curcumin analog: a

comparative study. J Med Food 2004; 7(4): 467-71.
[http://dx.doi.org/10.1089/jmf.2004.7.467] [PMID: 15671691]

[43]   Rukkumani R, Aruna K, Varma PS, Rajasekaran KN, Menon VP. Comparative effects of curcumin and an analog of curcumin on alcohol and PUFA induced oxidative stress. J Pharm Pharm Sci 2004; 7(2): 274-83.
[PMID: 15367386]

[44]   Kumar GSAKS, Shetty AK, Salimath PV. Modulatory effect of fenugreek seed mucilage and spent turmeric on intestinal and renal disaccharidases in streptozotocin induced diabetic rats. Plant Foods Hum Nutr 2005; 60(2): 87-91.
[http://dx.doi.org/10.1007/s11130-005-5104-5] [PMID: 16021836]

[45]   Venkatesan N, Punithavathi D, Arumugam V. Curcumin prevents adriamycin nephrotoxicity in rats. Br J Pharmacol 2000; 129(2): 231-4.
[http://dx.doi.org/10.1038/sj.bjp.0703067] [PMID: 10694226]

[46]   Farombi EO, Ekor M. Curcumin attenuates gentamicin-induced renal oxidative damage in rats. Food Chem Toxicol 2006; 44(9): 1443-8.
[http://dx.doi.org/10.1016/j.fct.2006.05.005] [PMID: 16814915]

[47]   Atsumi T, Murakami Y, Shibuya K, Tonosaki K, Fujisawa S. Induction of cytotoxicity and apoptosis and inhibition of cyclooxygenase-2 gene expression, by curcumin and its analog, alpha-diisoeugenol. Anticancer Res 2005; 25(6B): 4029-36.
[PMID: 16309195]

[48]   Chan MMY, Ho CT, Huang HI. Effects of three dietary phytochemicals from tea, rosemary and turmeric on inflammation-induced nitrite production. Cancer Lett 1995; 96(1): 23-9.
[http://dx.doi.org/10.1016/0304-3835(95)03913-H] [PMID: 7553604]

[49]   Neyrinck AM, Alligier M, Memvanga PB, *et al.* Curcuma longa extract associated with white pepper lessens high fat diet-induced inflammation in subcutaneous adipose tissue. PLoS One 2013; 8(11)e81252
[http://dx.doi.org/10.1371/journal.pone.0081252] [PMID: 24260564]

[50]   Kumar A, Dhawan S, Hardegen NJ, Aggarwal BB. Curcumin (Diferuloylmethane) inhibition of tumor necrosis factor (TNF)-mediated adhesion of monocytes to endothelial cells by suppression of cell surface expression of adhesion molecules and of nuclear factor-kappaB activation. Biochem Pharmacol 1998; 55(6): 775-83.
[http://dx.doi.org/10.1016/S0006-2952(97)00557-1] [PMID: 9586949]

[51]   Ejaz A, Wu D, Kwan P, Meydani M. Curcumin inhibits adipogenesis in 3T3-L1 adipocytes and angiogenesis and obesity in C57/BL mice. J Nutr 2009; 139(5): 919-25.
[http://dx.doi.org/10.3945/jn.108.100966] [PMID: 19297423]

[52]   Hong J, Bose M, Ju J, *et al.* Modulation of arachidonic acid metabolism by curcumin and related beta-diketone derivatives: effects on cytosolic phospholipase A(2), cyclooxygenases and 5-lipoxygenase. Carcinogenesis 2004; 25(9): 1671-9.
[http://dx.doi.org/10.1093/carcin/bgh165] [PMID: 15073046]

[53]   Leturque A, Brot-Laroche E, Le Gall M. GLUT2 mutations, translocation, and receptor function in diet sugar managing. Am J Physiol Endocrinol Metab 2009; 296(5): E985-92.
[http://dx.doi.org/10.1152/ajpendo.00004.2009] [PMID: 19223655]

[54]   Jung KK, Lee HS, Cho JY, *et al.* Inhibitory effect of curcumin on nitric oxide production from lipopolysaccharide-activated primary microglia. Life Sci 2006; 79(21): 2022-31.
[http://dx.doi.org/10.1016/j.lfs.2006.06.048] [PMID: 16934299]

[55]   Choi S, Choi Y, Choi Y, Kim S, Jang J, Park T. Piperine reverses high fat diet-induced hepatic steatosis and insulin resistance in mice. Food Chem 2013; 141(4): 3627-35.
[http://dx.doi.org/10.1016/j.foodchem.2013.06.028] [PMID: 23993530]

[56]　Kim SO, Kundu JK, Shin YK, *et al.* [6]-Gingerol inhibits COX-2 expression by blocking the activation of p38 MAP kinase and NF-kappaB in phorbol ester-stimulated mouse skin. Oncogene 2005; 24(15): 2558-67.
[http://dx.doi.org/10.1038/sj.onc.1208446] [PMID: 15735738]

[57]　Pal S, Bhattacharyya S, Choudhuri T, Datta GK, Das T, Sa G. Amelioration of immune cell number depletion and potentiation of depressed detoxification system of tumor-bearing mice by curcumin. Cancer Detect Prev 2005; 29(5): 470-8.
[http://dx.doi.org/10.1016/j.cdp.2005.05.003] [PMID: 16188398]

[58]　Garcea G, Berry DP, Jones DJL, *et al.* Consumption of the putative chemopreventive agent curcumin by cancer patients: assessment of curcumin levels in the colorectum and their pharmacodynamic consequences. Cancer Epidemiol Biomarkers Prev 2005; 14(1): 120-5.
[PMID: 15668484]

[59]　Chauhan DP. Chemotherapeutic potential of curcumin for colorectal cancer. Curr Pharm Des 2002; 8(19): 1695-706.
[http://dx.doi.org/10.2174/1381612023394016] [PMID: 12171541]

[60]　Volate SR, Davenport DM, Muga SJ, Wargovich MJ. Modulation of aberrant crypt foci and apoptosis by dietary herbal supplements (quercetin, curcumin, silymarin, ginseng and rutin). Carcinogenesis 2005; 26(8): 1450-6.
[http://dx.doi.org/10.1093/carcin/bgi089] [PMID: 15831530]

[61]　Lev-Ari S, Maimon Y, Strier L, Kazanov D, Arber N. Down-regulation of prostaglandin E2 by curcumin is correlated with inhibition of cell growth and induction of apoptosis in human colon carcinoma cell lines. J Soc Integr Oncol 2006; 4(1): 21-6.
[PMID: 16737669]

[62]　Li L, Braiteh FS, Kurzrock R. Liposome-encapsulated curcumin: *in vitro* and *in vivo* effects on proliferation, apoptosis, signaling, and angiogenesis. Cancer 2005; 104(6): 1322-31.
[http://dx.doi.org/10.1002/cncr.21300] [PMID: 16092118]

[63]　Ferreira N, Saraiva MJ, Almeida MR. Uncovering the Neuroprotective Mechanisms of Curcumin on Transthyretin Amyloidosis. Int J Mol Sci 2019; 20(6): 1287.
[http://dx.doi.org/10.3390/ijms20061287] [PMID: 30875761]

[64]　Pari L, Karthikesan K, Menon VP. Comparative and combined effect of chlorogenic acid and tetrahydrocurcumin on antioxidant disparities in chemical induced experimental diabetes. Mol Cell Biochem 2010; 341(1-2): 109-17.
[http://dx.doi.org/10.1007/s11010-010-0442-5] [PMID: 20339905]

[65]　Lucchesi AN, Freitas NT, Cassettari LL, Marques SF, Spadella CT. Diabetes mellitus triggers oxidative stress in the liver of alloxan-treated rats: a mechanism for diabetic chronic liver disease. Acta Cir Bras 2013; 28(7): 502-8.
[http://dx.doi.org/10.1590/S0102-86502013000700005] [PMID: 23842931]

[66]　Mohammed SA, Yaqub AG, Sanda KA, *et al.* Review on diabetes, synthetic drugs and glycemic effects of medicinal plants. J Med Plants Res 2013; 36: 2628-37.

[67]　Holt PR, Katz S, Kirshoff R. Curcumin therapy in inflammatory bowel disease: a pilot study. Dig Dis Sci 2005; 50(11): 2191-3.
[http://dx.doi.org/10.1007/s10620-005-3032-8] [PMID: 16240238]

[68]　Sathya S, Kokilavani R, Gurusamy K. Hypoglycemic effect of Gymnema sylvestre (retz.,) R.Br leaf in normal and alloxan induced diabetic rats. Anc Sci Life 2008; 28(2): 12-4.
[PMID: 22557305]

[69]　Mall GK, Mishra P, Prakash V. Antidiabetic and hypolipidemic activity of Gymnema sylvestre in alloxan-induced diabetic rats. Glob J Biotechnol Biochem 2009; 4(1): 37-42.

[70]　Racch PR, Rachh MR, Ghadiya NR, *et al.* Antihyperlipidemic activity of Gymenma sylvestre R. Br.

leaf extract on rats fed with high cholesterol diet. Int J Pharmacol 2010; 6(2): 138-41.
[http://dx.doi.org/10.3923/ijp.2010.138.141]

[71] Kang MH, Lee MS, Choi MK, Min KS, Shibamoto T. Hypoglycemic activity of Gymnema sylvestre extracts on oxidative stress and antioxidant status in diabetic rats. J Agric Food Chem 2012; 60(10): 2517-24.
[http://dx.doi.org/10.1021/jf205086b] [PMID: 22360666]

[72] Mallikarjuna G, Suguna R, Shridhar NB, Sathyanarayana ML, Byregowda SM, Ravikumar P. Efficacy of Gymnema sylvestre in the alleviation of streptozotocin-induced diabetes in patients. Int J Adv Biol Res 2013; 3(1): 51-7.

[73] Shafey AAME, El-Ezababi MM, Seliem MME, Ouda HHM, Ibrahim DS. Effect of Gymnema sylvestre R. Br. leaves extracts on certain physiological parameters of diabetic rats. J King Saud Univ Sci 2013; 25: 135-41.
[http://dx.doi.org/10.1016/j.jksus.2012.11.001]

[74] Raju MG, Satyanarayana S, Kumar E. Safety of Gliclazide with the aqueous extract of Gymnema Sylvestre on pharmacodynamic activity in Normal and alloxan-induced diabetic rats. American. J Phytomed Clin Therap 2014; 2(7): 901-9.

[75] Gopinathan S, Naveenraj D. Antidiabetic activity of Clerodendrum Phlomidis Linn. and Gymnema sylvestre Linn. In alloxan-induced diabetic rats - A comparative preclinical study. World. J Pharm Res 2014; 3: 1640-75.

[76] Singh K, Bandita D. Phytochemical evaluation and *in vitro* antioxidant activity of Gymnema sylvestre R. Br J Med Plant Stud 2014; 2(4): 19-23.

[77] Vaidy AS. Indian Medicinal Plants: A Compendium of 500 Species. Orient Longman Ltd Madras 1995; 4: 297.

[78] Agbor GA, Akinfiresoye L, Sortino J, Johnson R, Vinson JA. Piper species protect cardiac, hepatic and renal antioxidant status of atherogenic diet fed hamsters. Food Chem 2012; 134(3): 1354-9.
[http://dx.doi.org/10.1016/j.foodchem.2012.03.030] [PMID: 25005953]

[79] Agbor GA, Vinson JA, Sortino J, Johnson R. Antioxidant and anti-atherogenic activities of three Piper species on atherogenic diet fed hamsters. Exp Toxicol Pathol 2012; 64(4): 387-91.
[http://dx.doi.org/10.1016/j.etp.2010.10.003] [PMID: 21035316]

[80] Chonpathompikunlert P, Wattanathorn J, Muchimapura S. Piperine, the main alkaloid of Thai black pepper, protects against neurodegeneration and cognitive impairment in animal model of cognitive deficit like condition of Alzheimer's disease. Food Chem Toxicol 2010; 48(3): 798-802.
[http://dx.doi.org/10.1016/j.fct.2009.12.009] [PMID: 20034530]

[81] Wrba H, el-Mofty MM, Schwaireb MH, Dutter A. Carcinogenicity testing of some constituents of black pepper (*Piper nigrum*). Exp Toxicol Pathol 1992; 44(2): 61-5.
[http://dx.doi.org/10.1016/S0940-2993(11)80188-0] [PMID: 1617288]

[82] Bae GS, Kim MS, Jeong J, *et al.* Piperine ameliorates the severity of cerulein-induced acute pancreatitis by inhibiting the activation of mitogen activated protein kinases. Biochem Biophys Res Commun 2011; 410(3): 382-8.
[http://dx.doi.org/10.1016/j.bbrc.2011.05.136] [PMID: 21663734]

[83] Chatterjee S, Niaz Z, Gautam S, Adhikariv S, Variyar PS, Sharma A. Antioxidant activity of some phenolic constituents from green pepper (*Piper nigrum* L.) and fresh nutmeg mace. Food Chem 2007; 101(2): 515-23.
[http://dx.doi.org/10.1016/j.foodchem.2006.02.008]

[84] Atal S, Atal S, Vyas S, Phadnis P. Bio-enhancing effect of piperine with metformin on lowering the blood glucose level in alloxan-induced diabetic mice. Pharmacognosy Res 2016; 8(1): 56-60.
[http://dx.doi.org/10.4103/0974-8490.171096] [PMID: 26941537]

[85] Morais SM, Facundo VA, Bertini LM, Cavalcanti ESB. Chemical composition and larvicidal activity

of essential oils from Piper species. Biochem Syst Ecol 2007; 35(10): 670-5.
[http://dx.doi.org/10.1016/j.bse.2007.05.002]

[86] El Hamss R, Idaomar M, Alonso-Moraga A, Muñoz Serrano A. Antimutagenic properties of bell and black peppers. Food Chem Toxicol 2003; 41(1): 41-7.
[http://dx.doi.org/10.1016/S0278-6915(02)00216-8] [PMID: 12453727]

[87] Moumi SH. Isolation of Salmonella spp from raw meat, elucidation of their antibiotic susceptibility pattern and evaluation of the antimicrobial efficacy of Oregano (Origanum vulgare) and Black Sesame (Sesamum indicum). BRAC University 2018.

[88] Ramesh B, Saravanan R, Pugalendi KV. Influence of sesame oil on blood glucose, lipid peroxidation, and antioxidant status in streptozotocin diabetic rats. J Med Food 2005; 8(3): 377-81.
[http://dx.doi.org/10.1089/jmf.2005.8.377] [PMID: 16176150]

[89] Sani I, Sule FA, Warra AA, Bello F, Fakai IM, Abdulhamid A. Phytochemicals and mineral elements composition of white *Sesamum indicum* L. seed oil. Int. J. Nat. Tradit. Med. 2(2): 118-90. Sathya, S., R. Kokilavani and K. Gurusamy. 2008. Hypoglycemic effect of Gymnema sylvestre (retz.,) R.Br leaf in normal and alloxan-induced diabetic rats. J Anc Sci Life 2013; 28(2): 12-4.

[90] Akanya HO U L. Effect of *Sesamum indicum* (Linn) Seeds Supplemented Diets on Blood Glucose, lipid profiles and serum levels of enzymes in alloxan-induced diabetic rats J applied life sciences international 2015; 2(3): 134-44.

[91] Mallhi TH, Qadir MI, Ali M, Ahmad B, Khan YH, Rehman A. Review: Ajwa date (*Phoenix dactylifera*)- an emerging plant in pharmacological research. Pak J Pharm Sci 2014; 27(3): 607-16.
[PMID: 24811825]

[92] Joshua AM, Xin H, Huang N, Hu P. Phytomedicines as therapeutic interventions for hepatic encephalopathy. TMR Modern Herbal Medicine 2020; 3(1): 30-49.

[93] Yasin M, Ketema T, Bacha K. Physico-chemical and bacteriological quality of drinking water of different sources, Jimma zone, Southwest Ethiopia. BMC Res Notes 2015; 8: 541.
[http://dx.doi.org/10.1186/s13104-015-1376-5] [PMID: 26437931]

[94] Al-Farsi M, Alasalvar C, Morris A, Baron M, Shahidi F. Comparison of antioxidant activity, anthocyanins, carotenoids, and phenolics of three native fresh and sun-dried date (*Phoenix dactylifera* L.) varieties grown in Oman. J Agric Food Chem 2005; 53(19): 7592-9.
[http://dx.doi.org/10.1021/jf050579q] [PMID: 16159191]

[95] Saddiq AA, Bawazir AE. Antimicrobial activity of date palm (*Phoenix dactylifera*) pits extracts and its role in reducing the side effect of methylprednisolone on some neurotransmitter content in the brain, hormone testosterone in adulthood. Acta Hortic 2010; (882): 665-90.
[http://dx.doi.org/10.17660/ActaHortic.2010.882.74]

[96] Bilgari F, Alkarkhi AFM, Easa AM. Antioxidant activity and phenolic content of various date palm (*Phoenix dactylifera*) fruits from Iran. Food Chem 2008; 107: 1636-41.
[http://dx.doi.org/10.1016/j.foodchem.2007.10.033]

[97] Sarfraz M, Khaliq T, Khan JA, Aslam B. Effect of aqueous extract of black pepper and ajwa seed on liver enzymes in alloxan-induced diabetic Wister albino rats. Saudi Pharm J 2017; 25(4): 449-52.
[http://dx.doi.org/10.1016/j.jsps.2017.04.004] [PMID: 28579873]

[98] Arulselvan P, Fard MT, Tan WS, *et al.* Role of Antioxidants and Natural Products in Inflammation. Oxid Med Cell Longev 2016; 2016: 5276130-0.
[http://dx.doi.org/10.1155/2016/5276130] [PMID: 27803762]

[99] Friel H. Biopharmaceutical Monotargeting *versus* 'Universal Targeting' of Late-Onset Alzheimer's Disease Using Mixtures of Pleiotropic Natural Compounds. J Alzheimers Dis Rep 2019; 3(1): 219-32.
[http://dx.doi.org/10.3233/ADR-190127] [PMID: 31435619]

[100] Al-Shoaibi Z, Al-Mamary MA, Al-Habori MA, AlZubairi AS, Abdelwahab SI. *In vivo* antioxidant and hepatoprotective effects of palm date fruits (*Phoenix dactylifera*). Int J Pharmacol 2012; 7(1): 8733.

[101]   Huang P, Zheng N, Zhou H-b, *et al.* Curcumin inhibits BACE1 expression through the interaction between ER β and NFκB signaling pathway in SH-SY5Y cells. Mol Cell Biochem 2019; 15: 1-13.

[102]   Elberry AA, Mufti ST, Al-Maghrabi JA, *et al.* Anti-inflammatory and antiproliferative activities of date palm pollen (*Phoenix dactylifera*) on experimentally-induced atypical prostatic hyperplasia in rats. J Inflamm (Lond) 2011; 8(1): 40.
[http://dx.doi.org/10.1186/1476-9255-8-40] [PMID: 22195697]

[103]   Mohamed DA, Al-Okbi SY. *In vivo* evaluation of the antioxidant and anti-inflammatory activity of different extracts of date fruits in adjuvant arthritis. Pol J Food Nutr Sci 2004; 13(54): 397-402.

[104]   Eddine LS. Antioxidant, anti-inflammatory and diabetes-related enzyme inhibition properties of leaves extract from selected varieties of *Phoenix dactylifera* L. Innovare J Life Sci 2013; 1: 14-8.

[105]   Vayalil PK. Antioxidant and antimutagenic properties of aqueous extract of date fruit (*Phoenix dactylifera* L. Arecaceae). J Agric Food Chem 2002; 50(3): 610-7.
[http://dx.doi.org/10.1021/jf010716t] [PMID: 11804538]

[106]   Biglari F, AlKarkhi AFM, Easa MA. Antioxidant activity and phenolic content of various date palm (*Phoenix dactylifera*) fruits from Iran. Food Chem 2011; 107: 1636-41.
[http://dx.doi.org/10.1016/j.foodchem.2007.10.033]

[107]   Al-Qarawi AA, Abdel-Rahman H, Mousa HM, Ali BH, El-Mougy SA. Nephroprotective action of *Phoenix dactylifera.* in gentamicin-induced nephrotoxicity. Pharm Biol 2008; 4: 227-30.
[http://dx.doi.org/10.1080/13880200701739322]

[108]   Gupta SC, Kismali G, Aggarwal BB. Curcumin, a component of turmeric: from farm to pharmacy. Biofactors 2013; 39(1): 2-13.
[http://dx.doi.org/10.1002/biof.1079] [PMID: 23339055]

[109]   Gaddam A, Galla C, Thummisetti S, Marikanty RK, Palanisamy UD, Rao PV. Role of Fenugreek in the prevention of type 2 diabetes mellitus in prediabetes. J Diabetes Metab Disord 2015; 14(1): 74.
[http://dx.doi.org/10.1186/s40200-015-0208-4] [PMID: 26436069]

[110]   Goyal SNG, Chatterjee S. Investigating the therapeutic potential of T. Foeneum graceum L. as our defense mechanism against several human diseases. J Toxicol 2016; 1: 10.

[111]   Genet AG, Debebe YG, Nguse NA. Antidiabetic effect of Fenugreek seed powder solution (Trigonella foenu-graceum L.) on hyperlipidemia in diabetic patients. J Diabetes Res 2019; 1: 8.

CHAPTER 3

Anti-Diabetic and Anti-Hypertensive Potentials of Essential Oil Bearing Medicinal Plants

Farwa Nadeem[1], Muhammad Asif Hanif[1,*], Asma El Zerey-Belaskri[2], Muhammad Irfan Majeed[1] and Haq Nawaz[1]

[1] *Nano and Biomaterials Lab, Department of Chemistry, University of Agriculture, Faisalabad-38040-Pakistan*

[2] *Laboratoire de recherche Biodiversité végétale: conservation et valorisation, Faculté des Sciences de la nature et de la Vie, Université de Sidi Bel Abbes, Algérie*

Abstract: Medicinal plants have long been the area of great interest and a hot topic of current scientific investigations for the biochemists, chemists and pharmaceutics. These researches play an important role in discovering the new natural resources and developing the potential drugs for the treatment of various unknown diseases. These drugs are supposed to have more effectiveness and no side effects unlike most other synthetically produced modern drugs. In accordance with the World Health Organization (WHO), approximately four billion people constituting eight percent population of the world, use herbal based natural drugs for the majority of primary health care problems. Diabetes mellitus and hypertension are the two most common diseases that sometimes also coexist and enhance the chances of neuropathic disorders, brain strokes, retinopathic symptoms, peripheral vascular diseases and cardiac arrest. This chapter describes various medicinal plants having anti-diabetic and anti-hypertensive potentials along with their detailed mechanisms and mode of actions. Some potential anti-diabetic plants are alkanet, asthma weed, bamboo, basil, caraway, chirayita, coleus, cubeb, cumin, cypress, damask rose, fennel, fenugreek, fig, frangipani, ginseng, guava, henna, Indian globe thistle, Indian pennywort, ma-huang, moringa, olive, puncture vine, saffron, sweet lemon, tree turmeric, walnut, corn and tawa tawa. Anti-hypertensive plants discussed in this chapter include basil, black piper, coleus, curry leaf, puncture vine, sesame seed, yarrow, passion fruit, onion, garlic, celery, oat, barberry, black cumin, ylang ylang, garden cress, ginger and sweet lemon.

Keywords: Anti-diabetic, Anti-hypertensive, Brain Stroke, Cardiac Arrest, Essential oils, Medicinal Plants.

INTRODUCTION

Mother-nature has provided us a complete store-house of remedies in order to

---

* **Corresponding Author Muhammad Asif Hanif:** Nano and Biomaterials Lab, Department of Chemistry, University of Agriculture, Faisalabad-38040-Pakistan; E-mail: drmuhammadasifhanif@gmail.com

cure all sorts of ailments, proving to be catastrophic for human races. According to an estimate, a major portion of the world's population utilizes medicinal plants either in parts or as a whole plant [1]. Some additional medicinal uses of curative plants are recognized to learn more about the potential future perspective of medicinal plants. Medicinal remedies derived from plants, either by getting information through traditional knowledge or by exploring literature, are now being handed down generation after generation. Various pharmaceutical industries are now looking for some other natural alternative resources proven to be environmentally benign and potentially viable in nature. Nowadays, scientists are working to explore the potential anti-biotic, anti-oxidant, anti-microbial, anti-diabetic and crop protecting agents for the sustenance of all life forms on earth. Medicinal plants generally provide a great source of a wide variety of natural bioactive compounds including phenolics, nitrogenous compounds, terpenoids, vitamins and various other secondary plant metabolites showing potential bioactivities *e.g.*, anti-oxidants, anti-tumor, anti-inflammatory, anti-mutagenic, anti-bacterial, anti-carcinogenic and anti-viral activities [1].

Essential oils are the natural, complex, volatile aromatic compounds containing a number of structurally different organic constituents isolated from different scented plants having high commercial importance and extreme therapeutic potentials. Essential oils have extensively been used as a potential ingredient in order to enhance the functionality of a number of commercial products like green pesticides, cosmetic products, pharmaceuticals, perfumes, soft drinks and food stuff. Currently, global research is mainly focused on the development of eco-friendly techniques and innovative ideas for the extraction of essential oils and to stabilize them through proper encapsulation for bringing the natural products under the label of generally-recognized-as-safe. Essential oil is a biochemical product and a mixture of a large number of structurally related compounds, produced inside the cytoplasmic fluid and are then transported into intracellular space in the form of smaller droplets. These chemical compounds are highly volatile in nature and have a characteristic aroma. They are generally composed of a combination of aromatic and non-aromatic compounds having specific chemical composition and characteristic aroma [2].

Aromatic oils or scents contain approximately more than two hundred known complex chemical compounds having hydrogen, oxygen and carbon as the backbone of all complicated molecules. Essential oils can be broadly classified as (i) volatile and (ii) non-volatile components. Approximately 90 to 95 percent chemical constituents of essential oils such as alcohols, aliphatic compounds, esters, aldehydes, monoterpenes, sesquiterpenes and hydrocarbons along with their oxygenated derivative, are highly volatile in nature. Only 1 to 10 percent of molecules out of total weight are non-volatile in nature including hydrocarbons, sterols, waxes, fatty acids, carotenoids and flavonoids. Chemical composition of the essential oils significantly changes with the duration of the growth period, environmental conditions, harvesting time and extraction technique. Composition of an essential oil significantly varies by changing the plant source and chemical constituents can range from a few dozens to hundreds of complex molecules. Oxygenated derivatives of hydrocarbons are accountable for the flavors and fragrances while higher phenolic contents help to improve the antibacterial activities [3].

The aromatic oils contain natural anti-oxidants that restrict the free radical reactions of deoxyribonucleic acid (DNA), unsaturated lipids, amino acids and proteins. Human body is known to have a strong defense mechanism against free radicals abundantly found in most of the body cells. The balance between the amount of antioxidants and free radicals can only be achieved by an external supply of natural or synthetic anti-oxidants. Scented aromatic oils are richly supplied with phenolic compounds that significantly contribute to determining free radical scavenging activities and anti-oxidant potentials. Essential oils of thyme, oregano, nutmeg, clove, cinnamon and basil are known to have strong anti-oxidant and free radical scavenging potentials in DPPH radical assay [4]. Some essential oils have strong anti-bacterial potentials against a wide spectrum of disease-causing bacterial strains such as *Salmonella typhimurium*, *Staphylococcus aureus*, *Bacillus cereus*, *Shigella dysenteria*, *Escherichia coli*, *Salmonella typhimurium*, *Listeria innocua* and *Listeria monocytogenes*. The volatile essential oil of *Commiphora africana* is known to inhibit the various pathological bacterial strains such as *Helicobacter pylori*, *Candida albicans*, *Escherichia coli* and *Staphylococcus aureus* [4].

Essential oils are generally added as food flavors and also act as anti-fungal and anti-bacterial additives. Macro-dilution technique is helpful in accessing the anti-microbial potentials of essential oils. Similarly, significant inhibition in mycelial growth of fungi can be observed on applying different concentrations of varied essential oils on an experimental basis. Essential oil extracted from thyme, tea tree, cinnamon and catnip exhibits maximum anti-microbial potentials. Some recent evidences have indicated that *in-vitro* applications of essential oil of *Thymus schimperi* Ronniger can act as a strong anti-bacterial agent against wide spectrum pathogenic fungal isolates such as *Microsporum gypseum*, *Beauveria bassiana*, *Aspergillus minutus*, *Aspergillus tubingensis*, *Verticillium* sp. and *Penicillium chrysogenum* [4].

Diabetes mellitus is a severe endocrinological metabolic disorder, rapidly spreading across the globe. Major symptoms of diabetes mellitus are high blood glucose levels as a consequence of inadequate secretion of pancreatic insulin or poorly directed metabolization of glucose by target cells. This disease is further aggravated by or mainly associated with metabolic complications which can subsequently lead to death [5]. According to an estimate, the number of people suffering from diabetes has suddenly risen from 108 million to 422 million from the year 1980 to 2014. The global spread of diabetes in adults was 4.7% in 1980 which has reached up to 8.5% in the year 2014 more specifically in middle- and low-income countries. It is also a major cause of surgical cuts of the lower limb, heart stroke, kidney failure and vision loss along with night blindness. Approximately, 1.6 million deaths were directly caused by diabetes in 2016 which was about 2.2 million in the year 2012. Almost half of all the deaths are mainly attributed to extremely high blood glucose level even before the age of seventy, as per the reports of the World Health Organization released in 2016. In the year 2010, almost 285 million people suffered from diabetes at the age ranging from 20 to 79 years all over the world and this estimate is unfortunately expected to increase up to 438 million by 2030 [5].

High blood pressure also known as hypertension, is a serious global health issue, operationally defined as "resting systolic and diastolic blood pressure greater than 140 to 90 mmHg". Recently, the Joint National Committee on Prevention, Detection, Evaluation and Treatment of High Blood Pressure issued a guideline explaining that people having diastolic blood pressure between 80 to 89 and systolic blood pressure between 120 to 139 mmHg are ranked as "pre-hypertensive patients". The patients that fall in this category are more likely to develop frank hypertension thereby requiring proper clinical attention [6]. In accordance with the estimation, almost 26% population of the world is hypertensive and its further prevalence is expected to increase up to 29% by 2025 including even the developing nations of the world. High blood pressure is the third major cause of worldwide deaths after myocardial infarction and heart stroke [7].

One fourth adult population of the world is suffering from hypertension. According to an estimate, more than 75 million people of the United States are hypertensive and additionally, 50 million are above the prehypertensive range. More often, hypertension is also named as "the silent killer" and in most of the cases, underlying etiology of this disease remains unknown. In order to compete with this matter more appropriately, detailed studies of gene mutations must be ensured. The prevalence of this disease is dependent on many factors like improper lifestyle, routine activities, medications, kidney diseases, cholestrol metabolism, lipid oxidation and extra load on the autonomic nervous system. All these problems are caused by the lack of exercise, excessive drinking and abundant smoking. The multitude of genetic influences and imbalances in vascular endothelial growth factors (A, B and C), endothelin (1, 2 and 3), chloride-bicarbonate exchangers (1, 2 and 3), apolipoproteins (A1, A2, and C2-C4) and 11-β-hydroxysteroid dehydrogenases (B1 and B2) are also some of them. Hypertension causes renal infections, cerebral vascular problems and cardiovascular diseases [6].

Some recent investigations have shown that essential oil of neroli, majoram, ylang ylang and lavender possesses excellent therapeutic potentials for controlling the high blood pressure. Following natural essential oils have shown promising results against hypertension; (a) bergamot oil reduces the blood pressure and chances of heart attack (b) cedar wood essential oil can promote the relaxation and temporarily decrease the heart rate (c) citronella essential oil helps to ease the stress and this in turn can lower the blood pressure (d) clary sage essential oil can reduce the anxiety levels and thus lower the blood pressure (e) frankincense essential oil may reduce the stress levels and regulate the heart function (f) jasmine essential oil might ease a tense nervous system (g) helichrysum essential oil is believed to have hypotensive properties that act as a natural relaxant to reduce the blood pressure (h) lavender essential oil has calming properties that reduce the anxiety and heart rate (i) lemon essential oil is believed to relieve the stress, depression and helps in lowering the blood pressure naturally (j) lemon balm essential oil may decrease the blood pressure while protecting against heart palpitations, tachycardia and heart attacks (k) lime essential oil is said to have stress-reducing properties (l) neroli essential oil may have anti-hypertensive properties (m) calming effect and anti-inflammatory characteristics of rose essential oil help to relax the entire body to increase the blood circulation and lower the high blood pressure (n) sage essential oil may promote the weight loss through increasing the body's metabolism. Weight loss has been shown to have a positive influence on lowering the blood pressure (o) sweet marjoram essential oil may dilate the blood vessels to lower the high blood pressure (p) valerian essential oil may have powerful calming effects on the nervous system, which can lower the blood pressure, ease heart palpitations, ease insomnia, calm hyperactivity and reduce the nervous tension (q) yarrow essential oil is considered to be one of the top oils for improving the blood circulation and (r) ylang ylang essential oil may help to decrease the levels of cortisol (known as the "stress hormone") and lower the blood pressure [8]. Fig. (**1**) illustrates some factors related to high sugar level and high blood pressure along with their resulting consequences on the human body.

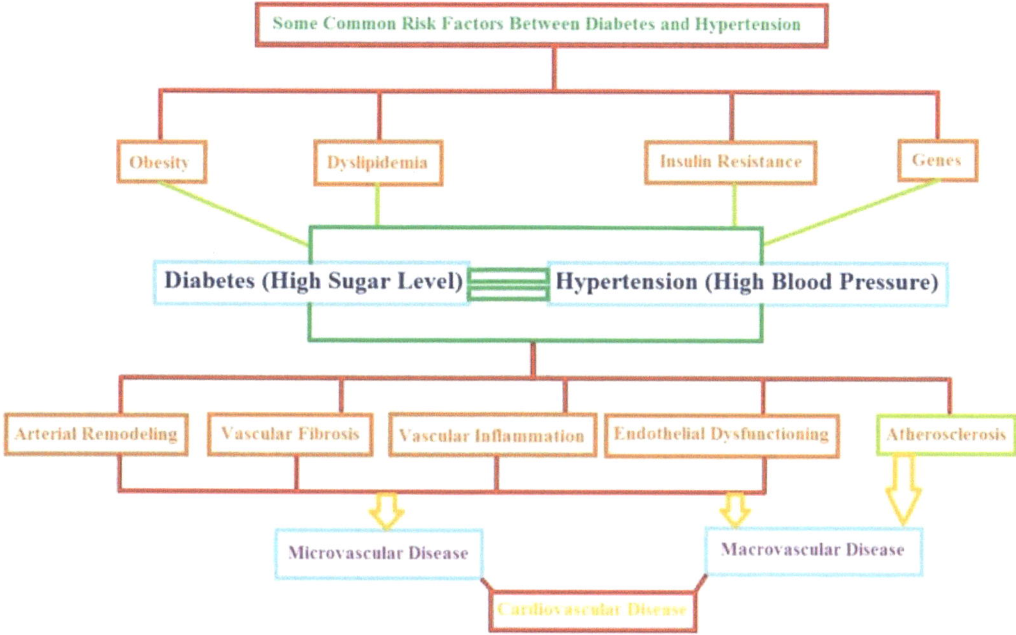

Fig. (1). Common risk factors of diabetes mellitus and hypertension.

BIOCHEMISTRY OF DIABETES MELLITUS

Diabetes mellitus is a combination of heterogeneous diseases having episodes of glucose intolerance. It is also known as "hyperglycemia" and characterized by the lack of insulin or defective insulin action. This disease is associated with defected regulatory system and improper storage of metabolic products such as proteins, carbohydrates and lipids. Classification of the diabetes mellitus is purely based on clinical presentations and aetiology. Till now, diabetes has been classified into four major types (i) type-I-diabetes (ii) type-II-diabetes (iii) gestational-diabetes and (iv) specific type of diabetes. Some of the destructive effects of diabetes mellitus include metabolic disorders, progressive complications and organ failure such as neuropathy, nephropathy and retinopathy. Diabetes mellitus is mostly accompanied by the risk of cerebrovascular, peripheral vascular and cardiovascular disorders. Numerous pathogenic processes are involved in the development of diabetes including destruction or degeneration of the pancreatic-β-cells which results in the lowered sensitivity of insulin action [5].

The word "diabetes" and "mellitus" are derived from Greek word where diabetes denotes "a passer through or a siphon" while mellitus stands for the "sweet". Generally, it was considered that urine produced by a diabetic patient is strongly attracted by the bees and flies as it releases an excess of sugar as a by-product.

Conventional method for the diagnosis of diabetes mellitus in ancient Chinese methods of treatment was observing the extent of attraction of ants towards the urine of a diabetic patient. However, till the medieval ages, European doctors were succeeded in developing a test for diabetes by testing the urine themselves similar to the sense occasionally depicted in Gothic beliefs [9]. In this method, a regular source of energy tends to be pre-requisite for each cell to work properly inside the human body. Glucose is the primary energy source of human body and all life forms on earth, which circulates the blood as a mobilizable fuel source [10]. Insulin is a pancreatic hormone that is mainly responsible for the regulation of blood glucose level. This hormone binds with the receptor sites located on the peripheral sides of cell membranes. It affords the entry of glucose inside the respiring cells and tissues through requisite channels. Catabolism of glucose into pyruvate is stimulated by the insulin through the process of glycolysis. It also upregulates the glycogenesis from lipogenesis and cytosolic glucose, that is mainly attributed by the excessive cytosolic acetyl-CoA and regular sugar. Such types of metabolic events are antagonistic to various metabolic events, triggered by the glucagon hormone. When the glucose level is at or below the normal threshold, glucose tends to remain in blood in spite of entering directly into the body cells [11].

Naturally, human body attempts to cope with the hyperglycemia through withdrawing excessive water from inside the cell and entering it into the bloodstream. Excessive sugar is then excreted into the urine. Therefore diabetic patients always feel constant thirst and drink an excess of water. Sometimes, diabetes also leads to polyuria where patient's cells try to get rid of extra glucose, subsequently resulting in glucosuria. In case if hyperglycemia prolongs, the cells of human body tend to devoid of glucose due to the lack of insulin. It ultimately forces the cells to seek alternative mobilizable energy resources. In this regard, human cells start the storage of fatty acids into the adipose tissues. However, these fats are not used as a fuel source for brain, kidney cortex and red blood cells. Red blood cells generally lack the mitochondria and so the beta-oxidation pathway. Fatty acids of normal cells usually cannot cross the blood-brain-barrier. In order to avail this energy, acetyl-CoA from catabolism of fatty acids are diverted to ketogenesis to generate the ketones that serve as an alternative fuel source for the cells and tissues. These ketonic bodies are then passed through the urine leading to the ketonuria, used to characterize diabetes mellitus. Ketosis is caused by the abnormal level of ketones in blood that further lowers the pH of blood leading to a condition called "ketoacidosis". It can even lead to coma and ultimately death [11].

BIOCHEMISTRY OF HYPERTENSION

Hypertension is the leading cause of diseases all across the globe. It is more prominent in African countries that are more likely to have undiagnosed causes of hypertension. The reasons for these complications include the number of genetic variations, salt stress and water retention. High blood pressure causes severe damage to smaller arteries found at the base of brain in a region called "vascular centrencephalon", a phylogenetically ancient part of the brain. Shorter arteries of internal capsule, cerebellum, brainstem, thalamus and basal ganglia are directly damaged by the high blood pressure resulting in hyaline degeneration and fibrinoid necrosis. These types of pathological symptoms are responsible for the lacunar infarctions, intracerebral hemorrhage and arteriole damage through immediate rupturing of blood vessels. Cerebral hemorrhages are perfused by the long arteries having a large number of branches acting as a step-down transformer. Hemorrhage and infarctions in the cortical regions of hemispheres are caused by the hypertension and amyloid angiopathy. Controlling hypertension markedly reduces the lacunar infarctions and preferably eliminates the intracerebral hemorrhage [12].

Proper regulation of the cerebral blood flow is ultimately required to maintain accurate brain functioning. Cerebral arteries are highly sensitive to slight variations in the normal blood pressure. Hypertension alters the arteries in a manner that impairs the ability of brain to tightly regulate the perfusions. Hypertension causes significant reductions in the diameter of lumen of cerebral arteries, often associated with the increase in wall-to-lumen ratio. Numerous circulating factors have commonly been implicated in mediating the inward artery remolding including the proinflammatory cytokines, angiotensin II, aldosterone and various other reactive species. Endothelium-dependent dilations, in response to epoxyeicosatrienoic acids and nitric oxide, are mostly impaired in hypertension. They ultimately increase the impaired dilations and myogenic tone. Dysfunctioning of iron channels constituting transient receptor potential V4 channels and calcium-activated potassium channels have mainly been associated with the impaired endothelial functioning in hypertensive models. Thorough understanding of the mechanism responsible for hypertension-associated vascular dysfunction is very much important due to the deep association of hypertension with increased risk of stroke, dementia and ischemic injury in the event of a stroke [12].

ANTI-DIABETIC PLANTS

Diabetes mellitus is an increasing cause of worldwide deaths at an alarming rate. Some recent statistics have shown that 34.2 million people (equivalent to 10.5%

of the world's population) have been diagnosed with diabetes mellitus in the year 2018. Some regional and global data regarding the prevalence of diabetes mellitus is in view that 9.3% of world's population (equal to 463 million people) is currently suffering from diabetes mellitus in 2019. As per the results released by "International Diabetes Federation Diabetes Atlas, 9th edition", this value is expected to reach upto 10.2% of world's population (equivalent to 578 million people) till the end of 2030 and almost 10.9% of global population density (equal to 700 million people) by 2045. Therefore prevention and control of diabetes mellitus are of extreme importance to ensure better living standards and to reduce the economic burden [13]. Some potential anti-diabetic and anti-hypertensive plants and their bioactive compounds are listed in Table **1**.

Alkanet (*Anchusa officinalis* L.)

Biguanides and sulfonylurea are the synthetic drugs used to reduce hyperglycemia in diabetes mellitus. These synthetic drugs have a number of side effects like hepatorenal disturbances and hyperglycemic coma and are not safe to use during pregnancy. In a recent study, roots extract of alkanet was found effective against diabetes. Anti-diabetic potentials of alkanet roots lowered the blood glucose level upto 23.3% in normal fasted rats when the dose was administered after every three hours [14].

Asthma Weed (*Euphorbia hirta* L.)

Anti-diabetic potential is one of the most important activities of asthma weed. Diabetes mellitus is a severe metabolic ailment that causes imperfections in the action and secretions of insulin. Chronic hyperglycemia is mainly relevant to the long term impairments [15]. Numerous experimental investigations have revealed that diabetes mellitus is concomitant with a significant decrease in anti-oxidant potential and a remarkable increase in the generation of free radicals [16]. Therefore, free radical species need to be scavenged for their anti-diabetic potentials. The floral extracts of asthma weed are expected to be anti-diabetic due to the presence of flavanoids, tannins and phenolic constituents. However, its exact mechanism and detailed mode of action are still unknown [17]. It is also known to reduce the side effects mainly related to the synthetic medicines.

Bamboo (*Bambusa arundinacea*)

Seeds of the *Bambusa arundinacea* were found to exhibit the anti-diabetic potentials when compared with standard glibenclamide. Anti-diabetic activity was evaluated through an *in-vitro* method by using α-amylase and α-glucosidase inhibition activity based on the colorimetric method. *Bambusa arundinacea*, by inhibiting α-amylase and α-glucosidase, reduces the digestion of carbohydrates which in turn reduces the blood glucose level. The presence of flavonoids in *Bambusa arundinacea* acts as an insulin mimetic to stimulate the peripheral tissues for increased glucose uptake and also regulates the rate-limiting enzymes. These enzymes are responsible for the anti-diabetic activity [18].

Basil (*Ocimum basilicum* L.)

Aqueous extracts of the basil are known to have strong anti-diabetic potentials when tested for hypoglycemia through an *in-vitro* investigation. Results of the entire study showed that these aqueous extracts also have anti-oxidative nature and possess enough potential to inhibit the α-glucosidase and α-amylase. Therefore, it has proven to be very effective in controlling the high blood sugar level in animals [19].

Caraway (*Carum carvi* L.)

Diabetes mellitus is the major cause of morbidity and mortality all across the globe. Naturally occuring caraway is known to have strong anti-hyperglycemic potentials. The aqueous extract of caraway is known to possess the strong anti-hyperglycemic effects in artificial streptozotocin-induced diabetic rats. Some anti-ulcerogenic agents have also been reported to found in the solvent extract and volatile essential oil of *Carum carvi* [20].

Chirayita (*Swertia chirayita*)

The ethanolic extracts of *Swertia chirayita* have found to be useful in normalizing the elevated blood sugar level, in experimentally induced diabetic animals. Chirayita is also a very effective medicine for a number of stomach related disorders and thus used for the treatment of diarrhea and dyspepsia. It helps to stimulate digestion and tends to maintain the sugar level of blood as it reduces the chances of hypoglycemia [21]. Alcoholic extract of this plant along with hexanic fraction showed excellent anti-diabetic potentials when tested on experimental albino rats. Hence, it was suggested that hexane fraction of this plant might not be able to lower the absorption of glucose in the intestine of experimental animals [22].

Coleus (*Coleus forskohlii*)

Coleus is a naturally existing plant that helps to maintain the composition of body [23]. It has proved to be a potential anti-diabetic agent of nature. It increases the level of cAMP in normal cells because of excessive production and release of insulin. In actual practice, cAMP activates the two major signaling paths of a β-cell which in turn helps to lower the elevated sugar level of the body. However, further research is still needed to explore the exact mechanism behind and their probable advantages and disadvantages for diabetic patients [24].

Cubeb (*Piper cubeba*)

The anti-lipid peroxidative and anti-hyperglycemic effects of the ethanolic extract of cubeb fruit were investigated in alloxan-induced diabetic mice. The level of glucose in blood, carbohydrates metabolizing enzymes, and grade of anti-oxidants and lipid peroxidation, were tested using colorimetric methods. Cubeb fruit ethanolic extract was orally administered to the mice and it showed potential anti-lipi--peroxidative and anti-hyperglycemic effects in the diabetic mice [25].

Cumin (*Cuminum cyminum*)

Natural cumin based medicines have proved to be more effective as compared to the glibenclamide for the treatment of diabetes mellitus [26]. Active chemical constituents of essential oil of cumin are known to inhibit the activity of aldose reductase and α-glycosidase [27]. Hyperlipidemia is an additional complication, mainly associated with diabetes mellitus. The oral administration of cumin preferably reduces the triglycerides, phospholipids, free fatty acids and plasma cholesterol, and body weight in alloxan-induced diabetic rats. Cumin decreased the level of liver cholesterol and serum in rats when added to the diet of hypercholesterolemic rats [28].

Cypress (*Cupressus sempervirens glauca*)

Ethanolic extracts of various cypress species were tested for their anti-diabetic potentials. This sugar-lowering activity was planned to be assessed by inducing the artificial symptoms of diabetes mellitus *via* serum biochemical analysis in fasting blood sugar tests, blood glutathione level test and alloxan test. The results of this experiment revealed that these extracts significantly lowered the blood sugar level even at minute dose concentrations. They also showed a remarkable increase in the level of glutathione due to their strong anti-oxidant potentials [29].

Damask Rose (*Rosa damascena* Mil.)

Damask rose extract is known to have non-competitive inhibitory effects for the enzyme α-glucosidase. Oral intake of the solvent extract of damask rose significantly reduces the blood glucose level when taken in a dose-dependent manner in a ratio of 100-1000 mg/kg of the body weight in normal and maltose induced diabetic rats. In this experimental investigation, postprandial glucose level was found to be decreased due to reduction in absorption of carbohydrates from small and large intestine. This suggests that damask rose can act as an anti-diabetic agent [30].

Fennel (*Foneiculum vulgare*)

Fennel essential oil potentially reduces the hypoglycemic effects and acts as a strong anti-oxidant of nature against streptozotocin-induced diabetic rats [31].

Fenugreek (*Trigonella foenum-groecum* L.)

Fenugreek is documented to have strong hypoglycemic effects more specifically in human beings and animals, suffering from type-I and type-II diabetes mellitus [32]. The results of an experimental study suggested that hypoglycemic effects can be mediated by stimulating the synthesis and secretion of insulin from β-pancreatic cells. However, the hypoglycemic effect can be slowed down by various environmental factors without even developing the risk of hypoglycemia [33]. High fibre fenugreek is a very effective diet in managing the blood glucose level [34]. Hence, the extract of fenugreek can lower the blood glucose level and kidney-to-body-weight ratio along with the significant improvements in hemorheological properties of diabetic rats [35]. In another study, it has been mentioned that the seeds of fenugreek (*Trigonella foenum-graecum*) are extensively used as anti-diabetic agents and this attribute of fenugreek is experimentally evidenced in a number of animal studies employing diabetic dogs, rabbits, mice and rats. Similarly, the oral intake of seeds and seed extracts has consistently shown the hypoglycemic effects [36].

Fig (*Ficus carica* L.)

Fig leaves are known to possess strong hypocholesterolemic potentials when used in the form of aqueous decoctions and chloroformic extracts. These extracts cause a significant decrease in the ratio of total cholesterol to high-density lipoprotein cholesterol. It also reduces the elevated blood sugar level and total cholesterol contents. Additionally, hepatocellular carcinomic cell lines and cell contents of the cholesterol help to decrease the level of blood cholesterol in streptozotocin-induced diabetic rats [37].

Frangipani (*Plumeria rubra* L.)

Solvent extract of the frangipani was subjected to an alloxan-induced diabetic rat in an experimental investigation to study the hypoglycemic effects of this plant extract at three different levels 100 mg/kg, 200 mg/kg and 400 mg/kg of body weight, respectively. Anti-diabetic potentials of frangipani were tested against standard drug glibenclamide. A significant reduction in blood glucose level was recorded, extending the applications of frangipani in modern pharmacological practices [38].

Ginseng (*Panax ginseng*)

Ginseng is an important herbal plant, used to maintain the blood glucose level. Anti-diabetic potentials of ginseng were studied in the patients suffering from diabetes type 2. It was reported that the daily dose of 100-200 mg of ginseng extract for 8 consecutive weeks, significantly reduced the blood glucose level and enhanced the physical performance [39]. In another study, almost 150 mg/kg of ginseng berry extract was injected for a period of 12 days in obese diabetic mice and results showed the improved blood glucose level [40]. Malonyl ginsenosides (MGR) are ginsenosides found in dried as well as fresh ginseng plants. The effect of MRG on diabetic rats was studied by different anti-diabetic tests. It was reported that 50-100 mg/kg dose per day significantly reduced the blood glucose level and improved the bodyweight of diabetic rats [41].

Guava (*Psidium guajava* L.)

In diabetes, either the production of insulin decreases or the body fails to respond to the produced insulin. In some severe cases, both conditions may occur simultaneously. Guava leaves are a potential anti-diabetic agent, as they reduce the blood glucose level and improve the plasma insulin [42, 43]. Guava decreases the damage, lipid oxidation and DNA breakage [44]. The aqueous extracts of this plant were reported to improve the glucose uptake by the cells due to the presence of phenolic compounds present in these extracts, responsible for showing the anti-diabetic activity [45]. Guava peels are also reported to reduce diabetes [46]. In another report, it was mentioned that the long-term use of guava peels resulted in a decrease of blood glucose level and improved plasma insulin [47]. In a comparative study, it was reported that guava leaves extracts showed a greater decrease in blood glucose levels than its peels [48].

Henna (*Lawsonia inermis* L.)

Polar leafy extracts of henna have been explored by different researchers for determining their anti-diabetic activities. Both in the basic and neutral media, the methanolic extracts obtained from the leaves were found to exhibit the hypoglycemic activity by a glucose oxidase assay. An ethanolic extract of henna leaves was administered to the euglycemic and diabetic rats. The results of this study showed the significant reductions in blood glucose levels of diabetic rats at the concentration of 200 mg/kg, compared to those treated with glibenclamide, a standard drug. It was further demonstrated that the ethanol leaf extract triggered a reduction in blood glucose, triglyceride, and total cholesterol concentrations ranging from 194 mg/dL to normal, 225.7±76.9 mg/dL and 148.9±55.3 mg/dL, respectively, in mice with an oral dose of 800 mg/kg [49].

Indian Globe Thistle (*Sphaeranthus indicus*)

Isobutylamide and steroidal glycoalkaloids extracted and isolated from the roots of globe thistle have proved to be potentially effective for the treatment of diabetes mellitus [50].

Indian Pennywort (*Centella asiatica*)

Methanolic and ethanolic extracts of the Indian pennywort were checked for their anti-diabetic potentials on alloxan-induced diabetic rats among which all alcoholic extracts were found to reduce the blood glucose level [51].

Ma-huang (*Ephedra gerardiana*)

Anti-diabetic potential is mainly attributed to the presence of five active glycans such as ephedran A, ephedran B, ephedran C, ephedran D and ephedran E. They all are responsible for lowering the blood glucose level in normal and alloxan-induced diabetic rats. Two compounds belonging to the family of epinephrine are found to be potent inhibitors of dipeptidyl peptidase-4. The names of these two compounds include (-)-ephedrine and (+)-pseudoephedrine. Both these compounds are reported to possess the hypoglycemic activity [52]. This anti-diabetic activity is expected to be proceeded by stimulating the release of epinephrine that results in the lowering of sugar level.

Moringa (*Moringa oleifera* L.)

Moringa leaves were checked for their anti-diabetic potentials in diabetic Wister and Goto-Kakizaki rats. The results of this experiment showed a significant decrease in the blood sugar level in experimental animals. However, changes in glucose levels were remarkably higher in Goto-Kakizaki rats as compared to the Wistar rats [53]. Anti-diabetic potentials were also tested with the aqueous leave extract of Moringa on total protein contents, glycemic control, urine sugar, haemoglobin, urine protein and body weight [54].

Olive (*Olea europaea* L.)

Leaves of the olives are strong anti-diabetic agents due to the presence of oleuropein and oleanolic acid [55]. In some recent experimental investigations, anti-diabetic potentials of the oleuropein and hydroxytyrosol were separately studied and results indicated that olive leaves have enough potential for reducing the oxidative stress mainly relevant to the pathological impediment of diabetes mellitus [56].

Puncture Vine (*Tribulus terrestris*)

Puncture vine is a rich source of natural saponins having strong hypoglycemic potentials [57]. It considerably lowers the level of serum glucose, serum cholesterol and serum triglyceride in alloxan-induced-diabetic rats. However, increase in the serum superoxide dismutase activity has been observed. Decoction of puncture vine tends to inhibit the gluconeogenesis in infected mice [58]. Ethanolic extract of this plant has found to lower the oxidative stress in streptozotocin-induced-diabetic rats by inhibiting the aldose reductases and α-glucosidase [59]. Similarly, post-prandial glucose level of the blood was substantially decreased in infected rats after the injection of saponins from the puncture vine. This is due to the dilation of coronary artery and enhanced coronary circulation. This plant is also recommended as a remedy for the cardiac complications, angina pectoris and elevated blood sugar level through the action of anti-oxidants [60].

Saffron (*Crocus sativus*)

To evaluate the effects of crocetin against the insulin resistance, dexamethasone (that causes insulin resistance) and dexamethasone plus crocetin were administered in the rats for 6 weeks. The dexamethasone plus crocetine treated group showed significantly lower levels of serum insulin, triglycerides, tumor necrosis factor-α (TNF-α), and free fatty acids as compared to the pure dexamethasone group. In case of insulin resistance, TNF-α is overexpressed, resulting in reduced glucose transporter 4 activity, causing decreased insulin-stimulated glucose absorption. In the crocetin-treated group, a reduction in TNF-α and serum insulin levels is the evidence of the role of crocetin against insulin resistance [61]. Furthermore, crocetin extracted from saffron works for insulin resistance and significantly decreases the level of free fatty acids, serum insulin, high density and low density cholesterol, serum triglycerides, blood pressure and epididymal in adipose tissues in crocetin induced experimental animals. However, fructose-induced experimental animals showed exactly opposite results against the insulin resistance [62].

Sweet Lemon (*Citrus limetta* Risso)

Methanolic extract of the fruit peel of sweet lemon showed strong anti-hyperglycemic potentials in streptozotocin-induced diabetic rats [63]. Citrus fruit peel is rich in flavanoids such as naringin and hesperidin. Both these flavonoids possess excellent hypoglycemic potentials and are mainly responsible for regulating the glucose regulating enzymes. Both naringin and hesperidin significantly lower the blood glucose level thereby increasing the concentration of glycogen and the rate of glycolysis. It can also lower the process of gluconeogenesis in liver. The presence of flavanoids in citrus peel extract is mainly responsible for the anti-hyperglycemic effects and anti-bacterial potentials.

Tree Turmeric (*Berberis aristata*)

In a recent experimental research, the effects of berberine were studied on some selected patients of diabetes mellitus. These patients were treated with oral administration of natural medicine for about three months, together with a helpful eating regime endorsed for a month [64]. With the passage of time, harmful effects of diabetes mellitus were disappeared and quality of patient's life was enhanced with noticeable fluctuations in the pulse rate and blood lipid level. The results of this study revealed that almost 60% patients were recovered from high blood sugar level. In addition, it was also observed that treatment with berberine prompted more advantageous pancreatic tissues as compared to the control group. Berberine is mainly related with the enhanced recovery and utilitarian recuperation of pancreatic β-cells [64].

Walnut (*Juglans regia* L.)

In a recent investigation, it has been found that diet rich in walnut seeds tends to reduce the blood sugar level in patients suffering with type-II diabetes mellitus [65]. However, dietary fats can significantly be influenced by excessive intake of walnut in order to induce the reductions in fasting levels of insulin. The walnut extract significantly inhibit the efficiency of α-glycosidase for both maltose and sucrose enzymes. However, no change has been observed in the level of insulin and expressions of glut-4-gene [66].

Corn (*Zea mays*)

Corn is a major source of numerous bioactive compounds such as anthocyanins including cyanidine-3-dimalonyl-glucoside, peonidine-3-glucoside and cyandin--glucoside. They are found in the leaves, seeds and purple cones of the flowers. These compounds show strong anti-oxidant, anti-cancer and anti-inflammatory potentials [67]. The use of corn kernels helps in the treatment of diabetes mellitus and hypertension due to the presence of phenolic phytoconstituents.

Tawa Tawa (*Euphorbia hirta*)

Some recent investigations have revealed that high blood glucose level is concomitant with the significant decrease in anti-oxidant potentials and generation of free radical species, making tawa tawa a best remedy. These free radicals are mainly scavenged for their anti-diabetic potentials. The floral extract of this plant is considered to be highly efficient due to the presence of phenolic compounds, flavonoid contents and tannins. However, its exact mechanism and mode of action is still unknown. Various other parts of this plant, also reduce the side effects, mainly relevant to the synthetic medicines [68].

Table 1. Potential anti-diabetic and anti-hypertensive plants and their bioactive components.

S. No.	Plants	Scientific Name	Plant Part	Bioactive Component	References
1	Alkanet	*Anchusa officinalis* L.	Roots	Naphthoquinone and alkannin	[69]
2	Asthma Weed	*Euphorbia hirta* L.	Weeds	Flavonol glycoside xanthorhamnin	[70]
3	Bamboo	*Bambusa arundinacea*	Stem	Tabashir	[71]

(Table 1) cont.....

S. No.	Plants	Scientific Name	Plant Part	Bioactive Component	References
4	Basil	*Ocimum basilicum* L.	Leaves	Linalool, methyl eugenol and methylchavicol	[72]
5	Caraway	*Carum carvi* L.	Seeds	Furfural, acetaldehyde, carveol, pinene, thujene, phellandrene, camphene, limonene, and carvone	[73]
6	Chirayita	*Swertia chirayita*	Whole plant	Undecanoic acid, 2-buten-2-one, camphor, 2-heptadecanone and cedral	[74]
7	Coleus	*Coleus forskohlii*	Different parts of plant	Diterpenes and forskolin	[75]
8	Cubeb	*Piper cubeba*	Leaves	Cubebic acid, cubeb-resin and cubebin	[76]
9	Cumin	*Cuminum cyminum*	Seeds	Cumin, cumin aldehyde and cumin alcohol	[77]
10	Cypress	*Cupressus sempervirens glauca*	Leaves	α-cadinol, α-pinene, manoyl oxide, sabinene, sandaracopimaradiene, p-pinene, two diterpenoids, one oxygenated sesquiterpene, mycene, bornyl acetate, carene, terpinolene, p-cymene, α-terpineol and terpinene	[78]
11	Damask Rose	*Rosa damascena* Mil.	Flower petals	Flavonoids, terpenes, anthocyanins and glycosides	[79]
12	Fennel	*Foneiculum vulgare*	Seeds	Fenchone and trans-anethole	[80]
13	Fenugreek	*Trigonella foenum-groecum* L.	Leaves and stem	Neryl acetate, camphor, β-pinene, β-caryophyllene, 2,5-dimethylpyrazine, geranial, 3-octen-2-one, α-selinene, 6-methyl-5-hepten-2-one, α-terpineol, α-pinene, α-campholenal, and γ-terpinene	[81]
14	Fig	*Ficus carica* L.	Fruit	(Z)-3-hexeny benzoate, n-nonanal, n-tetracosane, (E)-2-hexenal, n-hexadecanoic acid, n-docosane and phytol	[82]
15	Frangipani	*Plumeria rubra* L.	Leaves and flowers	n-tetradecanal, phenyl acetaldehyde, (E)-non-2-en-1-ol, limonene, cis-9-tricosene, γ-elemene, (E, E)-α-farnesene, octadecanal, n-nonanal, α-copaene and octadecanal	[83]
16	Ginseng	*Panax ginseng*	Leaves	Sesquiterpenes, phenolic compounds, polyacetylene and ginsenoside	[84]
17	Guava	*Psidium guajava* L.	Leaves	β-caryophyllene, α-pinene and 1,8-cineole	[85]
18	Henna	*Lawsonia inermis* L.	Leaves	α-limonene, β–limonene, β–myrcene and linalool	[86]

(Table 1) cont.....

S. No.	Plants	Scientific Name	Plant Part	Bioactive Component	References
19	Indian Globe Thistle	*Sphaeranthus indicus*	Roots and herb	23-dimethoxy-p-cymene, r-cadinol, (Z)-arteannuic alcohol, p-maaliene, caryophyllene oxide and 2.5-dimethoxy-p-cymene	[87]
20	Indian Pennywort	*Centella asiatica*	Whole plant	β-caryophyllene, α-humulene, trans--farnesene, germacrene-D and caryophyllene oxide	[88]
21	Ma-huang	*Ephedra gerardiana*	Herb	Ephedrine (E) alkaloids	[89]
22	Moringa	*Moringa oleifera* L.	Leaf	Hexacosane, pentacosane and heptacosane	[90]
23	Olive	*Olea europaea* L.	Fruit and leaves	Palmetic acid, Z-nerolidol, octacosane, caryophyllene oxide, tetracosane and 4-hydroxy-4-methyl-2-Pentanone	[91]
24	Puncture Vine	*Tribulus terrestris*	Leaves and fruits	Kaempferol, kaempferol-3-glucoside, kaempferol-3-rutinoside and tribuloside [kaempferol-3-β-d-(6″-p-coumaroyl) glucoside]	[92]
25	Saffron	*Crocus sativus*	Floral part	Crocin, crocetin, picrocrocin and safranal	[93]
26	Sweet Lemon	*Citrus limetta* Risso	Peel	D-Limonene, β-Myrcene and β-Linalool	[94]
27	Tree Turmeric	*Berberis aristata*	Root, bark and wood	Berberine, protoberberine and karachine	[95]
28	Walnut	*Juglans regia* L.	Fruit	α Pinene, β-Pinene, β-Myrcene, cymene, limonene, 1.8-cineol, α-terpinene, terpinolene, camphor, Myrtenol, Bornyl acetate, Eugenol, β-Bourbounene, β–caryophyllene, α-humelene, Geranyl acetate, β-farnesene, γ-Muurolene, Germacrene and curcumene	[96]
29	Corn	*Zea mays*	Seed	polyphenols, phenolic acids, flavonoids, anthocyanins, glycosides, carotenoids and polysaccharides	[97]
30	Tawa Tawa	*Euphorbia hirta*	Flower	Phenolic compounds, flavonoid contents and tannins	[68]

ANTI-HYPERTENSIVE PLANTS

High blood pressure or hypertension increases the risk of cerebrovascular and cardiovascular diseases. Hypertension is a dangerous disease due to its excessive prevalence and deep association with increased rate of morbidity and mortality in common people all around the world. Some recent researches have shown that prevalence of hypertension is expected to be increased by 7.2% till the end of 2030 starting from 2013. Complications arising due to the hypertension accounts for 9.4 million deaths all across the globe and is estimated to be increased upto 1.58 billion till 2025. In the year 2015, heart diseases and severe hypertension was the fourth major cause of deaths all over the world [98].

Basil (*Ocimum basilicum* L.)

Anti-hypertensive potentials of the basil extracts were tested on experimental animals affected by the renovascular hypertension. The results of this study indicated that basil possesses strong effects on cardiac hypertrophy, embryo transference and blood pressure. These effects are consistent with the effects of embryo-transfer-converting-enzyme that needs thorough investigation and detailed research [99].

Black piper (*Piper nigrum* L.)

Black piper is reported to possess the calcium channel blockade effects, responsible to cause the vasodilation and cardiac depression. These diseases provide the basis for low blood pressure. Piperine is further reported to be associated with the vasoconstriction, responsible for the significant decrease and slight increase in the blood pressure after drug administration. Hence, piperine does not allow the blood pressure to decrease beyond the specific limit; along with less side effects [100].

Coleus (*Coleus forskohlii*)

Coleus is known to have highly positive inotropic effects on the heart tissues. It helps to maintain the increased level of cAMP by decreasing the elevated blood pressure through vasodilation, in experimental animals. This plant has traditionally been used for the treatment of congestive heart failure, severe angina attack and intense hypertension. It basically lowers the blood pressure with slight increase in the contractility of heart muscles. This effect is considered to be due to the pronounced increase in levels of cAMP in normal cells. It causes the arterial relaxation and increases the contractions of heart muscles [101].

Curry Leaf (*Murraya koenigii* L.)

Curry leaves (*Murraya koenigii*) chutney supplementation showed promising anti-hypertensive activity in hypertensive subjects [102].

Puncture Vine (*Tribulus terrestris*)

Puncture vine is known to possess the strong anti-hypertensive potentials [103]. The solvent extract of this plant promotes the release of nitric oxide from endothelium and nerve endings. It remarkably reduces the effects of hypertension by increasing the production of angiotensin and relaxing the smooth muscles. It further alters the enzyme inhibition [104]. The extract of puncture vine enhances the production and release of nitroglycerine and prompts the relaxation by ensuring the proper functioning of pro-erectile. However, the exact mechanism behind lowering the high blood pressure is still unknown. Anti-hypertensive potentials of the aqueous extracts of this plant are mainly accredited to their inhibitory effects on angiotensin converting enzyme activity [105]. Treatment of rats with aqueous extracts of puncture vine has appreciably decreased the substantial acetylcholinesterase in all body tissues. Similarly, vasodilation of arterial smooth muscles in hypertension leads to the failure of relaxing effects in aorta of experimental animals along with repression in peristaltic movements of jejunum and ureter [103]. Remarkable improvements and significant dilations of coronary arteries have also been shown by its prolonged usage, without any side effect [106].

Sesame Seed (*Sesamum indicum* L.)

Sesamin and some of its potentially active metabolites can induce the anti-hypertensive effects in model experimental animals [107]. In a recent experimental investigation, it was found that consumption of sesame seed oil can reduce the oxidative stress and increase the activities of GPx, superoxide dismutase and catalase in hypertensive patients [108]. These results were in view that sesame oil consumption can enhance the defence mechanism in human beings. Sesame is also a useful prophylactic agent in the treatment of hypertension and cardiovascular hypertrophy [109]. In another experimental research, it was found that sesame seed oil is much better in reducing the elevated blood pressure in comparison with the nifedipine-a potential calcium channel blocker [110].

Yarrow (*Achillea wilhelmsii*)

Yarrow is a rich source of lactones, sesquiterpenes and natural flavonoids. It has been found to reduce the hypertension and high blood lipid level when tested on experimental specimens. In this experiment, double blind placebo controlled clinical trials were conducted in order to study the anti-hypertensive and anti-hyperlipidemic effects on the yarrow drops by considering the blood pressure, low density lipoproteins and high density lipoproteins as experimental parameters. The results were in view that yarrow can decrease the level of triglyceride after two months, low density lipoprotein and cholesterol after four months and high density lipoproteins after six months of medicinal administration. Moreover, significant decrease in systolic and diastolic blood pressure was also observed after the period ranging from two to six months [111].

Passion Fruit (*Passiflora edulis*)

Methanolic extracts of luteolin or rind of passion fruit constituting abundant polyphenols were found to reduce the systolic blood pressure in spontaneously hypertensive experimental animals. The quantitative analysis showed that the extracts constituting 20 μg/g luteolin and 41 μg/g of luteolin-6-C-glucoside have shown best results. This plant also contains γ-amino-butyric acid; responsible for the strong anti-hypertensive effects. Hence, it can be stated that high concentration of γ-amino-butyric acid is mainly responsible for the anti-hypertensive effects while some of the percentage is also contributed by vasodilatory effects of the polyphenols more specifically, luteolin [112].

Onion (*Allium cepa*)

Hydroalcoholic extracts of the onion peel have been reported to reduce the severe effects of hypertension when artificially induced by the aortic contractions and high fructose diet in an experimental research. The results showed that onion peel extract significantly reduced the aortic contractions induced by KCl in a concentration dependent manner. However, activity of onion peel extract was diminished or suppressed by removing the aortic endothelium. Inhibition of the synthesis of prostaglandin, cGMP and nitric oxide by indomethacin, methylene blue and L-NAME did not attenuate the activity of onion peel extract. The onion peel extract did not alter the rate of heart beat but reduced the extent of hypertension induced by the fructose. These results indicated that onion peel extract can reduce the aortic contractions *via* inhibition of calcium influx thereby affecting the extent of hypertension due to the anti-oxidant potentials, quercitin contents and inhibiting the calcium influx in vascular smooth muscle cells [113].

Garlic (*Allium sativum*)

Anti-hypertensive effects of garlic were elucidated in a recent research activity where two-kidney-one-clip Goldblatt model was used for induction of vasopressor agents like angiotensin-II and prostaglandins for pathological increase in blood pressure. The results of this experiment showed that single dose of garlic possesses maximum anti-hypertensive potentials after two to six hours of oral drug administration. However, residual effects of this medicine continued for upto twenty four hours. Multiple doses of garlic were found to be effective in restraining the expected rise in blood pressure which normally occurs in experimental animals. Making long story short, garlic (*Allium sativum*) possesses excellent anti-hypertensive potentials that can be used as a natural or supplementary remedy for the treatment of unilateral renovascular hypertension [114].

Celery (*Apium graveolens*)

Celery seed extract is known to have marvelous anti-hypertensive effects in normotensive or deoxycorticosterone-acetate-induced hypertensive experimental animals. Aqueous based ethanolic, methanolic and hexanoic extracts were intraperitoneally administered in experimental animals in order to check their effects on the rate of heart beat and blood pressure as compared to the spirnolactone as diuretic positive control. The appreciable amount of n-butylphthalide as strong anti-hypertensive constituent was also found to be evident. The results of whole study indicated that all these extracts significantly decreased the elevated blood pressure and increased the heart beat in a hypertensive rats without having any appreciable effect on the normotensive animals [115].

Oat (*Avena sativa* L.)

Hypertension is a severe pathological disorder and a clinical symptom, caused by the elevated blood pressure on the blood arteries. It also contributes in increased risk of cardiac arrest and endothelial injury. These symptoms are due to the infiltration of low density lipoproteins. Hypertension is known to accelerate the fatty streaks transformations in fibrous plaque by enhancing the proliferation of smooth muscles. Natural oat has recently been explored for its anti-hypertensive potentials by improving the insulinemic and glycemic profiles. The dietary approach to stop hypertension has demonstrated that a diet rich in whole grains, vegetables, fruits and low fat contents can lower the blood pressure and decrease the symptoms of hypertension [116].

Barberry (*Berberis vulgaris*)

Aqueous extracts of the fruit of barberry is a strong anti-hypertensive agent as shown by the deoxycorticosterone acetate-induced-hypertension activity. The obtained results were in view that vasodilatory and anti-hypertensive effects of the aqueous extracts of barberry were mainly endothelial-independent and can be used to treat the hypertension and endothelial dysfunctioning [117].

Black Cumin (*Nigella sativa*)

Seed extract of black cumin shows strong diuretic potentials, inhibits over activity of nervous system and enhances the production of nitric oxide in *in-vivo* studies. It also has many potential applications as an adjuvant anti-hypertensive agent for elderly population. In a recent research, some experimental organisms suffering from abnormal heart beat and elevated blood pressure were selected to be tested with seed extract of black cumin. Results of this study finally concluded that only slight changes in blood pressure were observed which proved that black cumin is only effective in reducing the blood pressure in elderly patient upto some extent [118].

Ylang-Ylang (*Cananga odorata* L.)

Ylang ylang has been reported for its efficiency on proper heart functioning including the rate of heart beat and normal blood pressure. Results of this study demonstrated that inhalation of ylang ylang can significantly lower the systolic and diastolic blood pressure and cause abnormal heart beat. However, some sedative effects of ylang ylang have also been reported in some research articles that further enhance its therapeutic value and medicinal applications [119].

Garden Cress (*Lapidium sativum* L.)

Anti-hypertensive and diuretic effects of the aqueous extracts of garden cress seeds have found to be beneficial in the spontaneously hypertensive and normotensive Wistar Kyoto rats. The results of this study showed that three weeks oral intake of this material significantly lowered the blood pressure and remarkably enhanced the excretion of various electrolytes without any change in excretion of water [120]. Similar results had also been found when diuretic effects of aqueous and methanolic extracts of the garden cress seeds were investigated in normal experimental animals more specifically rats [121].

Ginger (*Zingiber officinale*)

Ginger is a major ingredient of number of continental dishes and known to have high therapeutic potential. Ginger has numerous direct and indirect effects on the blood pressure and the rate of heart beat. Crude extract of the ginger can significantly lower the arterial blood pressure when taken in a dose dependent manner. It also exhibits the cardio-depressant potentials and cause spontaneous contractions in paired atria in experimental animals. Crude extract of the ginger can relax the phenylephrine induced vascular contractions at the dose concentration ten times higher than required for the potassium induced contractions [122]. Similarly, blocking effects of calcium showed that ginger can act as a membrane binder and regulator of an intracellular calcium channels. Crude extracts have more pronounced vasodilation potentials and can lower the blood pressure *via* blockade of voltage dependent calcium channels. Some other evidences are in support that aqueous extracts can also reduce the blood pressure through a dual inhibitory effect mediated by the stimulation of both muscarinic receptors and blockade calcium channels. It was also found that different components of ginger might have some opposite effects on the reactivity of blood vessels [123].

Sweet Lemon (*Citrus limetta* Risso)

Hesperidin and naringin are the major flavonoids of the fruit pulp and fruit peel of *Citrus limetta*. Therefore, due to the strong anti-hypertensive effects of the flavonoids, *Citrus limetta* fruit antagonizes the effects of angiotensin II [124]. Angiotensin II is a potent vasoconstrictor and is responsible for the immediate elevation of blood pressure due to its peptide nature. It is responsible for the cardiovascular diseases such as heart attack and stroke by causing the thrombosis (blood clotting). This antagonistic effect of *Citrus limetta* extract is considered to be a physiologic process, *i.e.*, without antagonizing the effects of any specific binding receptor.

CONCLUDING REMARKS

Hypertension (high blood pressure) and diabetes mellitus (elevated blood sugar level) are the two most deleterious diseases. These diseases are rapidly prevailing at alarming rate among both the genders, all across the globe. Hypertension is also known as a "silent killer" as most of the hypertensive patients does not even realize that they are hypertensive. Diabetes mellitus is the "biggest epidemic" of twenty first century. According to an estimate, 972 million people of the world are hypertensive while 415 million people are diabetic and this number is still increasing at rapid pace and expected to be further increased in near future.

Therefore, aroma compounds of essential oils have commonly been used in traditional system of medicines and advanced treatment processes. Starting from aromatherapy to allopathic system of medicines, bioactive compounds of essential oil are being used due to their unique chemical composition and extreme therapeutic potentials. Therefore, this chapter summarizes some of the commonly used anti-hypertensive and anti-diabetic plants with their major bioactive components.

CONSENT FOR PUBLICATION

Not applicable.

CONFLICT OF INTEREST

There is no conflict of interest declared.

ACKNOWLEDGEMENT

Declared none.

REFERENCES

[1]   Gupta S, Walia A, Malan R. Phytochemistry and pharmacology of cedrus deodera: an overview. Int J Pharm Sci Res 2011; 2(8): 2010.

[2]   Naeem A, Abbas T, Ali T, Hasnain A. Essential Oils: Brief Background and Uses. Ann Short Reports 2018; 1(1): 1006.

[3]   Nadeem F, Azeem MW, Jilani MI. Isolation of Bioactive Compounds from Essential Oils–A Comprehensive Review.

[4]   Saxena M, Saxena J, Nema R, Singh D, Gupta A. Phytochemistry of medicinal plants. J pharmacognosy and phytochem 2013; 1(6)

[5]   Piero M, Nzaro G, Njagi J. Diabetes mellitus-a devastating metabolic disorder Asian J biomedical and pharmaceut sci 2015; 5(40): 1.

[6]   Benos DJ. Biochemistry in medicine: hypertension minireview series. J Biol Chem 2010; 285(12): 8507-7.
        [http://dx.doi.org/10.1074/jbc.R109.025072] [PMID: 20118247]

[7]   Bromfield S, Muntner P. High blood pressure: the leading global burden of disease risk factor and the need for worldwide prevention programs. Curr Hypertens Rep 2013; 15(3): 134-6.
        [http://dx.doi.org/10.1007/s11906-013-0340-9] [PMID: 23536128]

[8]   Adefegha SA, Olasehinde TA, Oboh G. Essential oil composition, antioxidant, antidiabetic and antihypertensive properties of two Afromomum species. J Oleo Sci 2017; 66(1): 51-63.
        [http://dx.doi.org/10.5650/jos.ess16029] [PMID: 27928138]

[9]   Patlak M. New weapons to combat an ancient disease: treating diabetes. FASEB J 2002; 16(14): 1853.
        [http://dx.doi.org/10.1096/fj.02-0974bkt] [PMID: 12468446]

[10]   Piero M. Hypoglycemic effects of some Kenyan plants traditionally used in management of diabetes mellitus in eastern province 2006.

[11]   Belinda R. 2004.Gale Encyclopaedia of Alternative Medicine.

[12]   Girouard H. 2016.Hypertension and the Brain as an End-organ Target
       [http://dx.doi.org/10.1007/978-3-319-25616-0]

[13]   Pasupuleti VK, Anderson JW. Nutraceuticals, glycemic health and type 2 diabetes John Wiley & Sons
       2009.

[14]   Kumar N, Gupta AK. Wound-healing activity of Onosma hispidum (Ratanjot) in normal and diabetic
       rats. J Herbs Spices Med Plants 2010; 15(4): 342-51.
       [http://dx.doi.org/10.1080/10496470903507924]

[15]   Grover JK, Yadav S, Vats V. Medicinal plants of India with anti-diabetic potential. J Ethnopharmacol
       2002; 81(1): 81-100.
       [http://dx.doi.org/10.1016/S0378-8741(02)00059-4] [PMID: 12020931]

[16]   Naziroğlu M, Butterworth PJ. Protective effects of moderate exercise with dietary vitamin C and E on
       blood antioxidative defense mechanism in rats with streptozotocin-induced diabetes. Can J Appl
       Physiol 2005; 30(2): 172-85.
       [http://dx.doi.org/10.1139/h05-113] [PMID: 15981786]

[17]   Kumar S, Malhotra R, Kumar D. Antidiabetic and free radicals scavenging potential of Euphorbia
       hirta flower extract. Indian J Pharm Sci 2010; 72(4): 533-7.
       [http://dx.doi.org/10.4103/0250-474X.73921] [PMID: 21218075]

[18]   Umamaheswari S. 2016.Pharmacological Evaluation of Bambusa Arundinacea RETZ Roxb Seeds

[19]   El-Beshbishy H, Bahashwan S. Hypoglycemic effect of basil (Ocimum basilicum) aqueous extract is
       mediated through inhibition of α-glucosidase and α-amylase activities: an *in vitro* study. Toxicol Ind
       Health 2012; 28(1): 42-50.
       [http://dx.doi.org/10.1177/0748233711403193] [PMID: 21636683]

[20]   Lemhadri A, Hajji L, Michel J-B, Eddouks M. Cholesterol and triglycerides lowering activities of
       caraway fruits in normal and streptozotocin diabetic rats. J Ethnopharmacol 2006; 106(3): 321-6.
       [http://dx.doi.org/10.1016/j.jep.2006.01.033] [PMID: 16567073]

[21]   Kumar KS, Bhowmik D, Chiranjib B, Chandira M. Swertia chirata: A traditional herb and its
       medicinal uses. J Chem Pharm Res 2010; 2(1): 262-6.

[22]   Brahmachari G, Mondal S, Gangopadhyay A, *et al.* Swertia (Gentianaceae): chemical and
       pharmacological aspects. Chem Biodivers 2004; 1(11): 1627-51.
       [http://dx.doi.org/10.1002/cbdv.200490123] [PMID: 17191805]

[23]   Kavitha C, Rajamani K, Vadivel E. Coleus forskohlii A comprehensive review on morphology,
       phytochemistry and pharmacological aspects. J Med Plants Res 2010; 4(4): 278-85.

[24]   Ríos-Silva M, Trujillo X, Trujillo-Hernández B, *et al.* Effect of chronic administration of forskolin on
       glycemia and oxidative stress in rats with and without experimental diabetes. Int J Med Sci 2014;
       11(5): 448-52.
       [http://dx.doi.org/10.7150/ijms.8034] [PMID: 24688307]

[25]   Dhar ML, Dhar MM, Dhawan BN, Mehrotra BN, Ray C. Screening of Indian plants for biological
       activity: I. Indian J Exp Biol 1968; 6(4): 232-47.
       [PMID: 5720682]

[26]   Srinivasan K. Plant foods in the management of diabetes mellitus: spices as beneficial antidiabetic
       food adjuncts. Int J Food Sci Nutr 2005; 56(6): 399-414.
       [http://dx.doi.org/10.1080/09637480500512872] [PMID: 16361181]

[27]   Lee H-S. Cuminaldehyde: aldose reductase and α-glucosidase inhibitor derived from Cuminum
       cyminum L. seeds. J Agric Food Chem 2005; 53(7): 2446-50.
       [http://dx.doi.org/10.1021/jf048451g] [PMID: 15796577]

[28]   Sambaiah K, Srinivasan K. 1991.Effect of cumin, cinnamon, ginger, mustard and tamarind in induced
       hypercholesterolemic rats

[http://dx.doi.org/10.1002/food.19910350112]

[29]   Ahmad M, Saeed F, Noor Jahan M. Evaluation of insecticidal and antioxidant activity of selected medicinal plants. J Pharmacognosy and Photochem 2013; 2: 153-8.

[30]   Gholamhoseinian A, Fallah H, Sharifi far F. Inhibitory effect of methanol extract of Rosa damascena Mill. flowers on α-glucosidase activity and postprandial hyperglycemia in normal and diabetic rats. Phytomedicine 2009; 16(10): 935-41.
        [http://dx.doi.org/10.1016/j.phymed.2009.02.020] [PMID: 19380218]

[31]   Badgujar SB, Patel VV, Bandivdekar AH. Foeniculum vulgare Mill: a review of its botany, phytochemistry, pharmacology, contemporary application, and toxicology. BioMed Res Int 2014; 2014842674
        [http://dx.doi.org/10.1155/2014/842674] [PMID: 25162032]

[32]   Roberts KT. The potential of fenugreek (Trigonella foenum-graecum) as a functional food and nutraceutical and its effects on glycemia and lipidemia. J Med Food 2011; 14(12): 1485-9.
        [http://dx.doi.org/10.1089/jmf.2011.0002] [PMID: 21861724]

[33]   Puri D, Prabhu KM, Murthy PS. Mechanism of action of a hypoglycemic principle isolated from fenugreek seeds. Indian J Physiol Pharmacol 2002; 46(4): 457-62.
        [PMID: 12683221]

[34]   Wani SA, Kumar P. Fenugreek: A review on its nutraceutical properties and utilization in various food products. J Saudi Soc Agric Sci 2018; 17(2): 97-106.
        [http://dx.doi.org/10.1016/j.jssas.2016.01.007]

[35]   Xue W-L, Li X-S, Zhang J, Liu Y-H, Wang Z-L, Zhang R-J. Effect of Trigonella foenum-graecum (fenugreek) extract on blood glucose, blood lipid and hemorheological properties in streptozotocin-induced diabetic rats. Asia Pac J Clin Nutr 2007; 16 (Suppl. 1): 422-6.
        [PMID: 17392143]

[36]   Srinivasan K. Fenugreek and traditional antidiabetic herbs of Indian origin. Nutraceuticals. Glycemic Health and Type 2008; 2: 311-78.

[37]   Canal JR, Torres MD, Romero A, Pérez C. A chloroform extract obtained from a decoction of Ficus carica leaves improves the cholesterolaemic status of rats with streptozotocin-induced diabetes. Acta Physiol Hung 2000; 87(1): 71-6.
        [http://dx.doi.org/10.1556/APhysiol.87.2000.1.8] [PMID: 11032050]

[38]   Ahmed AS, Ahmed Q, Saxena AK, Jamal P. Evaluation of *in vitro* antidiabetic and antioxidant characterizations of Elettaria cardamomum (L.) Maton (Zingiberaceae), Piper cubeba L. f. (Piperaceae), and Plumeria rubra L. (Apocynaceae). Pak J Pharm Sci 2017; 30(1): 113-26.
        [PMID: 28603121]

[39]   Lakshmi T, Roy A, Geetha R. 2011.Panax ginseng–a universal panacea in the herbal medicine with diverse pharmacological spectrum–a review.

[40]   Attele AS, Zhou Y-P, Xie J-T, *et al.* Antidiabetic effects of Panax ginseng berry extract and the identification of an effective component. Diabetes 2002; 51(6): 1851-8.
        [http://dx.doi.org/10.2337/diabetes.51.6.1851] [PMID: 12031973]

[41]   Liu Z, Li W, Li X, *et al.* Antidiabetic effects of malonyl ginsenosides from Panax ginseng on type 2 diabetic rats induced by high-fat diet and streptozotocin. J Ethnopharmacol 2013; 145(1): 233-40.
        [http://dx.doi.org/10.1016/j.jep.2012.10.058] [PMID: 23147499]

[42]   Subramanian S, Banu HH, Ramya Bai RM, Shanmugavalli R. Biochemical evaluation of antihyperglycemic and antioxidant nature of Psidium guajava leaves extract in streptozotocin-induced experimental diabetes in rats. Pharm Biol 2009; 47(4): 298-303.
        [http://dx.doi.org/10.1080/13880200902748429]

[43]   Soman S, Rauf AA, Indira M, Rajamanickam C. Antioxidant and antiglycative potential of ethyl acetate fraction of Psidium guajava leaf extract in streptozotocin-induced diabetic rats. Plant Foods

Hum Nutr 2010; 65(4): 386-91.
[http://dx.doi.org/10.1007/s11130-010-0198-9] [PMID: 21120613]

[44]   Huang C-S, Yin M-C, Chiu L-C. Antihyperglycemic and antioxidative potential of Psidium guajava fruit in streptozotocin-induced diabetic rats. Food Chem Toxicol 2011; 49(9): 2189-95.
[http://dx.doi.org/10.1016/j.fct.2011.05.032] [PMID: 21679740]

[45]   Cheng FC, Shen SC, Wu JSB. Effect of guava (Psidium guajava L.) leaf extract on glucose uptake in rat hepatocytes. J Food Sci 2009; 74(5): H132-8.
[http://dx.doi.org/10.1111/j.1750-3841.2009.01149.x] [PMID: 19646046]

[46]   Rai PK, Rai NK, Rai A, Watal G. Role of LIBS in elemental analysis of Psidium guajava responsible for glycemic potential. Instrum Sci Technol 2007; 35(5): 507-22.
[http://dx.doi.org/10.1080/10739140701540230]

[47]   Shen SC, Cheng FC, Wu NJ. Effect of guava (Psidium guajava Linn.) leaf soluble solids on glucose metabolism in type 2 diabetic rats. Phytother Res 2008; 22(11): 1458-64.
[http://dx.doi.org/10.1002/ptr.2476] [PMID: 18819164]

[48]   Wu J-W, Hsieh C-L, Wang H-Y, Chen H-Y. Inhibitory effects of guava (Psidium guajava L.) leaf extracts and its active compounds on the glycation process of protein. Food Chem 2009; 113(1): 78-84.
[http://dx.doi.org/10.1016/j.foodchem.2008.07.025]

[49]   Badoni Semwal R, Semwal DK, Combrinck S, Cartwright-Jones C, Viljoen A. Lawsonia inermis L. (henna): ethnobotanical, phytochemical and pharmacological aspects. J Ethnopharmacol 2014; 155(1): 80-103.
[http://dx.doi.org/10.1016/j.jep.2014.05.042] [PMID: 24886774]

[50]   Girish C, Pradhan S. Herbal drugs on the liver. Liver Pathophysiology. Elsevier 2017; pp. 605-20.
[http://dx.doi.org/10.1016/B978-0-12-804274-8.00044-8]

[51]   Emran TB, Dutta M, Uddin MMN, Nath AK, Uddin MZ. Antidiabetic potential of the leaf extract of Centella asiatica in alloxaninduced diabetic rats. Jahangirnagar Uni J Bio Sci 2015; 4(1): 51-9.
[http://dx.doi.org/10.3329/jujbs.v4i1.27785]

[52]   Li WL, Zheng HC, Bukuru J, De Kimpe N. Natural medicines used in the traditional Chinese medical system for therapy of diabetes mellitus. J Ethnopharmacol 2004; 92(1): 1-21.
[http://dx.doi.org/10.1016/j.jep.2003.12.031] [PMID: 15099842]

[53]   Ndong M, Uehara M, Katsumata S, Suzuki K. Effects of oral administration of Moringa oleifera Lam on glucose tolerance in Goto-Kakizaki and Wistar rats. J Clin Biochem Nutr 2007; 40(3): 229-33.
[http://dx.doi.org/10.3164/jcbn.40.229] [PMID: 18398501]

[54]   Jaiswal D, Kumar Rai P, Kumar A, Mehta S, Watal G. Effect of Moringa oleifera Lam. leaves aqueous extract therapy on hyperglycemic rats. J Ethnopharmacol 2009; 123(3): 392-6.
[http://dx.doi.org/10.1016/j.jep.2009.03.036] [PMID: 19501271]

[55]   Sato H, Genet C, Strehle A, *et al.* Anti-hyperglycemic activity of a TGR5 agonist isolated from Olea europaea. Biochem Biophys Res Commun 2007; 362(4): 793-8.
[http://dx.doi.org/10.1016/j.bbrc.2007.06.130] [PMID: 17825251]

[56]   Jemai H, El Feki A, Sayadi S. Antidiabetic and antioxidant effects of hydroxytyrosol and oleuropein from olive leaves in alloxan-diabetic rats. J Agric Food Chem 2009; 57(19): 8798-804.
[http://dx.doi.org/10.1021/jf901280r] [PMID: 19725535]

[57]   Li M, Qu W, Wang Y, Wan H, Tian C. [Hypoglycemic effect of saponin from Tribulus terrestris]. Zhong Yao Cai 2002; 25(6): 420-2.
[PMID: 12583337]

[58]   Li M, Qu W, Chu S, Wang H, Tian C, Tu M. Effect of the decoction of tribulus terrestris on mice gluconeogenesis. Zhong Yao Cai 2001; 24(8): 586-8.
[PMID: 11715199]

[59]   Amin A, Lotfy M, Shafiullah M, Adeghate E. The protective effect of Tribulus terrestris in diabetes. Ann N Y Acad Sci 2006; 1084(1): 391-401.
[http://dx.doi.org/10.1196/annals.1372.005] [PMID: 17151317]

[60]   De B, Bhandari K, Singla RK, *et al.* Chemometrics optimized extraction procedures, phytosynergistic blending and *in vitro* screening of natural enzyme inhibitors amongst leaves of Tulsi, Banyan and Jamun. Pharmacogn Mag 2015; 11 (Suppl. 4): S522-32.
[http://dx.doi.org/10.4103/0973-1296.172956] [PMID: 27013789]

[61]   Xi L, Qian Z, Shen X, Wen N, Zhang Y. Crocetin prevents dexamethasone-induced insulin resistance in rats. Planta Med 2005; 71(10): 917-22.
[http://dx.doi.org/10.1055/s-2005-871248] [PMID: 16254822]

[62]   Xi L, Qian Z, Xu G, *et al.* Beneficial impact of crocetin, a carotenoid from saffron, on insulin sensitivity in fructose-fed rats. J Nutr Biochem 2007; 18(1): 64-72.
[http://dx.doi.org/10.1016/j.jnutbio.2006.03.010] [PMID: 16713230]

[63]   Arai Y, Watanabe S, Kimira M, Shimoi K, Mochizuki R, Kinae N. Dietary intakes of flavonols, flavones and isoflavones by Japanese women and the inverse correlation between quercetin intake and plasma LDL cholesterol concentration. J Nutr 2000; 130(9): 2243-50.
[http://dx.doi.org/10.1093/jn/130.9.2243] [PMID: 10958819]

[64]   Ni Y-x, Liu A-q, Gao Y-f, *et al.* Therapeutic effect of berberine on 60 patients with non-insulin dependent diabetes mellitus and experimental research. Chinese J Integrated Traditional and Western Med 1995; 1(2): 91-5.

[65]   Gillen LJ, Tapsell LC, Patch CS, Owen A, Batterham M. Structured dietary advice incorporating walnuts achieves optimal fat and energy balance in patients with type 2 diabetes mellitus. J Am Diet Assoc 2005; 105(7): 1087-96.
[http://dx.doi.org/10.1016/j.jada.2005.04.007] [PMID: 15983525]

[66]   Teimori M, Montasser Kouhsari S, Ghafarzadegan R, Hajiaghaee R. Study of hypoglycemic effect of Juglans regia leaves and its mechanism. Faslnamah-i Giyahan-i Daruyi 2010; 1(33): 57-65.

[67]   Huang B, Wang Z, Park JH, *et al.* Anti-diabetic effect of purple corn extract on C57BL/KsJ db/db mice. Nutr Res Pract 2015; 9(1): 22-9.
[http://dx.doi.org/10.4162/nrp.2015.9.1.22] [PMID: 25671064]

[68]   Baibado JT. Biological functions of the metabolites from Euphorbia hirta L. Int J Pharmaceutical and Biological Science Archive 2015; 3(1)

[69]   Shaheen A, Hanif MA, Rehman R, Jilani MI, Shikov A. Alkanet. Medicinal Plants of South Asia. Elsevier 2020; pp. 1-12.
[http://dx.doi.org/10.1016/B978-0-08-102659-5.00001-X]

[70]   Ijaz B, Hanif MA, Ayub MA, Hanif A, Mushtaq Z. Asthma Weed. Medicinal Plants of South Asia. Elsevier 2020; pp. 13-27.
[http://dx.doi.org/10.1016/B978-0-08-102659-5.00002-1]

[71]   Azeem MW, Hanif MA, Khan MM. Bamboo. Medicinal Plants of South Asia. Elsevier 2020; pp. 29-45.
[http://dx.doi.org/10.1016/B978-0-08-102659-5.00003-3]

[72]   Nadeem F, Hanif MA, Bhatti IA, Jilani MI, Al-Yahyai R. Basil. Medicinal Plants of South Asia. Elsevier 2020; pp. 47-62.
[http://dx.doi.org/10.1016/B978-0-08-102659-5.00004-5]

[73]   Javed R, Hanif MA, Rehman R, Hanif M, Tung BT. Caraway. Medicinal Plants of South Asia. Elsevier 2020; pp. 87-100.
[http://dx.doi.org/10.1016/B978-0-08-102659-5.00007-0]

[74]   Seher A, Hanif MA, Hanif M, Hanif A. Chirayita. Medicinal Plants of South Asia. Elsevier 2020; pp.

125-34.
[http://dx.doi.org/10.1016/B978-0-08-102659-5.00010-0]

[75] Nisar S, Hanif MA, Soomro K, Jilani MI, Kala CP. Coleus. Medicinal Plants of South Asia. Elsevier 2020; pp. 135-47.
[http://dx.doi.org/10.1016/B978-0-08-102659-5.00011-2]

[76] Ahmad H, Khera RA, Hanif MA, Ayub MA. Cubeb. Medicinal Plants of South Asia. Elsevier 2020; pp. 149-64.
[http://dx.doi.org/10.1016/B978-0-08-102659-5.00012-4]

[77] Chaudhry Z, Khera RA, Hanif MA, Ayub MA, Sumrra SH. Cumin. Medicinal Plants of South Asia. Elsevier 2020; pp. 165-78.
[http://dx.doi.org/10.1016/B978-0-08-102659-5.00013-6]

[78] Shaheen A, Hanif MA, Rehman R, Hanif A. Cypress. Medicinal Plants of South Asia. Elsevier 2020; pp. 191-205.
[http://dx.doi.org/10.1016/B978-0-08-102659-5.00015-X]

[79] Shabbir F, Hanif MA, Ayub MA, Jilani MI, Rahman S. Damask Rose. Medicinal Plants of South Asia. Elsevier 2020; pp. 217-30.
[http://dx.doi.org/10.1016/B978-0-08-102659-5.00017-3]

[80] Javed R, Hanif MA, Ayub MA, Rehman R. Fennel. Medicinal Plants of South Asia. Elsevier 2020; pp. 241-56.
[http://dx.doi.org/10.1016/B978-0-08-102659-5.00019-7]

[81] Sarwar S, Hanif MA, Ayub MA, Boakye YD, Agyare C. Fenugreek. Medicinal Plants of South Asia. Elsevier 2020; pp. 257-71.
[http://dx.doi.org/10.1016/B978-0-08-102659-5.00020-3]

[82] Saif S, Hanif MA, Rehman R, Hanif M, Khan O, Khan S. Figs. Medicinal Plants of South Asia. Elsevier 2020; pp. 273-86.
[http://dx.doi.org/10.1016/B978-0-08-102659-5.00021-5]

[83] Idrees S, Hanif MA, Ayub MA, Jilani MI, Memon N. Frangipani. Medicinal Plants of South Asia. Elsevier 2020; pp. 287-300.
[http://dx.doi.org/10.1016/B978-0-08-102659-5.00022-7]

[84] Mohsin MM, Hanif MA, Ayub MA, Dharmadasa R. Ginseng. Medicinal Plants of South Asia. Elsevier 2020; pp. 331-40.
[http://dx.doi.org/10.1016/B978-0-08-102659-5.00025-2]

[85] Irshad Z, Hanif MA, Ayub MA, Jilani MI, Tavallali V. Guava. Medicinal Plants of South Asia. Elsevier 2020; pp. 341-54.
[http://dx.doi.org/10.1016/B978-0-08-102659-5.00026-4]

[86] Rehmat S, Khera RA, Hanif MA, Ayub MA, Hussain AI. Henna. Medicinal Plants of South Asia. Elsevier 2020; pp. 355-68.
[http://dx.doi.org/10.1016/B978-0-08-102659-5.00027-6]

[87] Tariq N, Waheed A, Majeed MI, Hanif MA, Rehman R, Eddouks M. Indian Globe Thistle. Medicinal Plants of South Asia. Elsevier 2020; pp. 407-22.
[http://dx.doi.org/10.1016/B978-0-08-102659-5.00031-8]

[88] Yousaf S, Hanif MA, Rehman R, Azeem MW, Racoti A. Indian Pennywort. Medicinal Plants of South Asia. Elsevier 2020; pp. 423-37.
[http://dx.doi.org/10.1016/B978-0-08-102659-5.00032-X]

[89] Iqbal A, Khera RA, Hanif MA, Ayub MA, Zafar MN. Ma-Huang. Medicinal Plants of South Asia. Elsevier 2020; pp. 479-94.
[http://dx.doi.org/10.1016/B978-0-08-102659-5.00036-7]

[90]   Nadeem F, Hanif MA, Bhatti IA, Basra SMA. Moringa. Medicinal Plants of South Asia. Elsevier 2020; pp. 509-23.
[http://dx.doi.org/10.1016/B978-0-08-102659-5.00038-0]

[91]   Mushtaq A, Hanif MA, Ayub MA, Bhatti IA, Romdhane M. Olive. Medicinal Plants of South Asia. Elsevier 2020; pp. 541-55.
[http://dx.doi.org/10.1016/B978-0-08-102659-5.00040-9]

[92]   Hanif MA, Yousaf S, Rehman R, Hanif A, Nadeem R. Puncture Vine. Medicinal Plants of South Asia. Elsevier 2020; pp. 571-85.
[http://dx.doi.org/10.1016/B978-0-08-102659-5.00042-2]

[93]   Khan M, Hanif MA, Ayub MA, Jilani MI, Chatha SAS. Saffron. Medicinal Plants of South Asia. Elsevier 2020; pp. 587-600.
[http://dx.doi.org/10.1016/B978-0-08-102659-5.00043-4]

[94]   Iqbal A, Khera RA, Hanif MA, Ayub MA, Al-Sadi AM. Sweet Lemon. Medicinal Plants of South Asia. Elsevier 2020; pp. 617-30.
[http://dx.doi.org/10.1016/B978-0-08-102659-5.00045-8]

[95]   Shamim A, Nawaz H, Hanif MA, Jilani MI, Júnior UL. Tree Turmeric. Medicinal Plants of South Asia. Elsevier 2020; pp. 645-55.
[http://dx.doi.org/10.1016/B978-0-08-102659-5.00047-1]

[96]   Chudhary Z, Khera RA, Hanif MA, Ayub MA, Hamrouni L. Walnut. Medicinal Plants of South Asia. Elsevier 2020; pp. 671-84.
[http://dx.doi.org/10.1016/B978-0-08-102659-5.00049-5]

[97]   Nawaz H, Muzaffar S, Aslam M, Ahmad S. 2018.

[98]   Khader Y, Batieha A, Jaddou H, *et al.* Hypertension in Jordan: Prevalence, Awareness, Control, and Its Associated Factors. Int J Hypertens 2019; 20193210617
[http://dx.doi.org/10.1155/2019/3210617] [PMID: 31186953]

[99]   Umar A, Imam G, Yimin W, *et al.* Antihypertensive effects of Ocimum basilicum L. (OBL) on blood pressure in renovascular hypertensive rats. Hypertens Res 2010; 33(7): 727-30.
[http://dx.doi.org/10.1038/hr.2010.64] [PMID: 20448636]

[100]   Taqvi SIH, Shah AJ, Gilani AH. Blood pressure lowering and vasomodulator effects of piperine. J Cardiovasc Pharmacol 2008; 52(5): 452-8.
[http://dx.doi.org/10.1097/FJC.0b013e31818d07c0] [PMID: 19033825]

[101]   de Souza NJ, Dohadwalla AN, Reden J. Forskolin: a labdane diterpenoid with antihypertensive, positive inotropic, platelet aggregation inhibitory, and adenylate cyclase activating properties. Med Res Rev 1983; 3(2): 201-19.
[http://dx.doi.org/10.1002/med.2610030205] [PMID: 6345959]

[102]   Gaikwad P, Khan T, Nalwade V. Impact of curry leaves (Murraya koenigii) chutney supplementation on hypertensive subjects. Int J Food Nutr Sci 2013; 2: 68-72.

[103]   Karimi Jashni H, Malekzadeh Shiravani S, Hoshmand F. The effect of the Tribulus terrestris extract on spermatogenesis in the rat. Journal of Jahrom University of Medical Sciences 2011; 9(4): 8-13.
[http://dx.doi.org/10.29252/jmj.9.4.8]

[104]   Fatima L, Sultana A, Ahmed S, Sultana S. Pharmacological activities of Tribulus terrestris Linn: a systemic review. World J Pharm Pharm Sci 2015; 4(02): 136-50.

[105]   Sharifi AM, Darabi R, Akbarloo N. Study of antihypertensive mechanism of Tribulus terrestris in 2K1C hypertensive rats: role of tissue ACE activity. Life Sci 2003; 73(23): 2963-71.
[http://dx.doi.org/10.1016/j.lfs.2003.04.002] [PMID: 14519445]

[106]   Gauthaman K, Adaikan PG. Effect of Tribulus terrestris on nicotinamide adenine dinucleotide phosphate-diaphorase activity and androgen receptors in rat brain. J Ethnopharmacol 2005; 96(1-2):

127-32.
[http://dx.doi.org/10.1016/j.jep.2004.08.030] [PMID: 15588660]

[107]   Nakano D, Kwak C-J, Fujii K, *et al.* Sesamin metabolites induce an endothelial nitric oxide-dependent vasorelaxation through their antioxidative property-independent mechanisms: possible involvement of the metabolites in the antihypertensive effect of sesamin. J Pharmacol Exp Ther 2006; 318(1): 328-35.
[http://dx.doi.org/10.1124/jpet.105.100149] [PMID: 16597711]

[108]   Shasmitha R. Health Benefits of *Sesamum indicum*: A Short Review. Asian J Pharm Clin Res 2015; 8(6): 1-3.

[109]   Nakano D, Itoh C, Takaoka M, Kiso Y, Tanaka T, Matsumura Y. Antihypertensive effect of sesamin. IV. Inhibition of vascular superoxide production by sesamin. Biol Pharm Bull 2002; 25(9): 1247-9.
[http://dx.doi.org/10.1248/bpb.25.1247] [PMID: 12230131]

[110]   Sankar D, Sambandam G, Ramakrishna Rao M, Pugalendi KV. Modulation of blood pressure, lipid profiles and redox status in hypertensive patients taking different edible oils. Clin Chim Acta 2005; 355(1-2): 97-104.
[http://dx.doi.org/10.1016/j.cccn.2004.12.009] [PMID: 15820483]

[111]   Asgary S, Naderi GH, Sarrafzadegan N, Mohammadifard N, Mostafavi S, Vakili R. Antihypertensive and antihyperlipidemic effects of Achillea wilhelmsii. Drugs Exp Clin Res 2000; 26(3): 89-93.
[PMID: 10941601]

[112]   Ichimura T, Yamanaka A, Ichiba T, *et al.* Antihypertensive effect of an extract of Passiflora edulis rind in spontaneously hypertensive rats. Biosci Biotechnol Biochem 2006; 70(3): 718-21.
[http://dx.doi.org/10.1271/bbb.70.718] [PMID: 16556991]

[113]   Naseri MKG, Arabian M, Badavi M, Ahangarpour A. Vasorelaxant and hypotensive effects of Allium cepa peel hydroalcoholic extract in rat. Pak J Biol Sci 2008; 11(12): 1569-75.
[http://dx.doi.org/10.3923/pjbs.2008.1569.1575] [PMID: 18819643]

[114]   Al-Qattan KK, Alnaqeeb MA, Ali M. The antihypertensive effect of garlic (Allium sativum) in the rat two-kidney--one-clip Goldblatt model. J Ethnopharmacol 1999; 66(2): 217-22.
[http://dx.doi.org/10.1016/S0378-8741(98)00173-1] [PMID: 10433481]

[115]   Moghadam MH, Imenshahidi M, Mohajeri SA. Antihypertensive effect of celery seed on rat blood pressure in chronic administration. J Med Food 2013; 16(6): 558-63.
[http://dx.doi.org/10.1089/jmf.2012.2664] [PMID: 23735001]

[116]   Ahmad M, Dar Z, Habib M. A review on oat (Avena sativa L.) as a dual-purpose crop. Sci Res Essays 2014; 9(4): 52-9.
[http://dx.doi.org/10.5897/SRE2014.5820]

[117]   Fatehi-Hassanabad Z, Jafarzadeh M, Tarhini A, Fatehi M. The antihypertensive and vasodilator effects of aqueous extract from Berberis vulgaris fruit on hypertensive rats. Phytother Res 2005; 19(3): 222-5.
[http://dx.doi.org/10.1002/ptr.1661] [PMID: 15934023]

[118]   Rizka A, Setiati S, Lydia A, Dewiasty E. Effect of Nigella sativa seed extract for hypertension in elderly: a double-blind, randomized controlled trial. Acta Med Indones 2017; 49(4): 307-13.
[PMID: 29348380]

[119]   Jung D-J, Cha J-Y, Kim S-E, Ko I-G, Jee Y-S. Effects of Ylang-Ylang aroma on blood pressure and heart rate in healthy men. J Exerc Rehabil 2013; 9(2): 250-5.
[http://dx.doi.org/10.12965/jer.130007] [PMID: 24278868]

[120]   Maghrani M, Zeggwagh N-A, Michel J-B, Eddouks M. Antihypertensive effect of Lepidium sativum L. in spontaneously hypertensive rats. J Ethnopharmacol 2005; 100(1-2): 193-7.
[http://dx.doi.org/10.1016/j.jep.2005.02.024] [PMID: 15955648]

[121]   Behrouzian F, Razavi SM, Phillips GO. Cress seed (Lepidium sativum) mucilage, an overview. Bioactive Carbohydrates and Dietary Fibre 2014; 3(1): 17-28.
[http://dx.doi.org/10.1016/j.bcdf.2014.01.001]

[122]   Ody P. Dorling-Kinderesly Extraction and quantification o f sterols from Tribulus terrestras. Sida acuta burm F. and Tridax procumbens L. Int J Current Pharmaceutical Res 2000; 5: 95-7.

[123]   Thomson M, Al-Qattan KK, Al-Sawan SM, Alnaqeeb MA, Khan I, Ali M. The use of ginger (Zingiber officinale Rosc.) as a potential anti-inflammatory and antithrombotic agent. Prostaglandins Leukot Essent Fatty Acids 2002; 67(6): 475-8.
[http://dx.doi.org/10.1054/plef.2002.0441] [PMID: 12468270]

[124]   Touyz RM, Schiffrin EL. Signal transduction mechanisms mediating the physiological and pathophysiological actions of angiotensin II in vascular smooth muscle cells. Pharmacol Rev 2000; 52(4): 639-72.
[PMID: 11121512]

CHAPTER 4

Management of Diabetes Mellitus by Natural Products: Glucagon-like Peptide 1 Perspective

Ojaskumar D. Agrawal[1,2] and **Yogesh A. Kulkarni**[1,*]

[1] *Shobhaben Pratapbhai Patel School of Pharmacy & Technology Management, SVKM's NMIMS, V.L Mehta Road, Vile Parle (W), Mumbai – 400 056, India*

[2] *Vivekanand Education Society's College of Pharmacy, Chembur (E), University of Mumbai, Mumbai 400074, India*

Abstract: Diabetes Mellitus (DM) has become a major and serious health problem worldwide. To overcome this lifestyle disease, natural products can be explored systematically. These natural products act on various targets and show their effect in diabetic conditions. Out of this, GLP-1 Receptor is one of the promising targets. Cells in the small intestine secrete Incretin hormones upon nutrient ingestion. Glucagon-like peptide-1 (GLP-1) is a primary incretin hormone in metabolism that has a potent antihyperglycemic effect. Insulin will release, in the presence of hyperglycemia, GLP-1 stimulates the pancreas to release insulin, stops glucagon release, gastric emptying slows down and increases satiety by acting on the hypothalamus. Storage of GLP-1 is mainly in secretory granules of L cells, in small intestinal distal portion and colon. When the cells are activated, this peptide is released into the main bloodstream.GLP-1 secreted mainly upon the ingestion of oral glucose or the ingestion of a mixed meal. Other factors like neurotransmitters and intestinal hormones also affect GLP-1 secretion from the intestine. Considering the above-mentioned parameters, regulation and control of GLP-1 are necessary as GLP-1 secretion is hampered in T2DM.

The present chapter focuses on scientific information about natural products specifically acting as GLP- 1 Receptor Agonist (GLP-1 RA).

Keywords: Diabetes Mellitus, GLP-1 Receptor Agonist, Herbal Medicine, Insulinotropic, Natural Products.

INTRODUCTION

The number of individuals suffering from diabetes has reached 425 million. International Diabetes Federation data shows that in 2045 there will be 629 million people affected with diabetes. At the global level, India is going to be one

* **Corresponding author Yogesh A. Kulkarni:** Shobhaben Pratapbhai Patel School of Pharmacy & Technology Management, SVKM's NMIMS, V.L Mehta Road, Vile Parle (W), Mumbai – 400 056, India; E-mail: yogeshkulkarni101@yahoo.com

M. Eddouks (Ed.)

of the major countries having a large number of diabetic patients. Regular exercise and a healthy lifestyle can reduce the risk of this disease. The invention of a new drug molecule which is safer and better than the existing one, newer methodology and approach is need of an hour. All these invented drugs will help in reducing diabetes and its complications and as a result decrease in mortality and morbidity [1, 2].

Synthetic antidiabetic drugs have drawbacks like poor bioavailability, the too short or too long half-life, low therapeutic index, non – linear kinetics because of saturable clearance mechanism, on repeat, dosing increased clearance because of auto induction, multiple metabolites not covered by toxicity studies [1].

Considering the above points, there is utmost need to find out more efficacious, better and safer alternatives in the management of diabetes [2]. In recent years various natural products have been evaluated and proved for their beneficial effects in the management of diabetes.

In the ancient era, medicinal plants which are collected from the forest were only the basic source of drugs for all types of ailments. Hence more Weightage is given to these traditional and herbal drugs which can be used to treat all types of diseases. Thus medicinal natural products are playing a crucial role in the management of health care. Over twelve hundred medicinal plants have been identified and have been claimed as a remedy for diabetes and out of those, several hundred have been evaluated for the said treatment [3]. Several synthetic compounds have been discovered from medicinal plants like metformin, which was based on biguanide compound from plant *Galanga officinalis* [3]. Throughout the world, more than 400 plants, over 700 recipes and compounds have been broadly evaluated for T2D treatment [4]. In the human body, these natural products act on various targets and show their effects.

Glucagon-Like Peptide - 1

Upon oral glucose intake, gastrointestinal tract secretes incretin hormones [5]. These are gut peptides generally secreted after food intake and augment insulin secretion. Incretin hormones like Glucose-dependent insulinotropic polypeptide and Glucagon-Like Peptide -1 are secreted by upper K cells and lower enteroendocrine L cells of gut respectively.

Also, GLP-1 has different and multiple effects on different organs. GLP-1 is responsible for decreasing apatite which is linked with food intake and weight loss. GLP-1 is synthesized from the posttranslational modification of proglucagon, by Prohormone Convertase 1 (PC1). It stimulates Glucose Stimulated Insulin Secretion (GSIS) when glucose and free fatty acids are taken orally [6]. It has been reported that GLP-1 has insulinotropic action. High sugar intake results in increased GLP-1 secretion and ultimately in the stimulation of β-cells which secrets insulin. This proves that GLP-1 mimetics or its receptor agonists can be used for the management of diabetes [7].

Chemically, GLP-1 is available in two forms: GLP-1 (7–36) amide (80% of circulating GLP-1) and GLP-1 (7–37) amide. GLP-1 (1–36 amide) is predominantly secreted in the pancreas, whereas GLP-1 (1–37) is secreted in the ileum and hypothalamus [8 - 13].

Secretion of Incretin Hormones in Healthy Human Subjects

Carbohydrates like glucose and sucrose, starch; amino acids, triglycerides and proteins stimulate the secretion of GLP-1.

Proteins serve as a relatively weak stimulus for GLP-1 secretion. For this purpose, a minimum fixed rate of gastric emptying is required to have measurable secretion. Despite the distal location of secretory L cells in the gut, GLP-1 will be secreted immediately after ingestion of nutrients and meals [14].

Deacon and Holst identified that for degradation of GLP-1, dipeptidyl peptidase 4 (DPP-4) enzyme in plasma is responsible [15] and also showed that this degradation could be prevented by inhibiting enzyme DPP-4 [16]. GLP-1 has a very short half-life (<2 min) because of its speedy cleavage by Dipeptidyl peptidase-4 (DPP-4) [7]. Studies on pigs showed that practically it was possible to prevent degradation of GLP-1 by DPP-4 and this action showed a marked increase in insulin in response to glucose and GLP-1 [17].

GLP-1 affects levels of insulin and glucagon to decrease elevated blood sugar levels in two ways. First GLP-1 increases the body's natural insulin secretion in response to a meal and second GLP-1 lowers levels of the hormone glucagon after eating. Glucagon works opposite to insulin and raises blood sugar levels', so decreasing glucagon level helps to lower blood sugar. For insulin production, β-cell protection and β-cell proliferation, attenuating gastric emptying, reducing glucose secretion, decreasing appetite/weight, GLP 1 has a pivotal role [18, 19].

Various medicinal plants extracts have also reported increasing secretion of GLP-1. Natural products stimulate GLP-1 receptor on the enteroendocrine cells of GIT. As a result, depolarization of the enteroendocrine cell membrane by an increase in the level of intracellular calcium concentration and secretion of GLP-1 (Fig. **1**).

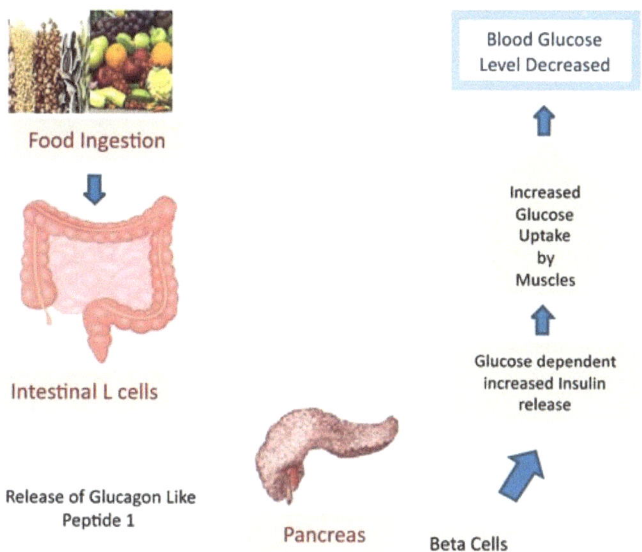

Fig. (1). Role of Incretin in Glucose Homeostasis.

1. Soybeans (*Glycine max,* Leguminosae)

Isoflavones are one of the important components of soy, which are responsible for the reduction of glucose in Type 2 diabetes [20]. It contains about 40% of protein and 20% cholesterol-free oil and is a popular food grain to combat protein and calorie deficiency [21]. Chang has reported that Soybean contains complex carbohydrates, protein, dietary fibre, oligosaccharides, phytosterol, saponin, lecithin, isoflavone, phytic acid, trypsin inhibitor, and minerals. Complex carbohydrates and dietary fibre contents contribute to low glycemic indexes, which benefit diabetic individuals and reduce the risk of developing diabetes [22].

Park and his researchers have found that Glyceollins a type of phytoalexins present in Soybeans was studied in 3T3L1 cell lines for antidiabetic effect by GLP-1 secretion. They reported that glyceollins could support the homeostasis by increasing β-cell function *via* GLP-1 release. Glyceollins also potentiated GLP-1 secretion to enhance insulinotropic actions in enteroendocrine cells [7] (Fig. **2**).

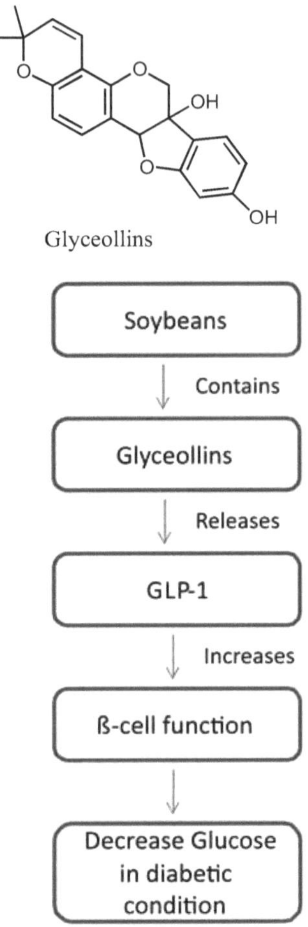

Fig. (2). Effect of *Glycine max* in diabetes.

2. Coffee (*Coffea arabica,* Rubiaceae)

Cafestol, a bioactive substance in coffee, increases glucose-stimulated insulin secretion *in vitro* and increases glucose uptake in human skeletal muscle cells [23].

McCarty has found that Chlorogenic acid and quinides are responsible for Reduction of intestinal glucose absorption through inhibition of glucose-6-phosphate translocase 1 and a subsequent increase in GLP-1 levels [24, 25]. He also reported that coffee increases the production of the incretin hormone glucagon-like peptide-1 (GLP-1), which is reported for its inhibitory effect of chlorogenic acid (the chief polyphenol in coffee) on glucose absorption. GLP-1 acts on β-cells, *via* cAMP-dependent mechanisms and increases activity of the transcription factor IDX-1 (islet/duodenum homeobox-1) [26], which is responsible for β-cell activity against excessive glucose [24]. Further Ong and Van have also reported that Chlorogenic acid improved glucose metabolism, *via* activation of AMPK [27, 28].

Campos-Florián has reported that coffee contains chlorogenic acid, which protects pancreatic beta cells and decreases intestinal absorption of glucose, increasing the levels of glucagon-like peptide-1 (GLP-1). They have also reported that the quinolactonas or quinides are present in coffee which in turn increases the uptake of glucose by peripheral tissues [29] (Fig. **3**).

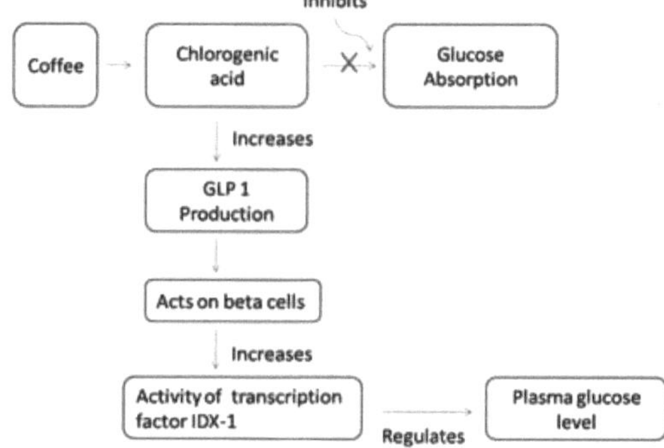

Fig. (3). Mechanism of action of *Coffea arabica*.

3. Bitter melon (*Momordica charantia,* Cucurbitaceae)

Bitter melon, cultivated in Asia, Africa, and South America, has been widely used in folk medicine as a treatment for diabetes. It has been reported to contain a bioactive constituent Polypeptide P, which has a structural similarity with insulin [30, 31]. Huang and co-researchers reported that, increase in *in-vitro* GLP-1 secretion in a murine enteroendocrine Secretin Tumor Cell line (STC-1), was dose-dependent. It was stimulated by water extract (WE), its fractions, and a bitter compounds-rich fraction of Bitter gourd [32, 33] (Fig. **4**).

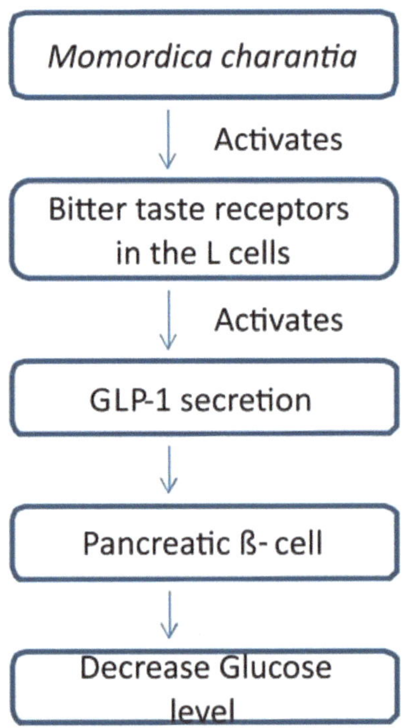

Fig. (4). Effect of *Momordica charantia* on Glucose level.

4. Gentian (*Gentiana scabra,* Gentianaceae)

Suhand coworkers found that root extract of Gentian contains loganic acid, gentiopicrin, trifloroside and rindoside, bitter iridoid glycosides. Gentian on the NCI-H716cells showed GLP-1 secretory activity. Secreting effect of Gentian is mediated by the G protein βγ-subunit and inositol triphosphate. In *db/db* mice, it was found that gentian is responsible for GLP-1 secretion [33, 34].

Shin and co-researchers showed that the GLP-1 secretion of the enteroendocrine L cell stimulated by *Gentiana scabra* extract through G - Protein-Coupled Receptor (GPCR) pathway. To confirm the results ELISA and microarray were also performed. Gentian was extracted with 95% ethanol and was fractionated using butanol, hexane and ethyl acetate. Results with differentiated NCI-H716 cells showed that ethyl acetate portion showed most efficacies for the GLP-1 receptor. This study provides an understanding of *Gentiana scabra* used as a therapeutic herbal medicine for type II diabetes [35] (Fig. **5**).

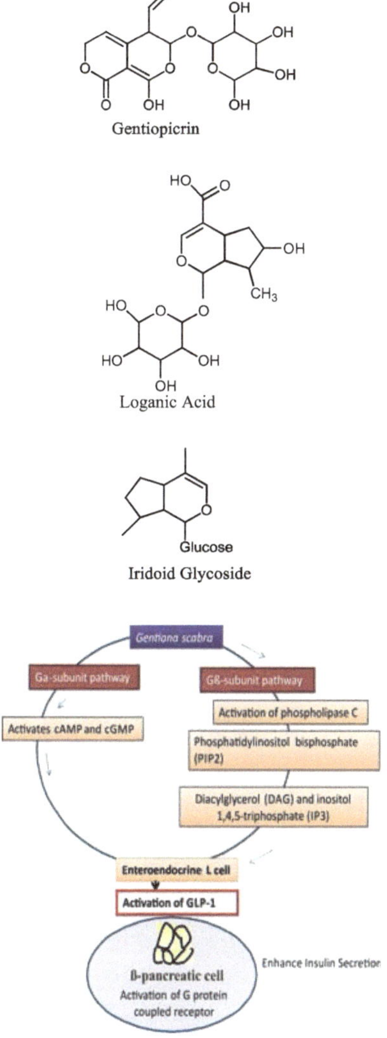

Fig. (5). Mechanism of Action of Gentiana scabra induced GLP-1 secretion activated *via* Gα and Gβγ-subunit pathway.

5. Chicory Roots (*Cichorium intybus,* Asteraceae)

The genus *Cichorium* (Asteraceae) commonly known as chicory contains six species majorly found in Asian and European countries. Genus *Cichorium* is widely used for many diseases ranging from a wound to diabetes [36]. It also has antihyperglycemic and antidyslipidemic effects and it also improved bowel movement [37, 38]. Various genotypes of *Cichorium* have also been thoroughly studied for its anti-diabetic activity. A study by Fouré and his co-workers have found that G12 and G35 genotype obtained from roasted roots of Cichorium have activity against satiety hormones and gut microbiota. They reported that GLP-1 secretion was found to increase by *in vitro* digestion of chicory G35 genotype [39].

Urı´as-Silvas and co-workers found that GLP-1 production in the colon was found to be increased by inulin-type fructans extracted from chicory roots which help in regulating appetite and glucose /lipid metabolism [40]. Cani has also reported that short-chain fructans derivative Reftilose (RAF) isolated from Chicory root increases inulin by the increasing portal and colonic secretion of GLP-1 (7-36) amide levels and the mice lacking GLP-1 receptor functionality did not respond to RAF in terms of regulation of food intake, glycaemia and fat mass development [41, 42].

Delzenne and co-researchers found that inulin-type fructans extracted from chicory root also help in modulating the production of peptides, such as incretins that are involved in the regulation of food intake and/or systemic effects. Regulation in food intake ultimately increases the colic and portal GLP-1 content [43].

Kok's study reported that supplementation of the diet with oligofructose (OFS) improved glucose disposal and decreased postprandial insulin level in rats. It increased GLP secretion, and thus GLP-1 concentration [44] (Fig. **6**).

6. Cinnamon (*Cinnamomum zeylanicum,* Lauraceae)

Cinnamaldehyde, which is Transient Receptor Potential Agonist 1 (TRPA1) [45], reported for decreased fasting plasma glucose and triglyceride levels [46]. Another finding supports that the present active constituent increases GLP-1 secretion and has a pivotal role in the effective control of Diabetes mellitus [47, 48]. Cinnamon dose 1 and 3 g was found to increase GLP-1 levels in humans [49] (Fig. **7**).

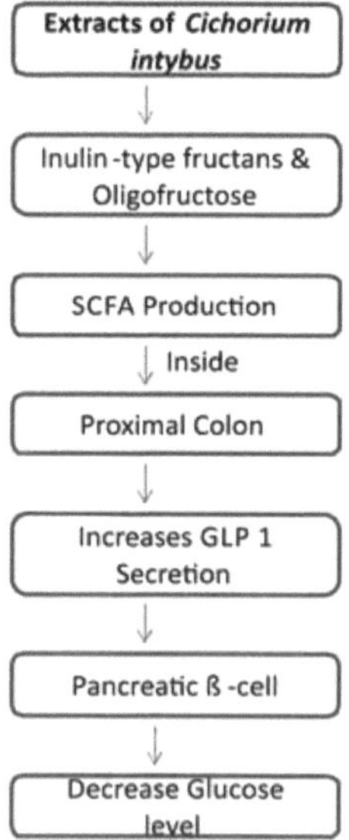

Fig. (6). Effect of *Cichorium intybus* on Glucose level.

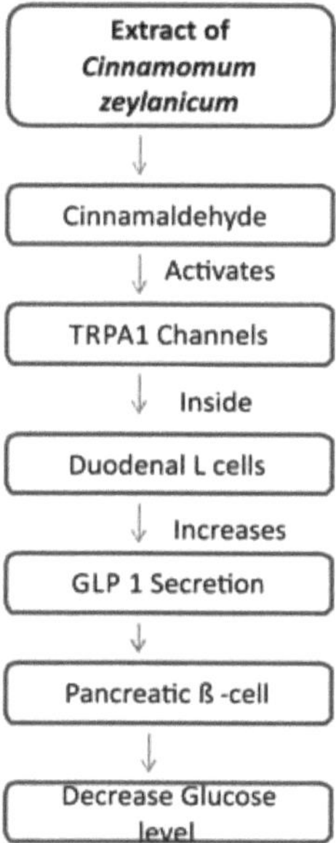

Fig. (7). Effect of *Cinnamomum zeylanicum* on Glucose level.

7. Gardenia fruit (*Gardenia jasminoides*, Rubiaceae)

Song and co-researchers have found that Geniposide is the active iridoid glucoside of Gardenia fruit. It has a considerable effect on the GLP-1 receptor and the secretion of insulin. Research suggests that insulin secretion has been induced by geniposide in the β-cells. The study also revealed that geniposide is responsible for insulin secretion in INS-1 cells [50].

The in-vitro study by Guo and coworkers showed that geniposide directly induced insulin secretion in INS-1 cells when it kept in the absence of glucose. This effect may be because of the activation of GLP-1R by geniposide, which regulates the concentration of Ca^{2+} through a signal pathway, or changes in the energy balance of INS-1 cells by altering ATP ratio and regulating the activity of ATP-sensitive K^+ channels. Many other reported literature also shows Geniposide with INS-1 cells enhances insulin secretion [50 - 53] (Fig. **8**).

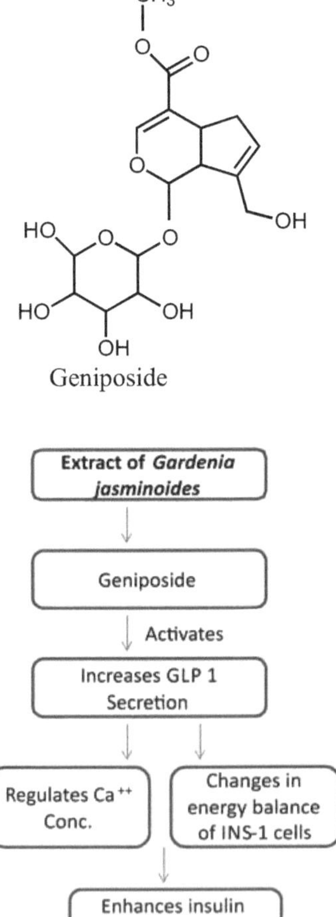

Fig. (8). Mechanism of action of *Gardenia jasminoides*.

8. Korean Pine Nut (*Pinus koraiensis*, Pinaceae)

Korean pine nut, an appetite suppressant acts by increasing satiety hormones (like GLP-1) and reducing food intake. Supplementary eating of free fatty acid with pine nut which contains triglycerides reported to increase GLP-1, satiety – inducing hormone when given postprandially. This study suggested that active content of pine nut may be acting as an appetite suppressant in overweight women [54 - 57].

9. A little dragon (*Artemisia dracunculus*, Asteraceae)

Ribnicky and co-workers have found that treatment with Tarralin (an ethanolic extract) in genetically diabetic KK-Ag mice, lowered elevated blood glucose levels significantly relative to control animals. In Streptozotocin-induced diabetic mice, Tarralin showed considerable reduction in blood glucose concentration relative to control [58]. The extract has reported augmenting the binding of GLP-1 to its receptor *in vitro*. This shows that Tarralin is bestowed with antihyperglycemic activity and has a prospective role in the management of diabetes [58, 59].

10. Mango (*Mangifera indica*, Anacardiaceae)

Mangoes belong to genus *Mangifera* which consists of about 30 species of tropical fruiting trees in the flowering plant family *Anacardiaceae*. According to Ayurveda, an Indian traditional system of medicine, varied medicinal properties are attributed to different parts of mango tree [60]. Methanolic extract of leaves of Mango has proven the increase in the GLP-1 concentration which results in a decrease in blood glucose level [61]. This effect may be possible because of the decrease in the intestinal absorption of the glucose. Yogisha and co-researchers have performed *an in-vitro* study on methanolic extract of *Mangifera indica* and concluded that methanolic extract of *M. indica* inhibited DPP-IV mediated degradation of GLP-1. *M. indica* methanolic extract exhibited a competitive type of enzyme inhibition. The result explains inhibitory activities on DPP IV and may have therapeutic potential on type 2 diabetes [62]. Further, Aderibigbe and co-researchers have also concluded that the aqueous extract of the leaves of *Mangifera indica* possesses hypoglycaemic activity. This action may be due to an intestinal reduction of the absorption of glucose [63, 64] (Fig. **9**).

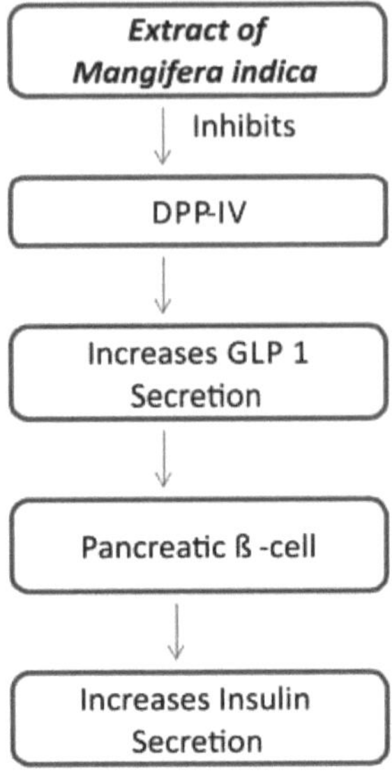

Fig. (9). Effect of *Mangifera indica* on Glucose level.

11. Wheat (*Triticumae stivum*, Poaceae)

GLP-1 is reported for its appetite suppression, insulin secretion and reducing insulin resistance activity [64, 65]. Freeland and co-researchers have concluded that wheat fibre intake increases plasma GLP-1 concentrations in hyperinsulinaemic subjects [66]. Massimino and researchers have performed the study on Dogs and demonstrated that fibre fermentability, independent of changes in fibre intake, modulates intestinal proglucagon GLP-1 secretion. Postprandial GLP-1 secretion was significantly greater when dogs consumed the HFF diet rather than the LFF diet [67].

12. Yacon Root (*Smallanthus sonchifolius*, Asteraceae)

South American plant Yakon has large tuberous roots considered as a fruit because of its juiciness and sweet taste [68]. Habib has found that 90 days of Yacon root flour treatment significantly increased GLP-1 content in the cecum of STZ-induced diabetic rats accompanied by an important cecal tissue enlargement [69, 70].

13. Pygeum (*Prunus africanum*, Rosaceae)

Pygeum africanum contains active constituents as Phytosterols, triterpenoids, aliphatic alcohols Stem bark [71]. Suleiman has found that half-life of GLP-1 was increased by the use of the extract of bark of *Prunus africana* in Wistar rat model. This extract increased insulin secretion by lowering DPP-4 activity [72, 73] (Fig. **10**).

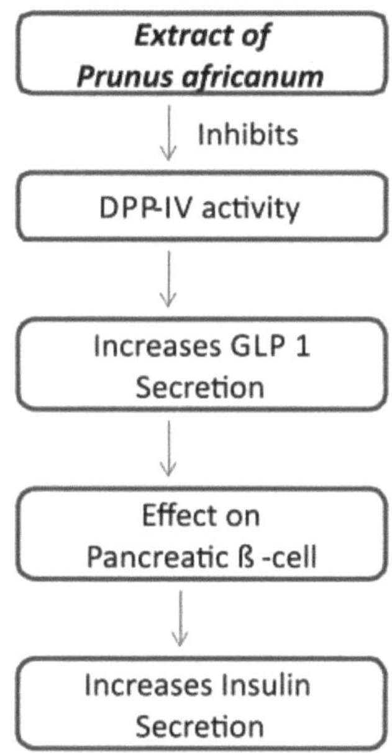

Fig. (10). Effect of Prunus *africanum* on Glucose level.

14. Turmeric (*Curcuma longa*, Zingiberaceae)

GLP-1 secretion in GLUTag cells was increased by curcumin, a yellow pigment, isolated from rhizomes of *Curcuma longa*.Ca^{2+}–Ca^{2+}/calmodulin dependent kinase II pathway is responsible for this secretion [74, 75]. These DPP-IV inhibitors can prevent inactivation of glucagon like peptide-1 (GLP-1), which then enhanced and prolonged the action of the endogenously released incretin hormone, and therefore insulin secretion is stimulated. It has been hypothesized that curcumin could act as an inhibitor (with lower affinity) on the same DPP-IV and demonstrated the possible interaction of curcumin with the enzyme by molecular interaction studies of this drug with DPP-IV [76 - 79] (Fig. **11**).

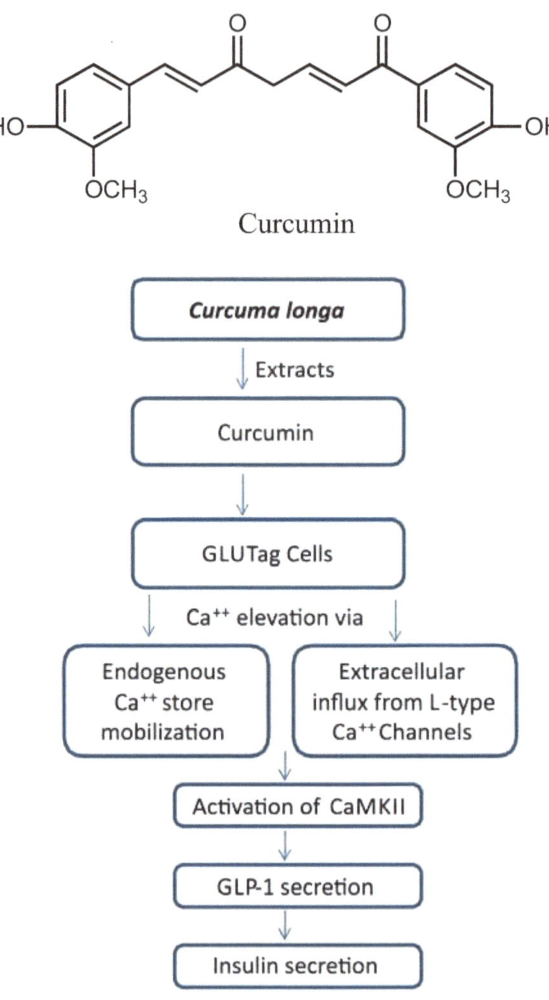

Fig. (11). Effect of *Curcuma longa* on Glucose level.

15. Barberry (*Berberis vulgaris,* Berberidaceae)

The Berberine as alkaloid can be found in the roots, rhizomes, and stem bark of *Berberis vulgaris* [80, 81]. It increases insulin secretion; as a result, it will stimulate glycolysis and GLP-1 in the rat model. It also inhibits DPP-4, which increases the concentration of GLP-1 [82, 83]. *In vitro* study performed by Yu and co-researchers have demonstrated that berberine may stimulate GLP-1 secretion from the NCI-H716 cells in a dose-dependent manner, accompanied by increased both cellular GLP-1 level and total GLP-1 content, which indicated that berberine may increase GLP-1 release as well as promote GLP-1 biosynthesis [84]. Yu's further studies showed that berberine stimulated GLP-1 secretion through activation of the bitter taste receptor TAS2R38. These findings provided evidence for the bitter taste receptor involved in the regulation of glucose homeostasis and can be used as a pharmacological target for developing anti-diabetic drugs [85]. Zhou's study showed that increased blood insulin and oxidative stress, decreased pancreatic insulin expression, β cells number, islet area and pancreas to body weight ratio, damaged β cells are apparent in streptozotocin-induced diabetic rats. Berberine exhibits significant insulin sensitization, insulin secretion and β cells regeneration as well as antioxidant activity in experimental rats [86]. In diabetic animals, berberine significantly, improved glucose tolerance, reduced body weight gain and adipose tissue mass [87]. Yin showed that Berberine is known as an AMP-activated protein kinase (AMPK) activator. Its insulin-independent hypoglycemic effect is related to inhibition of mitochondrial function, stimulation of glycolysis and activation of the AMPK pathway. Additionally, berberine may also act as α-glucosidase inhibitor. In the newly-diagnosed type 2 diabetic patients, berberine can lower blood insulin level *via* enhancing insulin sensitivity [88]. Despite valuable properties, the clinical use of berberine has been limited due to its poor intestinal absorption, low bioavailability and limited penetration [89] (Fig. **12**).

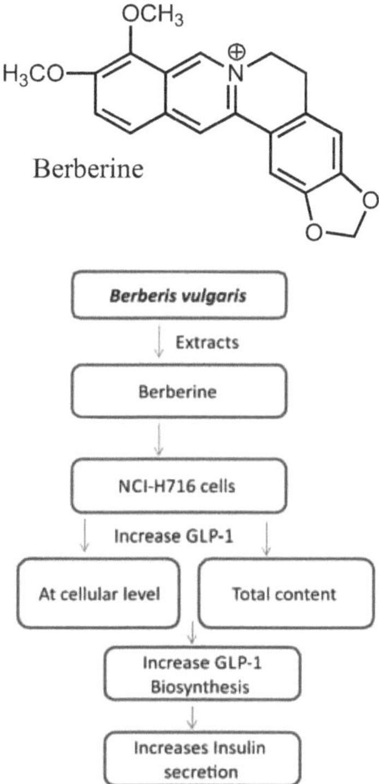

Fig. (12). Effect of *Berberis vulgaris* on Glucose level.

16. Agave (*Agave tequilana*, Agavaceae)

Results suggest that fermentable fructans from the various botanical origin and has a different chemical structure and augment the release of incretin peptides in the gut, with promising effects on fat mass development, body weight and glucose metabolism. This effect is shown by fructans which are obtained from *Agave tequilana* [3, 40, 90].

17. Olive oil (*Olea europaea*, Oleaceae)

Olive oil is a great source of healthy monounsaturated fats and polyphenol (plant-based micronutrients that are high in antioxidants). The greatest effect of olive oil by preventing and controlling type 2 diabetes [91]. Prieto and co-researchers have found that, in meal-trained rats, studies showed that the mean increment in plasma GLP-1 concentration is higher in rats with olive oil diet when compared to control diet. Relative to the initial value on the first day, higher body weight is reported on the fifth day in the animals fed the Olive oil compare to control diet. This showed that Olive oil contained diet helped in increasing GLP-1 concentration [92, 93]. Violi and researcher have studied and investigated that, 25 healthy subjects who were randomly allocated in a cross-over design to a Mediterranean-type meal added with or without Extra Virgin Olive Oil. Analysis of this study concluded that GLP-1 after Mediterranean-type lunch demonstrated that supplementation with Extra Virgin Olive Oil was associated with an increase of incretin [94]. Rocca and his scientist have reported the mechanism by which the Olive Oil diet enhanced GLP-1 secretion; a GLP-1 secreting L cell line was incubated for 24 h with either 100 mM oleic acid (MUFA) or 100 mM palmitic acid (SFA) and subsequently challenged with GIP, a known stimulator of the L cell. Preexposure to oleic acid but not to palmitic acid significantly increased GIP-induced GLP-1 secretion when compared with controls [93].

18. Grape-Seed (*Vitis vinifera*, Vitaceae)

González-Abuín from Spain found that the cafeteria diet decreased active GLP-1 plasma levels, which is attributed to a decreased intestinal GLP-1 production, linked to reducing colonic enteroendocrine cell populations. Such effects were prevented by Grape-seed procyanidin extract (GSPE). It has been reported to improve insulin resistance in cafeteria rats [95] (Fig. **13**).

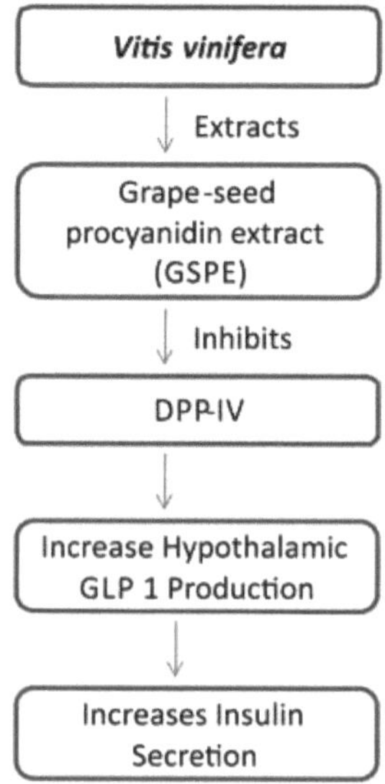

Fig. (13). Effect of *Vitis vinifera* on Glucose level.

19. Green Tea (*Camellia sinensis*, Theaceae)

A water-soluble polysaccharide arabinogalactan is isolated from green tea which contains Arabinose and Galactose. It possesses 1, 3- and 1, 6- linked galacto-pyranosyl residues. It will considerably increase insulin secretion in the *in-vitro* method by RIN-5F cells in Glucose-stimulated insulin secretion assay. This will regulate the transcription of GLP-1R and stimulates the protein level [96]. Planes-Munoz from Spain has used enteroendocrine cell line and incubated with digested and not digested green tea extracts measuring the secretion of GLP-1 by enzyme-linked immunosorbent assay (ELISA). The release of satiety hormones by the STC-1 cells showed similar or higher results for the same plant extracts compared to the positive controls [97].

20. Mate tea (*Ilex paraguariensis*, Aquifoliaceae)

Hussein and co-researchers have reported that aqueous infusion of mate tea exhibited a significant increase in GLP-1 levels compared with the control group. Active phytoconstituents like alpha-linolenic acid and 3, 5-Odicaffeoyl-D-quinic acid and matesaponin showed significant increase in GLP-1 levels [98].

21. Butyrate and Propionate

Butyrate and Propionate are the predominant Short-chain fatty acids in the gut lumen in humans and rodents and are present at high mM levels [99]. Lin and co-researchers have found that these short-chain fatty acids are metabolites formed by dietary carbohydrates. They have also reported that oral administration of sodium butyrate in mice significantly increased plasma levels of GLP-1. Reports suggested that stimulation of GLP-1 by butyrate secretion from L cells is partially mediated by free fatty acid receptors 3 (FFAR3) [100]. Psichas and researchers have demonstrated that intra-colonic administration of propionate stimulates the concurrent release of GLP-1 in rodents and demonstrated *in vitro*, and for the first time *in vivo*, that free fatty acid receptor 2 deficiency impairs Short-chain fatty acid-induced gut hormone secretion.

Propionate stimulated the secretion of GLP-1 from wild-type primary murine colonic crypt cultures. This effect was significantly attenuated in cultures from FFA2 mice. Intra-colonic infusion of propionate elevated GLP-1 levels in jugular vein plasma in rats and portal vein plasma in both rats and mice. However, propionate did not significantly stimulate gut hormone release in FFA2 mice [101 - 104] (Fig. **14**).

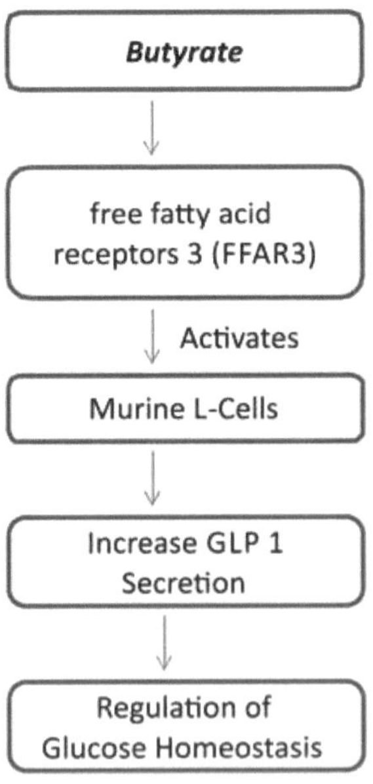

Fig. (14). Effect of *Butyrate* on Glucose level.

22. Palatinose Disaccharide

Palatinose (6-O-D-glucopyranosyl-D-fructose, isomaltulose) is a naturally-occurring disaccharide that gives honey-like sweetness. Its caloric value is 4 kcal/g, the same as that of sucrose. It is composed of alpha-1, 6-linked glucose and fructose. Commercial isomaltulose is produced from sucrose by enzymatic rearrangement [105, 106]. It is particularly suitable as a non-cariogenic sucrose replacement and is favorable in products for diabetics and prediabetic dispositions [107]. Ang and researcher have reported that the enhanced GLP-1 secretion observed after isomaltulose ingestion caused inhibition of glucagon release, which resulted in the enhancement of the insulin-to-glucagon ratio, which in turn increased insulin action [108]. Tohur Hira and co-researcher has studied the effect of Palatinose and sucrose in conscious rats, GLP-1 and glucose were measured. Secondly, GLP-1 and glucose were measured after jejunal or ileal administration of each sugar in anaesthetized rats. Finally, they observed the effect of these sugars on GLP-1 secretion. GLP-1 secretion was remarkably increased after administration of Palatinose in conscious rats, compared with sucrose [109]. Also, the same researcher has reported that it is a slowly digested disaccharide; Palatinose (isomaltulose) is used as a non-carcinogenic sugar and as an alternative to sucrose in the diet. They have also studied the direct effect of GLP-1 secretion on GLUTag, a murine GLP producing cell line, using several sugars. Palatinose has given good results when analyzed with sucrose to enhance portal GLP-1 level when given in conscious rats [109]. Maeda and co-researcher have designed a double-blind, placebo-controlled study. Whereby they have given palatinose and sucrose samples to 10 healthy male participants. Blood samples were obtained before the ingestion of the samples. Total GLP-1 was measured after the solid-phase preparation of the specimens using a total GLP-1 RIA Kit. Statistical analysis showed that GLP-1 potentiates insulin secretion glucose-dependently, protects and promotes pancreatic β-cell growth, and inhibits glucagon secretion. This study reported that GLP-1 secretion is significantly stimulated by palatinose intake [106].

23. Whey protein

Dairy products have reported having an insulinogenic effect on healthy subjects. Protein fraction is responsible for the insulin-releasing ability of dairy products. Whey has shown to augment insulin release in healthy subjects. *In-vitro* studies suggested that whey protein produces its insulinogenic effect by increasing plasma concentrations of GLP-1 [110]. Santos-Hernández and co-researcher studied whey protein expression in STC-1 cells in gastrointestinal digests as persuader of secretion of GLP-1. *In vitro* digests were distinguished and characterized by peptide, protein and content of free amino acid. However, whey protein intestinal digests have increased release of GLP-1. Also, their findings demonstrated that the extent of protein hydrolysis during digestion plays an important role in GLP-1 secretion [111]. Chaudhary and coauthors have found that hydrolysates of whey protein as well as fermentates of *Lactobacillus helveticus* induced the proglucagon, pro-GIP and CCK expression and secretion of GLP-1 in STC-1 (pGIP/Neo) cells. Fermentates obtained from *Lactobacillus helveticus* milk showed higher potential for GLP-1 induction [112]. Giezenaar and co-workers have reported that hydrolyzed whey-protein and a saline control were infused intraduodenally for 60 min in 10 younger and 10 older healthy men in a randomized, double-blind fashion. Results of this study showed that the concentration of GLP-1 was increased [113]. In another study, Giezenaar has reported that 16 healthy older (eight men, eight women) and 16 younger (eight men, eight women) adults were studied on three occasions in which they ingested 30 g (120 kcal) or 70 g (280 kcal) whey protein, or a flavoured-water control drink (~2 kcal). At regular intervals, concentration was measured and it was found that GLP-1 concentrations were dose-dependently increased by the whey protein ingestion [114].

24. Fructose

On healthy human volunteers, fructose intake caused a rise in blood glucose, plasma insulin and GLP-1. Similar studies were conducted by Kuhre and group on mouse and rat with fructose stimulating GLP-1 secretion. To prove this hypothesis, Kuhre used GLUTage cells as a model for L cells. It is a murine cell line, in this cell fructose is metabolized and stimulates GLP-1 secretion in a Dose-Dependent Manner by ATP-Sensitive Potassium Channel. The increase in GLP-1 release without an increase in the glucagonotropic hormone proved that fructose may be one of the agonists for GLP-1 secretion. In clinical studies, volunteers to consume 75 g of fructose, it resulted in a modest elevation in blood glucose, GLP-1 and insulin [115, 116]. Ritzel and co-researcher have reported that Ileal perfusion with fructose caused a significant elevation of plasma GLP-1 within 20 min. This was independent of sodium chloride since fructose dissolved in distilled water increased GLP-1 about 18-fold [117]. Nuttall *et al.*, research reported that Fructose is known to have modest effects on plasma glucose, insulin and GIP concentrations in normal subjects, although in patients with non-insuli--dependent diabetes it has a marked stimulatory effect on insulin secretion [118]. Kong's study normal subjects demonstrated that oral fructose stimulates GLP-1 secretion, but also demonstrated that the response is much less than those to equicaloric glucose load [119].

25. Peanut (*Arachis hypogaea*, Fabaceae)

Natural phytoalexin Resveratrol (3, 4', 5-trihydroxytrans-stilbene), which is major phytochemicals obtained from plants belonging to genus Arachis and Grapevines. In animal models, it helped to decrease the high blood sugar [120]. Animal studies have also shown that it can reduce oxidative stress. Waget and co-researchers found that in Resveratrol treatment at dose 60 mg/kg significantly reduced glucose intolerance and increased active GLP-1 levels in high-fat diet diabetic mice and showed antidiabetic effect [121]. *In vivo* studies showed that administration of Resveratrol for few weeks increased portal vein concentration of Glucagon-like peptide-1 [121]. Although few researchers found controversial results in clinical trials, which showed that there is no significant change in the GLP-1 levels due to Peanut administration for a few weeks [122]. Another randomized controlled trial showed that administration of Resveratrol for 5 weeks did not affect GLP-1 secretion in type 2 diabetes [123].

Resveratrol

CONCLUSION

As diabetes has become a global problem worldwide, there is an unmet need for new therapies for the management of diabetes. Many drugs for diabetes from the synthetic origin are in various phases of the drug discovery programme. GLP-1 regulates glucose homeostasis through the control of insulin release from the pancreas. Thus, GLP-1 related drugs are important for the treatment of diabetes. Many natural products have been studied for their possible effects on GLP 1 in diabetic conditions. Majority studies report an increase in GLP levels due to various natural products in diabetes. There is a need to explore these natural products as a treatment option in diabetes by using systematic investigations focusing on molecular mechanisms, preclinical studies and clinical investigations.

CONSENT FOR PUBLICATION

Not applicable.

CONFLICT OF INTEREST

There is no conflict of interest declared.

ACKNOWLEDGEMENT

Declared none.

REFERENCES

[1]   Vaz JA, Patnaik A. Diabetes mellitus: Exploring the challenges in the drug development process. Perspect Clin Res 2012; 3(3): 109-12. http://www.pubmedcentral.nih.gov/articlerender.fcgi?artid=348 7225&tool=pmcentrez&rendertype=abstract [Internet].
[http://dx.doi.org/10.4103/2229-3485.100660] [PMID: 23125962]

[2]   Safavi M, Foroumadi A, Abdollahi M. The importance of synthetic drugs for type 2 diabetes drug discovery. Expert Opin Drug Discov 2013; 8(11): 1339-63. http://www.tandfonline.com/doi/full/ 10.1517/17460441.2013.837883 [Internet].
[http://dx.doi.org/10.1517/17460441.2013.837883] [PMID: 24050217]

[3]   Chang C, Lin Y, Bartolome A, Chen Y-C, Chiu S-C, Yang W-C. Herbal Therapies for Type 2 Diabetes Mellitus: Chemistry, Biology, and Pote...: EBSCOhost. Evidence-Based Complement Altern Med [Internet]. 2013;2013:1–33. http://web.b.ebscohost.com.ezproxy.think.edu.au/ehost/pdfviewer/ pdfviewer?sid=c049c6b6-7b8f-4672-8838-059fb794dac7@sessionmgr120&vid=1&hid=118

[4]   Singh J, Cumming E, Manoharan G, Kalasz H, Adeghate E. Medicinal Chemistry of the Anti-Diabetic Effects of Momordica Charantia: Active Constituents and Modes of Actions. Open Med Chem J [Internet]. 2011 [cited 2018 Sep 28];5(Suppl 2):70–7. https://pdfs.semanticscholar.org/a713/7f968f8 a92474117ca 40d8297f0145846ec5.pdf

[5]   Holst JJ. From the Incretin Concept and the Discovery of GLP-1 to Today's Diabetes Therapy. Front Endocrinol (Lausanne) [Internet]. 2019 Apr 26 [cited 2019 May 29];10:260. www.frontiersin.org

[6]   Hirasawa A, Tsumaya K, Awaji T, Katsuma S, Adachi T, Yamada M, *et al.* Free fatty acids regulate gut incretin glucagon-like peptide-1 secretion through GPR120. Nat Med [Internet]. 2005 Jan 26 [cited 2018 Sep 16];11(1):90–4. http://www.nature.com/articles/nm1168
[http://dx.doi.org/10.1038/nm1168]

[7]   Park S, Ahn IS, Kim JH, Lee MR, Kim JS, Kim HJ. Glyceollins, one of the phytoalexins derived from soybeans under fungal stress, enhance insulin sensitivity and exert insulinotropic actions. J Agric Food Chem 2010; 58(3): 1551-7.
[http://dx.doi.org/10.1021/jf903432b] [PMID: 20067288]

[8]   Gupta V. Glucagon-like peptide-1 analogues: An overview. Indian J Endocrinol Metab 2013; 17(3): 413-21.http://www.ijem.in/text.asp?2013/17/3/413/111625 [Internet].
[http://dx.doi.org/10.4103/2230-8210.111625] [PMID: 23869296]

[9]   Underwood CR, Garibay P, Knudsen LB, *et al.* Crystal structure of glucagon-like peptide-1 in complex with the extracellular domain of the glucagon-like peptide-1 receptor. J Biol Chem 2010; 285(1): 723-30.
[http://dx.doi.org/10.1074/jbc.M109.033829] [PMID: 19861722]

[10]   Song G, Yang D, Wang Y, *et al.* Human GLP-1 receptor transmembrane domain structure in complex with allosteric modulators. Nature 2017; 546(7657): 312-5.

[http://dx.doi.org/10.1038/nature22378] [PMID: 28514449]

[11]   Jazayeri A, Rappas M, Brown AJH, *et al.* Crystal structure of the GLP-1 receptor bound to a peptide agonist. Nature 2017; 546(7657): 254-8. [Internet].
[http://dx.doi.org/10.1038/nature22800] [PMID: 28562585]

[12]   Green B, Gault V, O'Harte F, Flatt P. Structurally Modified Analogues of Glucagon-Like Peptide-1 (GLP-1) and Glucose-Dependent Insulinotropic Polypeptide (GIP) As Future Antidiabetic Agents. Curr Pharm Des [Internet]. 2004 Nov 1 [cited 2019 May 29];10(29):3651–62. http://www.eureka select.com/openurl/content.php?genre=article&issn=1381-6128&volume=10&issue=29&spage=3651

[13]   Holst JJ. The incretin system in healthy humans: The role of GIP and GLP-1. Metabolism 2019; 96: 46-55.
[http://dx.doi.org/10.1016/j.metabol.2019.04.014] [PMID: 31029770]

[14]   Nauck MA, Meier JJ. Incretin hormones: Their role in health and disease. Diabetes, Obes Metab [Internet]. 2018 Feb [cited 2019 May 29];20:5–21. http://www.ncbi.nlm.nih.gov/pubmed/29364588

[15]   Deacon CF, Johnsen AH, Holst JJ. Degradation of glucagon-like peptide-1 by human plasma *in vitro* yields an N-terminally truncated peptide that is a major endogenous metabolite *in vivo*. J Clin Endocrinol Metab [Internet]. 1995 Mar 1 [cited 2019 May 29];80(3):952–7. https://academic.oup.com/ jcem/article-lookup/doi/10.1210/jcem.80.3.7883856

[16]   Deacon CF, Nauck MA, Toft-Nielsen M, Pridal L, Willms B, Holst JJ. Both subcutaneously and intravenously administered glucagon-like peptide I are rapidly degraded from the NH2-terminus in type II diabetic patients and in healthy subjects. Diabetes [Internet]. 1995 Sep 1 [cited 2019 May 29];44(9):1126–31. http://www.ncbi.nlm.nih.gov/pubmed/7657039

[17]   Deacon CF, Hughes TE, Holst JJ. Dipeptidyl peptidase IV inhibition potentiates the insulinotropic effect of glucagon-like peptide 1 in the anesthetized pig. Diabetes [Internet]. 1998 May 1 [cited 2019 May 29];47(5):764–9. http://www.ncbi.nlm.nih.gov/pubmed/9588448
[http://dx.doi.org/10.2337/diabetes.47.5.764]

[18]   Nadkarni P, Chepurny OG, Holz GG. Regulation of Glucose Homeostasis by GLP-1.Progress in Molecular Biology and Translational Science. NIH Public Access 2014; pp. 23-65. http://www.ncbi. nlm.nih.gov/pubmed/24373234 Internet [cited 2019 Jan 20]

[19]   Knop F, Vilsboll T, Holst J. Incretin-Based Therapy of Type 2 Diabetes Mellitus. Curr Protein Pept Sci [Internet]. 2009 Feb 1 [cited 2019 May 29];10(1):46–55. http://www.eurekaselect.com/openurl/ content.php?genre=article&issn=1389-2037&volume=10&issue=1&spage=46

[20]   Mueller NT, Odegaard AO, Gross MD, *et al.* Soy intake and risk of type 2 diabetes in Chinese Singaporeans [corrected]. Eur J Nutr 2012; 51(8): 1033-40. http://www.pubmedcentral.nih.gov/ articlerender.fcgi?artid=3480546&tool=pmcentrez&rendertype=abstract [corrected]. [Internet].
[http://dx.doi.org/10.1007/s00394-011-0276-2] [PMID: 22094581]

[21]   Deshpande SD, Bal S, Ojha TP. Physical Properties of Soybean. Vol. 56. J Agric Eng Res 1993; 89-98.
[http://dx.doi.org/10.1006/jaer.1993.1063]

[22]   Chang JH, Kim MS, Kim TW, Lee SS. Effects of soybean supplementation on blood glucose, plasma lipid levels, and erythrocyte antioxidant enzyme activity in type 2 diabetes mellitus patients. Nutr Res Pract 2008; 2(3): 152-7.
[http://dx.doi.org/10.4162/nrp.2008.2.3.152] [PMID: 20126600]

[23]   Mellbye FB, Jeppesen PB, Shokouh P, Laustsen C, Hermansen K, Gregersen S. Bioactive Substance in Coffee, Has Antidiabetic Properties in KKAy Mice. J Nat Prod [Internet]. 2017 Aug 25 [cited 2018 Jun 30];80(8):2353–9. http://www.ncbi.nlm.nih.gov/pubmed/28763212

[24]   McCarty MF. A chlorogenic acid-induced increase in GLP-1 production may mediate the impact of heavy coffee consumption on diabetes risk. Med Hypotheses [Internet]. 2005 Jan [cited 2018 Jun 30];64(4):848–53. http://intl.elsevierhealth.com/journals/mehy

[25]   Shearer J, Farah A, de Paulis T, *et al.* Quinides of roasted coffee enhance insulin action in conscious rats. J Nutr 2003; 133(11): 3529-32.
[http://dx.doi.org/10.1093/jn/133.11.3529] [PMID: 14608069]

[26]   Miller CP, McGehee RE Jr, Habener JF. IDX-1: a new homeodomain transcription factor expressed in rat pancreatic islets and duodenum that transactivates the somatostatin gene. EMBO J 1994; 13(5): 1145-56.
[http://dx.doi.org/10.1002/j.1460-2075.1994.tb06363.x] [PMID: 7907546]

[27]   Ong KW, Hsu A, Tan BKH. Anti-diabetic and anti-lipidemic effects of chlorogenic acid are mediated by ampk activation. Biochem Pharmacol [Internet]. 2013 [cited 2018 Nov 14];85(9):1341–51.
[http://dx.doi.org/10.1016/j.bcp.2013.02.008]

[28]   van Dam RM. Coffee and type 2 diabetes: from beans to beta-cells. Nutr Metab Cardiovasc Dis 2006; 16(1): 69-77.
[http://dx.doi.org/10.1016/j.numecd.2005.10.003] [PMID: 16399494]

[29]   Campos-Florián J, Bardales-Valdivia J, Caruajulca-Guevara L, Cueva-Llanos D. Anti-diabetic effect of Coffea arabica, in alloxan-induced diabetic rats. Emir J Food Agric 2013; 25(10): 772-7.
[http://dx.doi.org/10.9755/ejfa.v25i10.16409]

[30]   Cefalu W, Ye J, Wang Z. Efficacy of Dietary Supplementation with Botanicals on Carbohydrate Metabolism in Humans 2008. http://www.eurekaselect.com/openurl/content.php?genre= article&issn=1871-5303&volume=8&issue=2&spage=78
[http://dx.doi.org/10.2174/187153008784534376]

[31]   Joseph B, Jini D. Antidiabetic effects of Momordica charantia (bitter melon) and its medicinal potency. Asian Pac J Trop Dis 2013; 3(2): 93-102.
[http://dx.doi.org/10.1016/S2222-1808(13)60052-3]

[32]   Huang TN, Lu KN, Pai YP, Hsu C, Huang CJ. Role of GLP-1 in the hypoglycemic effects of wild bitter gourd. Evidence-based Complement Altern Med 2013.
[http://dx.doi.org/10.1155/2013/625892]

[33]   Mccarthy T, Green BD, Calderwood D, Gillespie A, Cryan JF, Giblin L, *et al. In vitro* intestinal tissue models: General introduction. Impact Food Bioact Heal Vitr Ex Vivo Model 2015; 1: 239-44.

[34]   Suh HW, Lee KB, Kim KS, *et al.* A bitter herbal medicine Gentiana scabra root extract stimulates glucagon-like peptide-1 secretion and regulates blood glucose in db/db mouse. J Ethnopharmacol 2015; 172: 219-26. [Internet].
[http://dx.doi.org/10.1016/j.jep.2015.06.042] [PMID: 26129938]

[35]   Shin M, Suh H, Lee K, Kim K, Yang HJ, Choi E, *et al.* Gentiana scabra extracts stimulate glucagon-like peptide-1 secretion *via* G protein-coupled receptor pathway. 2012;6:114–9.
[http://dx.doi.org/10.1007/s13206-012-6202-8]

[36]   Street RA, Sidana J, Prinsloo G. Cichorium intybus: Traditional uses, phytochemistry, pharmacology, and toxicology. Evid Based Complement Alternat Med 2013; 2013579319
[http://dx.doi.org/10.1155/2013/579319] [PMID: 24379887]

[37]   Nishimura M, Ohkawara T, Kanayama T, Kitagawa K, Nishimura H, Nishihira J. Effects of the extract from roasted chicory (Cichorium intybus L.) root containing inulin-type fructans on blood glucose, lipid metabolism, and fecal properties. J Tradit Complement Med 2015; 5(3): 161-7.
[http://dx.doi.org/10.1016/j.jtcme.2014.11.016] [PMID: 26151029]

[38]   Carazzone C, Mascherpa D, Gazzani G, Papetti A. Identification of phenolic constituents in red chicory salads (Cichorium intybus) by high-performance liquid chromatography with diode array detection and electrospray ionisation tandem mass spectrometry. Food Chem 2013; 138(2-3): 1062-71. [Internet].
[http://dx.doi.org/10.1016/j.foodchem.2012.11.060] [PMID: 23411215]

[39]   Fouré M, Dugardin C, Foligne B, Hance P, Cadalen T, Delcourt A, *et al.* Chicory roots for prebiotics

and appetite regulation: a pilot study in mice. J Agric Food Chem [Internet]. 2018;acs.jafc.8b01055. http://pubs.acs.org/doi/10.1021/acs.jafc.8b01055

[40]   Urías-Silvas JE, Cani PD, Delmée E, Neyrinck A, López MG, Delzenne NM. Physiological effects of dietary fructans extracted from Agave tequilana Gto. and Dasylirion spp. Br J Nutr 2008; 99(2): 254-61.
[http://dx.doi.org/10.1017/S0007114507795338] [PMID: 17711612]

[41]   Cani PD, Knauf C, Iglesias MA, Drucker DJ, Delzenne NM, Burcelin R. Improvement of Glucose Tolerance and Hepatic Insulin Sensitivity by Oligofructose Requires a Functional Glucagon-Like Peptide 1 Receptor. Diabetes [Internet]. 2006 May 1 [cited 2018 Nov 14];55(5):1484-90. http://diabetes.diabetesjournals.org/content/diabetes/55/5/1484.full.pdf

[42]   Cani PD, Daubioul CA, Reusens B, Remacle C, Catillon G, Delzenne NM. Involvement of endogenous glucagon-like peptide-1(7-36) amide on glycaemia-lowering effect of oligofructose in streptozotocin-treated rats. J Endocrinol 2005; 185(3): 457-65.
[http://dx.doi.org/10.1677/joe.1.06100] [PMID: 15930172]

[43]   Delzenne NM, Cani PD, Daubioul C, Neyrinck AM. Impact of inulin and oligofructose on gastrointestinal peptides. Br J Nutr 2005; 93(S1) (Suppl. 1): S157-61. http://www.journals. cambridge.org/abstract_S0007114505000929 [Internet].
[http://dx.doi.org/10.1079/BJN20041342] [PMID: 15877889]

[44]   Kok NN, Morgan LM, Williams CM, Roberfroid MB, Thissen J-P, Delzenne NM. Insulin, glucagon-like peptide 1, glucose-dependent insulinotropic polypeptide and insulin-like growth factor I as putative mediators of the hypolipidemic effect of oligofructose in rats. J Nutr 1998; 128(7): 1099-103.http://www.ncbi.nlm.nih.gov/pubmed/9649591 [Internet].
[http://dx.doi.org/10.1093/jn/128.7.1099] [PMID: 9649591]

[45]   Emery EC, Diakogiannaki E, Gentry C, *et al.* Stimulation of GLP-1 secretion downstream of the ligand-gated ion channel TRPA1. Diabetes 2015; 64(4): 1202-10.
[http://dx.doi.org/10.2337/db14-0737] [PMID: 25325736]

[46]   Allen RW, Schwartzman E, Baker WL, Coleman CI, Phung OJ. Cinnamon use in type 2 diabetes: an updated systematic review and meta-analysis. Ann Fam Med 2013; 11(5): 452-9.www.ebscohost.com [Internet].
[http://dx.doi.org/10.1370/afm.1517] [PMID: 24019277]

[47]   Lu T, Sheng H, Wu J, Cheng Y, Zhu J, Chen Y. Cinnamon extract improves fasting blood glucose and glycosylated hemoglobin level in Chinese patients with type 2 diabetes. Nutr Res 2012; 32(6): 408-12. [Internet].
[http://dx.doi.org/10.1016/j.nutres.2012.05.003] [PMID: 22749176]

[48]   Akilen R, Tsiami A, Devendra D, Robinson N. Glycated haemoglobin and blood pressure-lowering effect of cinnamon in multi-ethnic Type 2 diabetic patients in the UK: a randomized, placebo-controlled, double-blind clinical trial. Diabet Med 2010; 27(10): 1159-67.
[http://dx.doi.org/10.1111/j.1464-5491.2010.03079.x] [PMID: 20854384]

[49]   Hlebowicz J, Hlebowicz A, Lindstedt S, *et al.* Effects of 1 and 3 g cinnamon on gastric emptying, satiety, and postprandial blood glucose, insulin, glucose-dependent insulinotropic polypeptide, glucagon-like peptide 1, and ghrelin concentrations in healthy subjects. Am J Clin Nutr 2009; 89(3): 815-21.
[http://dx.doi.org/10.3945/ajcn.2008.26807] [PMID: 19158209]

[50]   Song X, Guo M, Wang T, Wang W, Cao Y, Zhang N. Geniposide inhibited lipopolysaccharide-induced apoptosis by modulating TLR4 and apoptosis-related factors in mouse mammary glands. Life Sci 2014; 119(1-2): 9-17. [Internet].
[http://dx.doi.org/10.1016/j.lfs.2014.10.006] [PMID: 25445441]

[51]   Guo LX, Xia ZN, Gao X, Yin F, Liu JH. Glucagon-like peptide 1 receptor plays a critical role in geniposide-regulated insulin secretion in INS-1 cells. Acta Pharmacol Sin 2012; 33(2):

237-41.http://www.nature.com/doifinder/10.1038/aps.2011.146 [Internet].
[http://dx.doi.org/10.1038/aps.2011.146] [PMID: 22101168]

[52]   Xiao W, Li S, Wang S, Ho CT. Chemistry and bioactivity of Gardenia jasminoides. Yao Wu Shi Pin Fen Xi 2017; 25(1): 43-61. [Internet].
[http://dx.doi.org/10.1016/j.jfda.2016.11.005] [PMID: 28911543]

[53]   Liu J, Yin F, Xiao H, Guo L, Gao X. Glucagon-like peptide 1 receptor plays an essential role in geniposide attenuating lipotoxicity-induced β-cell apoptosis. Toxicol In Vitro 2012; 26(7): 1093-7.
[http://dx.doi.org/10.1016/j.tiv.2012.07.004] [PMID: 22819839]

[54]   Pasman WJ, Heimerikx J, Rubingh CM, *et al.* The effect of Korean pine nut oil on *in vitro* CCK release, on appetite sensations and on gut hormones in post-menopausal overweight women. Lipids Health Dis 2008; 7: 10.
[http://dx.doi.org/10.1186/1476-511X-7-10] [PMID: 18355411]

[55]   Gutzwiller J-P. Interaction between GLP-1 and CCK-33 in inhibiting food intake and appetite in men. AJP Regul Integr Comp Physiol [Internet]. 2004;287(3):R562–7.   http://ajpregu.physiology.org/cgi/doi/10.1152/ajpregu.00599.2003

[56]   Gutzwiller J, Göke B, Drewe J, Hildebrand P, Ketterer S, Handschin D, *et al.* Glucagon-like peptide-1 : a potent regulator of food intake in humans Glucagon-like peptide-1 : a potent regulator of food intake in humans. 1999;(October 2005):81–6.

[57]   Xie K, Miles EA, Calder PC. A review of the potential health benefits of pine nut oil and its characteristic fatty acid pinolenic acid. J Funct Foods 2016; 23: 464-73. [Internet].
[http://dx.doi.org/10.1016/j.jff.2016.03.003]

[58]   Ribnicky DM, Poulev A, Watford M, Cefalu WT, Raskin I. Antihyperglycemic activity of Tarralin, an ethanolic extract of Artemisia dracunculus L. Phytomedicine 2006; 13(8): 550-7. http://linkinghub.elsevier.com/retrieve/pii/S0944711305002102 [Internet].
[http://dx.doi.org/10.1016/j.phymed.2005.09.007] [PMID: 16920509]

[59]   Aggarwal S, Shailendra G, Ribnicky DM, Burk D, Karki N, Wang Q, *et al.* HHS Public Access. 2016; 98–105.

[60]   Shah KA, Patel MB, Patel RJ, Parmar PK. Mangifera indica (mango). Pharmacogn Rev 2010; 4(7): 42-8.http://www.phcogrev.com/text.asp?2010/4/7/42/65325 [Internet].
[http://dx.doi.org/10.4103/0973-7847.65325] [PMID: 22228940]

[61]   Madhuri AS, Mohanvelu R. Evaluation of Antidiabetic Activity of Aqueous Extract of Mangifera Indica Leaves in Alloxan Induced Diabetic Rats 2017; 10(2): 1029-35.

[62]   Yogisha S, Raveesha KA. Dipeptidyl Peptidase IV inhibitory activity of Mangifera indica. J Nat Prod 2010; 3: 76-9.

[63]   Aderibigbe AO, Emudianughe TS, Lawal BAS. Antihyperglycaemic effect of Mangifera indica in rat. Phytother Res 1999; 13(6): 504-7.
[http://dx.doi.org/10.1002/(SICI)1099-1573(199909)13:6<504:AID-PTR533>3.0.CO;2-9]   [PMID: 10479762]

[64]   Aderibigbe AO, Emudianughe TS, Lawal BAS. Evaluation of the antidiabetic action of Mangifera indica in mice. Phyther Res [Internet]. 2001 Aug;15(5):456–8. http://doi.wiley.com/10.1002/ptr.859
[http://dx.doi.org/10.1002/ptr.859]

[65]   Rask E, Olsson T, Söderberg S, *et al.* Impaired incretin response after a mixed meal is associated with insulin resistance in nondiabetic men. Diabetes Care 2001; 24(9): 1640-5. http://care.diabetesjournals.org/cgi/doi/10.2337/diacare.24.9.1640 [Internet].
[http://dx.doi.org/10.2337/diacare.24.9.1640] [PMID: 11522713]

[66]   Freeland KR, Wilson C, Wolever TMS. Adaptation of colonic fermentation and glucagon-like peptide-1 secretion with increased wheat fibre intake for 1 year in hyperinsulinaemic human subjects. Br J Nutr 2010; 103(1): 82-90.

[http://dx.doi.org/10.1017/S0007114509991462] [PMID: 19664300]

[67]   Massimino SP, McBurney MI, Field CJ, *et al.* Fermentable dietary fiber increases GLP-1 secretion and improves glucose homeostasis despite increased intestinal glucose transport capacity in healthy dogs. J Nutr 1998; 128(10): 1786-93.
[http://dx.doi.org/10.1093/jn/128.10.1786] [PMID: 9772150]

[68]   Seminario J. Juan seminario miguel valderrama [Internet]. 1997 [cited 2018 Nov 12]. http://cipotato.org/wp-content/uploads/2014/07/Yacon_Fundamentos_password.pdf

[69]   Habib NC, Honoré SM, Genta SB, Sánchez SS. Hypolipidemic effect of Smallanthus sonchifolius (yacon) roots on diabetic rats: biochemical approach. Chem Biol Interact 2011; 194(1): 31-9. [Internet].
[http://dx.doi.org/10.1016/j.cbi.2011.08.009] [PMID: 21907189]

[70]   Caetano BFR, de Moura NA, Almeida APS, Dias MC, Sivieri K, Barbisan LF. Yacon (Smallanthus sonchifolius) as a food supplement: Health-promoting benefits of fructooligosaccharides. Nutrients 2016; 8(7)E436
[http://dx.doi.org/10.3390/nu8070436] [PMID: 27455312]

[71]   Simon JE, Koroch AR, Acquaye D, Jefthas E, Juliani R, Govindasamy R. Medicinal Crops of Africa 2007.www.asnapp.org

[72]   Nazrul Islam M. Insulinotropic Effect of Herbal Drugs for Management of Diabetes Mellitus: A Congregational Approach 2016. https://www.omicsonline.com/open-access/insulinotropic-effect-of-herbal-drugs-for-management-of-diabetesmellitus-a-congregational-approach-2090-4967-1000138.php?aid=84367
[http://dx.doi.org/10.4172/2090-4967.1000142]

[73]   Singh R, Bhat GA, Sharma P. GLP-1 secretagogues potential of medicinal plants in management of diabetes. J Pharmacogn Phytochem [Internet] 2015; 4(1): 197-202. http://www.phytojournal.com/archives/?year=2015&vol=4&issue=1&part=D&ArticleId=568

[74]   Takikawa M, Kurimoto Y, Tsuda T. Curcumin stimulates glucagon-like peptide-1 secretion in GLUTag cells *via* Ca2+/calmodulin-dependent kinase II activation. Biochem Biophys Res Commun 2013; 435(2): 165-70. [Internet].
[http://dx.doi.org/10.1016/j.bbrc.2013.04.092] [PMID: 23660191]

[75]   Kato AM, Nishikawa S, Ikehata A, Tani T, Takahashi T, Imaizumi A, *et al.* Submitted to Food and Function section in Mol. Nutr. Food Res. Curcumin improves glucose tolerance via stimulation of glucagon-like peptide-1 secretion 2016; 10-25.

[76]   Antonyan A, De A, Vitali LA, Pettinari R, Marchetti F, Gigliobianco MR, *et al.* Evaluation of (arene)Ru(II) complexes of curcumin as inhibitors of dipeptidyl peptidase IV. Biochimie [Internet]. 2014 Apr 1 [cited 2018 Nov 11];99(1):146–52. https://www.sciencedirect.com/science/article/pii/S0300908413004306?via%3Dihub

[77]   Istyastono EP. Docking Studies of Curcumin As a Potential Lead Compound To Develop Novel Dipeptydyl Peptidase-4 Inhibitors. 2009;9(1):132–6.

[78]   Nauck MA, Vardarli I, Deacon CF, Holst JJ, Meier JJ. Secretion of glucagon-like peptide-1 (GLP-1) in type 2 diabetes: what is up, what is down? Diabetologia [Internet]. 2011 Jan 25 [cited 2018 Nov 11];54(1):10–8. http://link.springer.com/10.1007/s00125-010-1896-4

[79]   Gullo F, Ceriani M, D'Aloia A, Wanke E, Constanti A, Costa B, *et al.* Plant polyphenols and exendin-4 prevent hyperactivity and TNF-α release in LPS-treated *in vitro* neuron/astrocyte/microglial networks. Front Neurosci [Internet]. 2017 [cited 2018 Nov 11];11(SEP):500. www.frontiersin.org

[80]   Chen XW, Di YM, Zhang J, Zhou ZW, Li CG, Zhou SF. Interaction of herbal compounds with biological targets: A case study with berberine. Sci World J. 2012;2012.
[http://dx.doi.org/10.1100/2012/708292]

[81]   Cicero AFG, Tartagni E. Antidiabetic properties of berberine: from cellular pharmacology to clinical

effects. Hosp Pract (1995). 2012;40(2):56–63.
[http://dx.doi.org/10.3810/hp.2012.04.970]

[82]   Imanshahidi M, Hosseinzadeh H. Pharmacological and therapeutic effects of Berberis vulgaris and its active constituent, berberine 2008.http://doi.wiley.com/10.1002/ptr.2399
[http://dx.doi.org/10.1002/ptr.2399]

[83]   Imenshahidi M, Hosseinzadeh H. Berberis Vulgaris and Berberine : An Update Review. 2016.

[84]   Yu Y, Liu L, Wang X, Liu XX, Liu XX, Xie L, *et al.* Modulation of glucagon-like peptide-1 release by berberine: *In vivo* and *in vitro* studies. Biochem Pharmacol [Internet]. 2010 Apr 1 [cited 2018 Nov 11];79(7):1000–6. https://www.sciencedirect.com/science/article/pii/S0006295209009812

[85]   Yu Y, Hao G, Zhang Q, Hua W, Wang M, Zhou W, *et al.* Berberine induces GLP-1 secretion through activation of bitter taste receptor pathways. Biochem Pharmacol [Internet]. 2015 Sep 15 [cited 2018 Nov 11];97(2):173–7. https://www.sciencedirect.com/science/article/pii/S0006295215003822

[86]   Zhou J, Zhou S, Tang J, Zhang K, Guang L, Huang Y, *et al.* Protective effect of berberine on beta cells in streptozotocin- and high-carbohydrate/high-fat diet-induced diabetic rats. Eur J Pharmacol [Internet]. 2009 Mar 15 [cited 2018 Nov 11];606(1–3):262–8. https://www.sciencedirect.com/science/article/pii/S001429990900020X

[87]   Pirillo A, Catapano AL. Berberine, a plant alkaloid with lipid- and glucose-lowering properties: From *in vitro* evidence to clinical studies. Atherosclerosis [Internet]. 2015 Dec 1 [cited 2018 Nov 11];243(2):449–61. https://www.sciencedirect.com/science/article/pii/S0021915015301416

[88]   Yin J, Ye J, Jia W. Effects and mechanisms of berberine in diabetes treatment 2012. https://www.sciencedirect.com/science/article/pii/S2211383512000871
[http://dx.doi.org/10.1016/j.apsb.2012.06.003]

[89]   Raju M, Kulkarni YA, Wairkar S. Therapeutic potential and recent delivery systems of berberine: A wonder molecule. J Funct Foods [Internet]. 2019 Oct [cited 2019 Sep 3];61:103517. https://linkinghub.elsevier.com/retrieve/pii/S1756464619304414

[90]   Mancilla-Margalli NA, López MG. Water-soluble carbohydrates and fructan structure patterns from Agave and Dasylirion species. J Agric Food Chem 2006; 54(20): 7832-9. https://pubs.acs.org/doi/10.1021/jf060354v [Internet].
[http://dx.doi.org/10.1021/jf060354v] [PMID: 17002459]

[91]   Garg A. High-monounsaturated-fat diets for patients with diabetes mellitus: a meta-analysis 1998.https://academic.oup.com/ajcn/article/67/3/577S-582S/4666084
[http://dx.doi.org/10.1093/ajcn/67.3.577S]

[92]   Prieto PG, Cancelas J, Villanueva-Peñacarrillo ML, Valverde I, Malaisse WJ. Effects of an olive oil-enriched diet on plasma GLP-1 concentration and intestinal content, plasma insulin concentration, and glucose tolerance in normal rats. Endocrine 2005; 26(2): 107-15.
[http://dx.doi.org/10.1385/ENDO:26:2:107] [PMID: 15888922]

[93]   Rocca AS, LaGreca J, Kalitsky J, Brubaker PL. Monounsaturated fatty acid diets improve glycemic tolerance through increased secretion of glucagon-like peptide-1. Endocrinology 2001; 142(3): 1148-55.https://academic.oup.com/endo/article-lookup/doi/10.1210/endo.142.3.8034 [Internet].
[http://dx.doi.org/10.1210/endo.142.3.8034] [PMID: 11181530]

[94]   Violi F, Loffredo L, Pignatelli P, *et al.* Extra virgin olive oil use is associated with improved post-prandial blood glucose and LDL cholesterol in healthy subjects. Nutr Diabetes 2015; 5(7): e172-7. [Internet].
[http://dx.doi.org/10.1038/nutd.2015.23] [PMID: 26192450]

[95]   González-Abuín N, Martínez-Micaelo N, Blay M, Ardévol A, Pinent M. Grape-seed procyanidins prevent the cafeteria-diet-induced decrease of glucagon-like peptide-1 production. J Agric Food Chem 2014; 62(5): 1066-72.
[http://dx.doi.org/10.1021/jf405239p] [PMID: 24410268]

[96]   Wang H, Shi S, Bao B, Li X, Wang S. Structure characterization of an arabinogalactan from green tea and its anti-diabetic effect. Carbohydr Polym 2015; 124: 98-108. [Internet].
[http://dx.doi.org/10.1016/j.carbpol.2015.01.070] [PMID: 25839799]

[97]   Planes-Muñoz D, López-Nicolás R, González-Bermúdez CA, Ros-Berruezo G, Frontela-Saseta C. *In vitro* effect of green tea and turmeric extracts on GLP-1 and CCK secretion: the effect of gastrointestinal digestion. Food Funct [Internet]. 2018 [cited 2018 Oct 8];9(10):5245–50.
http://xlink.rsc.org/?DOI=C8FO01334A

[98]   Hussein GME, Matsuda H, Nakamura S, *et al.* Mate tea (Ilex paraguariensis) promotes satiety and body weight lowering in mice: involvement of glucagon-like peptide-1. Biol Pharm Bull 2011; 34(12): 1849-55.
[http://dx.doi.org/10.1248/bpb.34.1849] [PMID: 22130241]

[99]   Bergman EN. Energy contributions of volatile fatty acids from the gastrointestinal tract in various species 1990.http://www.physiology.org/doi/10.1152/physrev.1990.70.2.567
[http://dx.doi.org/10.1152/physrev.1990.70.2.567]

[100] Lin HV, Frassetto A, Kowalik EJ Jr, *et al.* Butyrate and propionate protect against diet-induced obesity and regulate gut hormones *via* free fatty acid receptor 3-independent mechanisms. PLoS One 2012; 7(4)e35240
[http://dx.doi.org/10.1371/journal.pone.0035240] [PMID: 22506074]

[101] Psichas A, Sleeth ML, Murphy KG, Brooks L, Bewick GA, Hanyaloglu AC, *et al.* The short chain fatty acid propionate stimulates GLP-1 and PYY secretion *via* free fatty acid receptor 2 in rodents. Int J Obes (Lond) [Internet]. 2015 Mar [cited 2018 Oct 14];39(3):424–9. http://www.ncbi.nlm.nih.gov/pubmed/25109781

[102] Ichimura A, Hasegawa S, Kasubuchi M, Kimura I. Free fatty acid receptors as therapeutic targets for the treatment of diabetes 2014.http://journal.frontiersin.org/article/10.3389/fphar.2014.00236/abstract
[http://dx.doi.org/10.3389/fphar.2014.00236]

[103] Tolhurst G, Heffron H, Lam YS, Parker HE, Habib AM, Diakogiannaki E, *et al.* Short-chain fatty acids stimulate glucagon-like peptide-1 secretion *via* the G-protein-coupled receptor FFAR2. Diabetes [Internet]. 2012 Feb 1 [cited 2019 Mar 31];61(2):364–71. http://www.ncbi.nlm.nih.gov/pubmed/22190648

[104] D'Alessio D. Intestinal hormones and regulation of satiety: The case for CCK, GLP-1, PYY, and Apo A-IV. In: Journal of Parenteral and Enteral Nutrition [Internet]. John Wiley & Sons, Ltd; 2008 [cited 2019 Mar 31]. p. 567–8. http://doi.wiley.com/10.1177/0148607108322401

[105] Shyam S, Ramadas A, Chang SK. Isomaltulose: Recent evidence for health benefits. J Funct Foods [Internet]. 2018 Sep [cited 2018 Oct 11];48:173–8. https://linkinghub.elsevier.com/retrieve/pii/S1756464618303372

[106] Maeda A, Miyagawa J-I, Miuchi M, Nagai E, Konishi K, Matsuo T, *et al.* Effects of the naturally-occurring disaccharides, palatinose and sucrose, on incretin secretion in healthy non-obese subjects. J Diabetes Investig [Internet]. 2013 May 6 [cited 2018 Oct 11];4(3):281–6. http://www.ncbi.nlm.nih.gov/pubmed/24843667

[107] Lina BAR, Jonker D, Kozianowski G. Isomaltulose (Palatinose®): a review of biological and toxicological studies. Food Chem Toxicol [Internet]. 2002 Oct [cited 2018 Oct 11];40(10):1375–81. http://linkinghub.elsevier.com/retrieve/pii/S0278691502001059

[108] Ang M, Linn T. Comparison of the effects of slowly and rapidly absorbed carbohydrates on postprandial glucose metabolism in type 2 diabetes mellitus patients: a randomized trial 2014.https://academic.oup.com/ajcn/article/100/4/1059/4576450
[http://dx.doi.org/10.3945/ajcn.113.076638]

[109] Hira T, Muramatsu M, Okuno M, Hara H. GLP-1 secretion in response to oral and luminal palatinose (isomaltulose) in rats. J Nutr Sci Vitaminol (Tokyo) 2011; 57(1): 30-5. http://www.ncbi.nlm.nih.gov/

pubmed/21512288 [Internet].
[http://dx.doi.org/10.3177/jnsv.57.30] [PMID: 21512288]

[110] Salehi A, Gunnerud U, Muhammed SJ, Östman E, Holst JJ, Björck I, *et al.* The insulinogenic effect of whey protein is partially mediated by a direct effect of amino acids and GIP on β-cells 2012.http://www.nutritionandmetabolism.com/content/9/1/48
[http://dx.doi.org/10.1186/1743-7075-9-48]

[111] Santos-Hernández M, Tomé D, Gaudichon C, Recio I. Stimulation of CCK and GLP-1 secretion and expression in STC-1 cells by human jejunal contents and *in vitro* gastrointestinal digests from casein and whey proteins. Food Funct [Internet]. 2018 [cited 2018 Oct 9];9(9):4702–13. http://xlink.rsc.org/?DOI=C8FO01059E

[112] Chaudhari DD, Singh R, Mallappa RH, Rokana N, Kaushik JK, Bajaj R, *et al.* Evaluation of casein & whey protein hydrolysates as well as milk fermentates from Lactobacillus helveticus for expression of gut hormones. Indian J Med Res [Internet]. 2017 [cited 2018 Oct 10];146(3):409–19. http://www.ncbi.nlm.nih.gov/pubmed/29355150

[113] Giezenaar C, Luscombe-Marsh ND, Hutchison AT, Standfield S, Feinle-Bisset C, Horowitz M, *et al.* Dose-dependent effects of randomized intraduodenal whey-protein loads on glucose, gut hormone, and amino acid concentrations in healthy older and younger men 2018.www.mdpi.com/journal/nutrients
[http://dx.doi.org/10.3390/nu10010078]

[114] Giezenaar C, Hutchison AT, Luscombe-Marsh ND, Chapman I, Horowitz M, Soenen S. Effect of age on blood glucose and plasma insulin, glucagon, ghrelin, CCK, GIP, and GLP-1 responses to whey protein ingestion. Nutrients [Internet]. 2017 [cited 2018 Oct 10];10(1). www.anzctr.org.au

[115] Kuhre RE, Gribble FM, Hartmann B, Reimann F, Windelov JA, Rehfeld JF, *et al.* Fructose stimulates GLP-1 but not GIP secretion in mice, rats, and humans. AJP Gastrointest Liver Physiol [Internet]. 2014;306(7):G622–30. http://ajpgi.physiology.org/cgi/doi/10.1152/ajpgi.00372.2013

[116] Laughlin MR. Normal Roles for Dietary Fructose in Carbohydrate Metabolism 2014.www.mdpi.com/journal/nutrients
[http://dx.doi.org/10.3390/nu6083117]

[117] Ritzel U, Fromme A, Ottleben M, Leonhardt U, Ramadori G. Release of glucagon-like peptide-1 (GLP-1) by carbohydrates in the perfused rat ileum. Acta Diabetol [Internet]. 1997 Apr 3 [cited 2018 Oct 4];34(1):18–21. http://link.springer.com/10.1007/s005920050059

[118] Nuttall FQ, Gannon MC, Burmeister LA, Lane JT, Pyzdrowski KL. The metabolic response to various doses of fructose in type II diabetic subjects 1992. http://linkinghub.elsevier.com/retrieve/pii/0026049592902102
[http://dx.doi.org/10.1016/0026-0495(92)90210-2]

[119] Kong M-F, Chapman I, Goble E, Wishart J, Wittert G, Morris H, *et al.* Effects of oral fructose and glucose on plasma GLP-1 and appetite in normal subjects. Peptides [Internet]. 1999 Jun [cited 2018 Oct 3];20(5):545–51. http://linkinghub.elsevier.com/retrieve/pii/S0196978199000066

[120] Sobolev VS, Khan SI, Tabanca N, Wedge DE, Manly SP, Cutler SJ, *et al.* Biological Activity of Peanut (Arachis hypogaea) Phytoalexins and Selected Natural and Synthetic Stilbenoids. Maedler K, editor. J Agric Food Chem [Internet]. 2011 Mar 9;59(5):1673–82. http://dx.plos.org/10.1371/journal.pone.0020700

[121] Waget T-M, Klopp A, Serino P, Vachoux M, Dao TMA, Waget A, *et al.* Resveratrol increases glucose induced GLP-1 secretion in mice: A mechanism which contributes to the glycemic control. PLoS One [Internet]. 2011 [cited 2018 Oct 2];6(6):20700. www.plosone.org

[122] Reis CEG, Ribeiro DN, Costa NMB, Bressan J, Alfenas RCG, Mattes RD. Acute and second-meal effects of peanuts on glycaemic response and appetite in obese women with high type 2 diabetes risk: A randomised cross-over clinical trial 2013.
[http://dx.doi.org/10.1017/S0007114512004217]

[123]   Thazhath SS, Wu T, Bound MJ, Checklin HL, Standfield S, Jones KL, *et al.* Administration of resveratrol for 5 wk has no effect on glucagon-like peptide 1 secretion, gastric emptying, or glycemic control in type 2 diabetes: a randomized controlled trial 2016. https://academic.oup.com/ajcn/article/103/1/66/4569302
[http://dx.doi.org/10.3945/ajcn.115.117440]

CHAPTER 5

Terpenes and Terpenoids in Management of Diabetes & Cardiovascular Diseases

Kaveri M. Adki[1], Ankit P. Laddha[1], Manisha J. Oza[1,2], Anil Bhanudas Gaikwad[3] and Yogesh A. Kulkarni[1,*]

[1] *Shobhaben Pratapbhai Patel School of Pharmacy & Technology Management, SVKM's NMIMS, V.L. Mehta Road, Vile Parle (W), Mumbai-400056, India*

[2] *SVKM's Dr. Bhanuben Nanavati College of Pharmacy, Vile Parle (W), Mumbai 400056, India*

[3] *Department of Pharmacy, Birla Institute of Technology and Science, Pilani, Pilani Campus Pilani- 333031, Rajasthan, India*

Abstract: Diabetes mellitus is a chronic metabolic disorder and is one of the major leading causes of death worldwide. According to the World Health Organisation, the burden of diabetes has increased almost two-fold in 2014 compared to 1980 in low- and middle-income countries. Uncontrolled levels of glucose in the blood are because of improper insulin secretion or insulin action which is associated with abnormalities in metabolic, genetic and hemodynamic systems. The term cardiovascular disease is used for all types of disorders associated with heart and blood vessels. Many researchers are trying to develop new therapeutic approaches for the treatment of diabetes and cardiovascular disease. Herbal medicines are one of the oldest and alternative therapeutic treatment options for diabetes and hypertension. Around 1200 traditional medicinal plants have been used for their beneficial effects on diabetes. These plants are rich in alkaloids, glycosides, flavonoids, polyphenols and terpenoids. Terpenoids are a diverse category of cyclic compounds obtained naturally from the isoprene unit. Among all reported natural products, about 60% of compounds are from terpenoids. More than 40,000 terpenoids are isolated from secondary metabolites of plants. Most of them are of plant dietary origin. Plants produce terpenoids as a secondary metabolite. More than hundreds of new terpenoid structures are reported every year for their activity in many disease conditions like cancer, malaria, inflammation, and a variety of infectious diseases. Various reports have shown that terpenoids are beneficial in the treatment of diabetes and cardiovascular diseases. The chapter is focused on terpenoids and their role in the treatment and management of diabetes and cardiovascular diseases.

Keywords: Arjunolic acid, Cardiovascular diseases, Corosolic acid, Diabetes, Glycyrrhetinic acid, Ginsenoside, Lupeol, Limonene, Pomolic acid, Terpenoids, Ursolic acid.

---

* **Corresponding author Yogesh A. Kulkarni:** Shobhaben Pratapbhai Patel School of Pharmacy & Technology Management, SVKM's NMIMS, V.L. Mehta Road, Vile Parle (W), Mumbai-400056, India; E-mail: yogeshkulkarni101@yahoo.com

M. Eddouks (Ed.)

INTRODUCTION

Diabetes mellitus (DM) is a chronic endocrine disease with a severe impact on modern global health. Diabetes occurs either when the pancreas does not produce the required amount of insulin or when the body cannot use the insulin produced by the pancreas. Blood glucose levels are mainly monitored by insulin. Hyperglycemia is an effect of uncontrolled diabetes. Continuous hyperglycemia leads to damage to nerves and blood vessels. World health organization (WHO) has classified diabetes into six types as type 1, type 2, hybrid forms of diabetes, other specific types, unclassified diabetes and hyperglycemia first detected during pregnancy. Type 1 diabetes mainly occurs due to β-cell destruction. Type 1 diabetes is immune-mediated and there is an absolute deficiency of insulin. The onset of type 1 is common in children and adults. Type 2 diabetes is the most common. Type 2 diabetes mainly occurs due to insulin resistance and various degrees of β-cell destruction. Type 2 diabetes is associated with overweight and obesity. Hybrid forms of diabetes are subdivided into two categories as slowly evolving, immune-mediated diabetes of adults and ketosis-prone type 2 diabetes. Slowly evolving, immune-mediated diabetes of adults is similar to type 1 but mainly due to metabolic syndrome of glutamic acid decarboxylase autoantibody and ketosis-prone type 2 diabetes is due to ketosis and insulin deficiency. Other specific types of diabetes have again classified into seven subdivisions including Monogenic diabetes (single gene defects of β-cell function or insulin action), Diseases of the exocrine pancreas (any defect to pancreas like inflammation, trauma and tumor), Endocrine disorders (over secretion of hormones that are insulin antagonists), Drug- or chemical-induced (impairment of insulin secretion or action due to medicines and chemicals), Infection-related diabetes (associated with viruses having direct β-cell destruction property), Uncommon specific forms of immune-mediated diabetes and other genetic syndromes sometimes associated with diabetes (due to chromosomal and any genetic disorders). Unclassified diabetes in this category of diabetes does not fit in any above classification. Hyperglycaemia first detected during pregnancy is subdivided into two types as follows diabetes mellitus in pregnancy (type 1 or type 2 diabetes diagnosed for the first time during pregnancy) and gestational diabetes mellitus (hyperglycemia below the diagnostic thresholds for diabetes in pregnancy). Diagnosis criteria for diabetes have been updated by the WHO in 2019. The person is said to be diabetic if 2-hour post-load plasma glucose equal to or more than 11.1 mmol/L, fasting plasma glucose equal to or more than 7.0 mmol/L or HbA1c equal to or more than 48 mmol/mol. Criteria for a pregnant woman are with 1-hour post-load plasma glucose equal to or more than 10.0 mmol/L, 2-hour post-load plasma glucose 8.5–11.0 mmol/L or fasting plasma glucose 5.1–6.9 mmol/L [1]. It is estimated that around 422 million people living with diabetes in 2014 this prevalence almost doubled since 1980 in low- and middle-income countries. The WHO also reported that 1.5 million deaths occurred due to diabetes and 2.2 million deaths occurred due to hyperglycemia in 2012 [2].

Cardiovascular Diseases (CVDs) are one of the leading causes of death in the world. CVDs include conditions like hypertension, angina (chest pain due to decreased blood flow to the heart), arrhythmia (irregular heartbeats), heart attack (blockage to the heart's blood vessel) and heart failure. According to the WHO, around 17.9 million people died from CVDs in 2018. Out of this, 85% of deaths are due to heart attack and heart failure. CVDs affect equally in men and women. It is estimated that 23.6 million people will die from CVDs by 2030 [3].

DM is responsible for the development of vascular diseases. The major risk factors include modern lifestyle, junk food, less physical activities, obesity, genetic factors, physical and mental stress [4].

Interconnection between Diabetes and Cardiovascular Diseases

Persistent hyperglycemia causes activation of molecular pathways like polyol, hexosamine, advanced glycation end products (AGEs) and protein kinase C (PKC), which may damage vital organs like brain, eyes, kidney and heart. Hyperglycemia alters cellular, sub-cellular and molecular mechanisms mainly by upregulating the pro-inflammatory biomarkers like interleukins, cytokines, transforming growth factor-β (TGF-β) and nuclear factor kappa B (NF-κB) [5].

About 50% of diabetics, either type 1 or 2 have chances to develop CVDs. The prevalence of CVDs in diabetes may vary with age, sex, basal mass index, presence of kidney disease and others. Hyperglycemia may lead to impairment in systolic and diastolic functions of the heart in diabetic patients independent of the presence of coronary heart disease [6]. Clinical and epidemiologic data from the last two decades have shown that the prevalence of hypertension and heart failure in diabetes is very high. It is predicted that the rate of mortality and morbidity is around 27 per 1000 diabetic patients per year compared to those without diabetes [7, 8].

Scientists are working to understand the exact mechanism of CVDs in diabetics. The literature revealed that continuous functional and metabolic alterations lead to prompt irreversible changes in heart of diabetics. The altered metabolism is associated with increased oxygen consumption in myocardial tissue and increased concentrations of free fatty acids (FFA) in the serum. The excess FFA uptake and hyperglycemia leads to dysfunction of mitochondria present in the heart. This leads to increased calcium sensitivity in cardiomyocyte and abnormality in contractile and regulatory protein expressions in diabetics. It is also reported that reduced activity of calcium pump and the rate of calcium removal of sarcoplasmic reticulum from the cytoplasm is responsible for cardiac diastolic dysfunction. Hyperglycemia causes structural alterations in diabetics, basically by glycation of numerous macromolecules that results in decreased elasticity of blood vessels and myocardial dysfunction. Hyperglycemia hampers the histoarchitecture of endothelial cells by alteration of nitric oxide production, reduction in vessel density and enhancing tissue permeability. The Renin-angiotensin-aldosterone system (RAAS) is activated during the early stages of DM. Uncontrolled hyperglycemia leads to the activation of RAAS, which stimulates the aggregation factors of CVDs and kidney function [9].

These reports suggest that multiple mechanisms are involved in the impairment of systolic and diastolic function in diabetics. Therefore, the combination therapy of diabetes and CVDs may help to prevent and reduce mortality in diabetic patients [10].

In 2016, Brunstrom and Carlberghave studied the effect of antihypertensive agents on mortality and cardiovascular morbidity in diabetic patients with different blood pressure levels. A randomized controlled trial was conducted on more than 100 diabetic patients with antihypertensive agents against placebo control for more than 12 months. Antihypertensive agents used in this study were verapamil, valsartan, nifedipine, perindopril, ramipril, *etc.* The results showed that, if systolic blood pressure was more than 140-150 mm of Hg, antihypertensive treatment reduced the risk of end-stage renal disease, myocardial infarction, stroke, and cardiovascular mortality. Metaregression analysis of this study has shown that antihypertensive treatment has the potential to reduce the risk of mortality and cardiovascular morbidity in diabetic patients with systolic blood pressure more than 140 mm of Hg [11]. Current clinical data has shown that sodium-glucose cotransporter 2 inhibitor empagliflozin treatment has lowered the hospitalization of diabetic patients suffering from heart failure and cardiovascular risk [7]. These reports suggested that the combinational treatment of diabetes and CVDs has the potential to decrease mortality in diabetic patients [10].

For thousands of years, herbal medicines are used in various traditional systems of medicine to manage and treat diabetes and hypertension. Although synthetic medicines are developed as antidiabetic and antihypertensive agents, their utilization has been questioned due to side effects on other vital organs. In this regard, natural product research has gained importance due to lesser side effects and safety profiles compared to synthetic drugs [12]. Terpenoids are a structurally diverse group of natural products. Terpenoids are also known as isoprenoids. Many *in vitro* preclinical and clinical studies reported that terpenoids have a wide array of potentially important pharmacological activities including antidiabetic and antihypertensive agents. Many medicinal plants possess hypoglycemic, hypotensive, lipid-lowering and immunomodulation properties due to their rich terpenoid content. Different procedures have been reported to increase extraction, isolation, and purification of many important terpenoids such as lycopene, farnesene, astaxanthin and taxadiene [13]. The discovery of novel terpenoids can aid chemical diversity and its medical applications to the world [14].

This chapter provides the utilization of terpenoids from various plants useful in diabetes, hypertension, dyslipidemia and other CVDs.

Terpenoids

Terpenes are the biggest class of secondary metabolites. Terpenes are simple hydrocarbons, basically consists of isoprene units (C_5). Terpenoids are derivatives of terpenes with a slight change in oxidized methyl group and other functional groups. Various plants produce numerous terpenoids. Terpenoids are basically involved in primary and secondary metabolism, hence helps in the growth and development of plants. Some terpenoids play an important role in the interaction of the plant with the biotic and abiotic environment [15]. More than 20,000 plant terpenoids have been identified and many are being discovered continuously [16]. Plant terpenoids play a crucial role in primary and secondary metabolism. In primary metabolism, they help in physiological, structural and metabolic functions such as chloroplast pigments, hormones, electron transport chain and post-translational modifications of protein molecules. Terpenoids play a diverse role in plant secondary metabolism like defense and communication with other organisms like a physical and chemical barrier, phytoalexins, antibiotics, antifeedants, repellents, toxins and attractants for fruit dispersing animals and pollinators [17]. Terpenoids are classified according to their number of C_5 units.

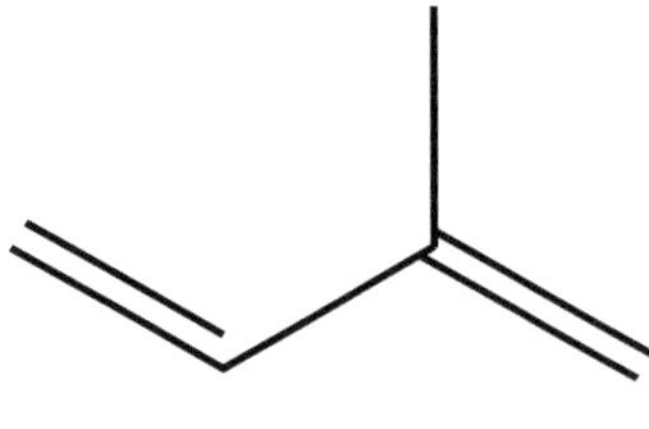

Isoprene unit

Isoprene Unit

In addition to these classes, many irregular terpenoid derivatives are also present in plants. Terpenoids are specifically involved in plant signaling, defense, and reproduction. For centuries, a plant containing terpenoids has been used by humans as traditional medicines. Terpenoids are extensively used as food, pharmaceuticals, essence, flavor, vitamins, print inks, cosmetics, and industrial resins. Nowadays, plant terpenoids are explored as an alternative to petroleum material. Terpenoids have great variation in their structure, hence they exhibit a wide range of biological activity. Terpenoids are reported as an anti-inflammatory, antioxidant, antidiabetic, antihypertensive, antibacterial, anti-malarial and anticancer activity. Taxol and its derivatives are used as anticancer agents and artemisinin and its derivatives used as antimalarial agents [18].

Hemiterpenes

Hemiterpenes are the simplest form of terpenoids. It consists of only one C_5 unit and the molecular formula is C_5H_8. These are secreted mainly from the leaves of plants conifers, oaks and herbs like *Hamamelis japonica* and *Archangelica officinalis*. Angelic, tiglic, senecioic, isovaleric acids are some of the known hemiterpenes [13].

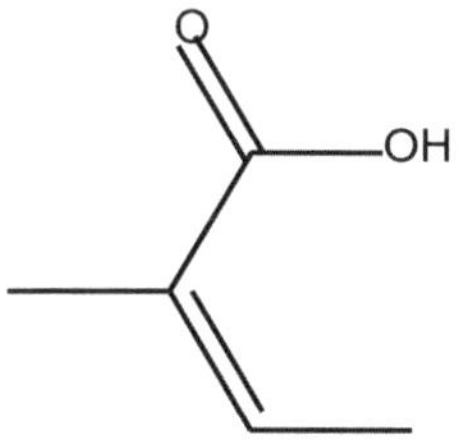

Angelic acid

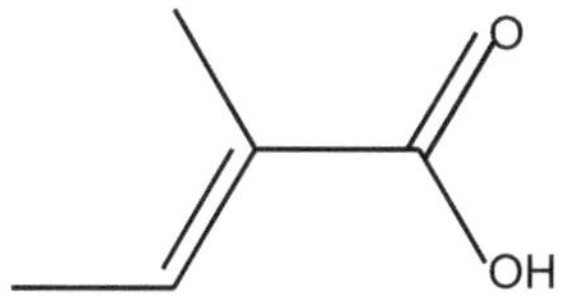

Tiglic acid

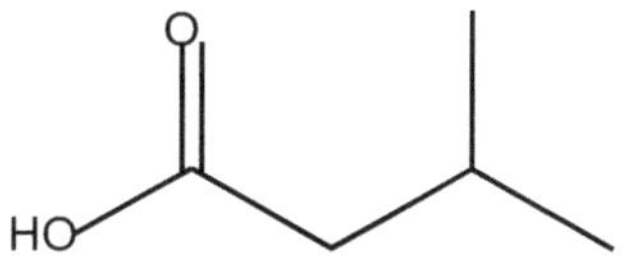

Isovaleric acid

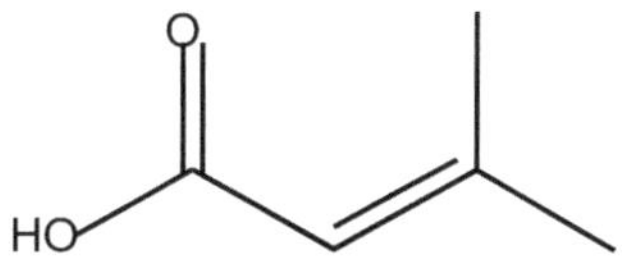

Senecioic acid

Monoterpenes

Monoterpenes consist of two C_5 units with the molecular formula $C_{10}H_{16}$. These are majorly found in fixed and essential oils of plants. Monoterpenes can be divided based on their structures as acyclic, monocyclic and bicyclic compounds. Monoterpenes have a strong odor and aroma. Hence, monoterpene-based oil mixtures are used as a fragrance in the perfume and cosmetic industries. Monoterpenes are reported for their antibacterial and antitumor activities. Limonene, thymol, myrcene, citral, carvone are the few examples of monoterpenoids. Recently, 9-OH-isoegomaketone [(2E)-1-(3-furanyl)--

-OH-4-Me-2-penten-1-one was isolated from leaves of plant *Perilla frutescens* var. crispa. This compound was reported for nitric oxide inhibitory activity in lipopolysaccharide (LPS)-activated RAW 264.7 (macrophage) cell line with IC_{50} value 14.4 µM [19].

Limonene

Thymol

Myrcene

Citral

Sesquiterpenes

Sesquiterpenes consist of three C_5 units and the molecular formula is $C_{15}H_{24}$. These are majorly found in latex producing plants. Structurally, these terpenes are present in the form of linear, bicyclic or tricyclic form. Sesquiterpenes are reported for their anti-insecticidal and antimicrobial activities. Farnesol, β-Bisabolene, α-Zingiberene, and β-Santalol are few examples of sesquiterpenoids. Artemisinin is a sesquiterpene lactone found in roots and shoots of plant *Artemisia annua* shoots [20]. Drimenin from plant *Drimys winteri* was reported for antidepressant activity [21].

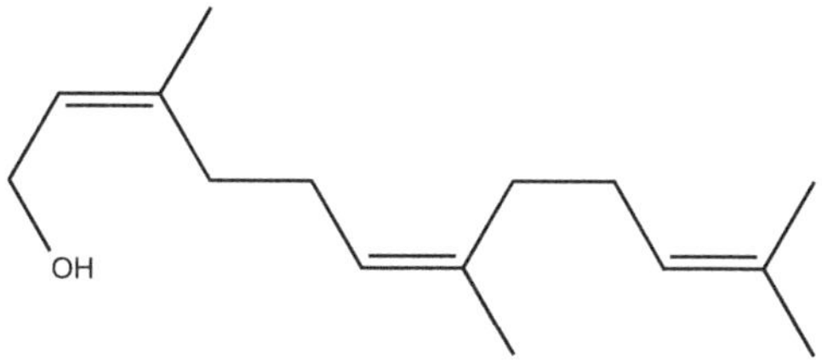

Farnesol

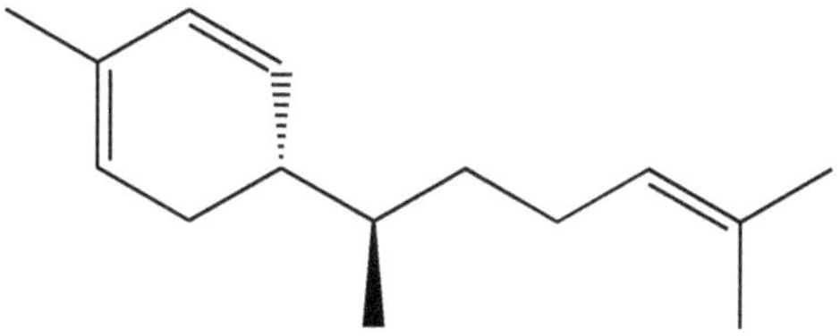

alpha-Zingiberene

Diterpenes

Diterpenes consist of four C_5 units and the molecular formula is $C_{20}H_{32}$. Diterpenes are reported for vast varieties of important biological activities. These have anti-inflammatory, antifungal, antimicrobial and anticancer activities. Phytol, grayanotoxin, abietic acid, and taxol are few examples of diterpenoids. Eleganolone, forskolin, marrubenol, cephinoids H and I and 14-deoxyandrographolide have an effect on cardiovascular activity. Genkwanine P and laurifolioside isolated from buds of *Wikstroemia chamaedaphne* were reported for anti-hepatitis B virus activities [22]. Nicaeenin F isolated from the latex of plant *Euphorbia nicaeensis*has reported for anticancer activity in cancer cell lines [23].

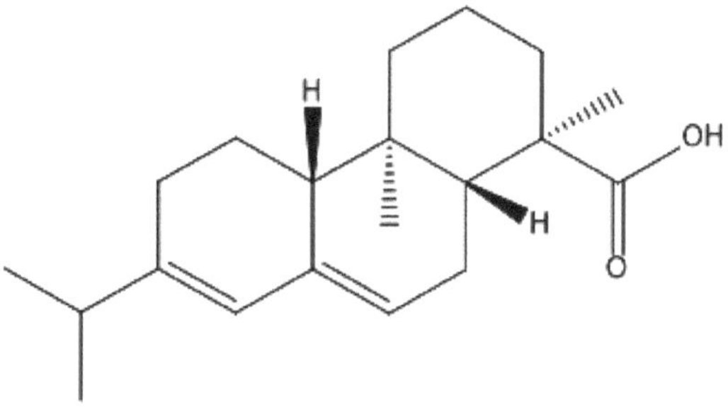

Abietic acid

Sesterpenes

Sesterpenes consists of five C_5 units and the molecular formula is $C_{25}H_{40}$. These are majorly found in plants, fungus, marine organisms and insects. Sesterpenes are reported for anti-inflammatory, antifungal, antimicrobial and anticancer activities. Manoalide, Nitiol and Leucosceptrine are few examples of sesterpenoids. Cybastacines A and B isolated from *Nostoc* and *Cyanobacterium* species were reported for antibiotic activity [24]. Scalarane sesterpenes isolated from mushroom species *Pleurotus ostreatus* and *Scleroderma areolatum* was reported for antiprotozoal activity [25].

Manoalide

Nitiol

Triterpenes

Triterpenes consist of six C_5 units and the molecular formula is $C_{30}H_{48}$. Triterpenes have complex structure due to the presence of methyl groups, which can undergo oxidation and give rise to alcohols, carboxylic acids, and aldehydes. Triterpenes have also shown the presence of glycosylation sites which leads to the production of triterpene glycoside "saponins". Squalene, α-amyrin, ursolic acid, and oleanolic acid are a few examples of triterpenoids. Recently, Xuedanencins H and G isolated from tubers of *Hemsleya penxianensis* and Cyclocariols A isolated from leaves of *Cyclocarya paliurus* reported for cytotoxic activity on different human cell lines. Polyporenic acid B from fruiting bodies of *Famitopsis palustris,* Pardinol B from *Tricholoma pardinum* [26, 27].

Tetraterpenes

Tetraterpenes consists of eight C_5 units and the molecular formula is $C_{40}H_{64}$. Carotenoids like lycopene, lutein, β-carotene, natural rubber and zeaxanthin are few examples of tetraterpenoids. These are normally present in flowers and fruits of higher plants [13].

Lycopene

Polyterpenes

Polyterpenes consist of more than eight C_5 units and the molecular formula is $(C_5H_8)_n$, where n>8. These are polymeric isoprenoids hydrocarbons. These are comparatively higher molecular weight polymers majorly found in rubbers. Balata from *Mimusops balata* and Guttapercha from *Palaquium gutta* are few examples of polyterpenes [13].

Meroterpenes

Meroterpenes have a partial terpenoid skeleton. Meroterpenes are partially biosynthesized from the mevalonate (MEV) pathway and are widely derived from bacteria, fungi, animals, and plants. Amestolkolide B isolated from mangrove endophytic fungus *Talaromyces amestolkiae* reported for anti-inflammatory property in LPS-induced inflammation in RAW 264.7 cell lines [28]. Spiroapplanatumines G from *Ganoderma applanatum* has been reported for its anticancer activity [29].

Table 1. Some known plant terpenoid compounds along with their uses.

Sr. No.	Plants	Terpenoids	Use	Ref
1	*Lagerstroemia speciose*	Corosolic acid	Antidiabetic	[30]
2	*Agrimoniapilosa Ledeb*	1β, 2β, 3β, 19α-tetrahydroxy-12-en-28-oic acid	Antidiabetic	[31]
3	*Lagerstroemia speciosa*	Arjunolic acid	Antidiabetic	[32]

(Table 1) cont.....

Sr. No.	Plants	Terpenoids	Use	Ref
4	*Panax ginseng*	Ginsenoside Rh2	Antidiabetic	[33]
5	*Eclipta prostrata*	6/6/6/6-fused tetracyclic triterpenoid	Antidiabetic	[34]
6	*Parmentiera cereifera*	Cycloart-23-ene-3β, 25-diol	Cardioprotective	[35]
7	*Leonotis leonurus*	Marrubiin	Cardioprotective	[36]
8	*Ginkgo biloba*	Ginkgolides A and B,	Cardioprotective	[37]

Biosynthesis of Terpenoids

Plant terpenoids have been reported for its chemical diversity, which is due to terpenoid synthase and modifying enzymes that are involved in stabilization of carbocation intermediates, rearrangement, and stereochemistry. Hence, terpenoids can be volatile or non-volatile, cyclic or acyclic, hydrophilic or lipophilic, chiral or achiral [38].

The vast diversity of plant terpenoids is due to the pathway that biosynthesizes them and complex structures. Plant terpenoids can be studied by traditional and biotechnological methods. The traditional method involves extraction, isolation, structural elucidation and identification of target for its biological activity. The biotechnological study of terpenoids includes the gene sequencing to discover a set of genes encoding enzymes involved in terpenoid biosynthesis. A combination of these two methods can be used for a comprehensive understanding of the biosynthetic origin, chemistry, and biology of various terpenoids.

Terpenes are majorly produced in specialized cells like glandular trichomes, scent-releasing epidermal cells that are present near resin ducts. Biosynthesis of terpenoids is mostly regulated by diurnal cycles, growth or developmental stage, hormones and pathogen infection.

Two C_5 unit containing compounds isopentenyl pyrophosphate (IPP) and dimethylallyl pyrophosphate (DMAPP) are known as universal precursors to terpenoids. These precursors originate from mevalonate (MEV) and 2C-methy--D-erytritol-4-phosphate (MEP) pathway. Eukaryotic organisms majorly biosynthesize terpenoids by the MEV pathway. MEV pathway is present in the endoplasmic reticulum and MEP pathway present in plastids of plants [39]. MEV pathway provides C_5 units for sesquiterpenes biosynthesis and the MEP pathway provides DMAPP and IPP for the biosynthesis of hemi, mono, and diterpene [40]. MEV pathway was discovered in yeast and animals. It was considered that IPP was synthesized *via* MEV from acetyl-CoA and then isomerized to DMAPP in eukaryotes. The MEV pathway was the only biosynthetic pathway for the synthesis of terpenoids in plants during 1993. Recently, it was discovered that the nonstandard MEV pathway in archaeal species involves phosphorylation of isopentenyl phosphate in *Methanocaldococcus jannaschii* [41]. Rohmer in 1993, reported an alternate pathway for the biosynthesis of terpenoids that do not originate from acetyl-CoA. This pathway was further elucidated in 2002 and named as 2C-methyl-D-erytritol-4-phosphate (MEP) pathway. MEP pathway is present in plants and bacteria [42]. The literature also provided evidence that there is a certain amount of crosstalk between the MEV and MEP pathway. Hence, plants have an enormous capacity to synthesize massive amounts of diverse terpenoids *via* a combination of these two pathways Fig. (**1**). For example, tocopherols are biosynthesized by isoprenoids and shikimic acid pathways, which produces homogentisic acid phytyl diphosphate. These two molecules combine and lead to the production of tocopherols [43].

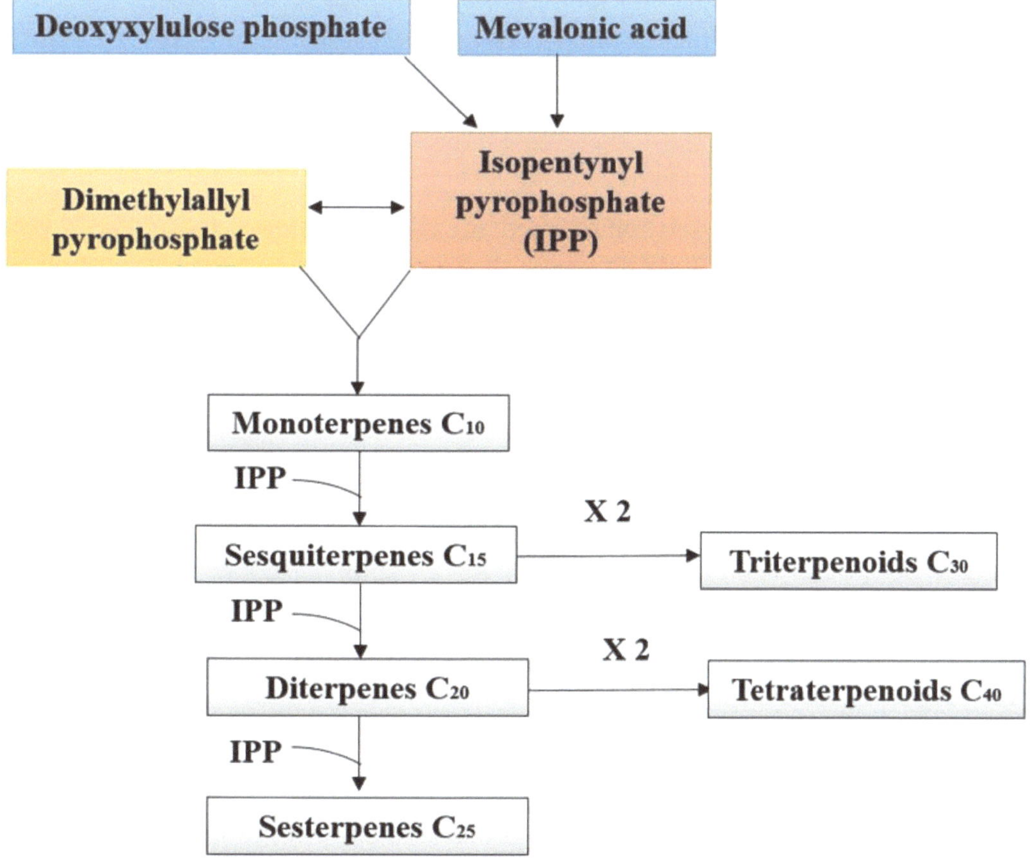

Fig. (1). Biosynthesis of terpenoids.

Terpenoids in Diabetes and Cardiovascular Diseases

1. Lupeol

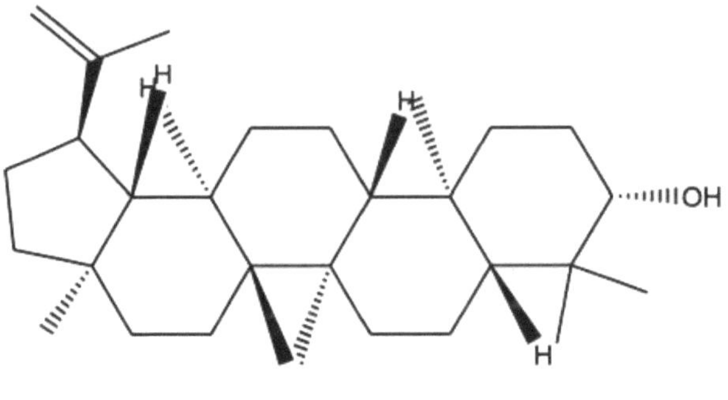

Lupeol is a pentacyclic triterpenoid found in *Gymnema, Glycyrrhiza* and *Crataegus* species. It is also found in plants like *Aegle marmelos, Camellia sinensis, Sapium ellipticum, Terminalia serica, Pueraria lobata, Malus pumila, Crataeva nurvala, Centella asiatica, Prosopis cineraria, Gentiana kuroo* and *Olea europaea.*

Lupeol in Diabetes

In 2003, Kamalakkanan and group studied the role of aqueous extract of *Aegle marmelos* fruits in streptozotocin (STZ)-induced diabetic rat model. Female albino wistar rats were treated orally with 250 mg/kg aqueous extract for 1 month. The study reported that aqueous extract of *Agegle marmelos* fruits decreased glucose and glycosylated hemoglobin levels in plasma. It also increased insulin and liver glycogen levels. The antidiabetic activity of *Aegle marmelos* may be due to the presence of lupeol [44].

Methanolic and hydroethanolic extract of plant *Gentiana kuroo* at the dose of 250 and 500 mg/kg body weight has been reported for its antidiabetic activity in STZ-induced diabetic rats. The plasma glucose levels in diabetic rats were significantly lowered by these extracts. Extracts have also reduced the levels of low-density lipoproteins, cholesterol, triglycerides, creatinine, alkaline phosphatase, serum glutamate pyruvate transaminase, and serum glutamate oxaloacetate transaminase. The extract showed a protective effect on pancreatic β-cells in diabetic rats. Further extracts were characterized by liquid chromatography and mass spectroscopy (LC-MS). The study proved that the antidiabetic activity of methanolic and hydroethanolic extract of plant *Gentiana kuroo* Royle is due to the presence of lupeol [45].

In vitro and *in vivo* antidiabetic activity of lupeol was studied by Soni and group in 2018. The lupeol was extracted from stem bark if *Prosopis cineraria.* The effect of oral treatment of chloroform extract of this plant was studied in STZ-induced diabetic rats at a dose of 50 and 100 mg/kg for 21 days. The study reported that lupeol significantly lowered blood glucose, glycosylates hemoglobin, lipid profile markers. Additionally, it also lowered serum insulin level, serum lipid profiles and liver glycogen content in a dose-dependant manner. In *in vitro* study, chloroform extract was significantly reduced α-amylase activity with an IC_{50} value of 40.29 µg/ml. The chloroform extract was characterized for the presence of lupeol by various analytical tools [46].

Naturally occurring lupeol and its allylic oxidative derivatives are reported for antidiabetic activity *in vitro* assay using L6 skeletal muscle cell lines. Lupeol and its derivatives at 10 µM concentration showed significant stimulation of glucose uptake. This stimulation is associated with activation of the IRS-1/PI3-K/A-T-dependent signaling pathway and translocation of glucose transporter 4 in L6 cells [47].

Lupeol was isolated from *Aegle marmelos* leaves and its novel derivatives were synthesized. Lupeol at a dose of 100 mg/kg body weight have shown antihyperglycemic activity in sucrose challenged STZ-induced diabetic rats. Lupeol and its derivatives at the dose of 50 mg/kg body weight showed a significant reduction in triglyceride, cholesterol levels in dyslipidemic hamster model [48].

Sapium ellipticum was reported for antidiabetic activity at a dose of 400 and 800 mg/kg body weight in the STZ-induced diabetes rat model. Diabetic animals were treated with *Sapium ellipticum* extract twice a daily oral dose for 21 days. *Sapium ellipticum* extract significantly reduced fasting blood glucose and showed improvement in plasma and pancreatic insulin levels. Histopathology study showed the regeneration of pancreatic beta cells in diabetic rats. Further, the antidiabetic activity of *Sapium ellipticum* extract was confirmed for the presence of lupeol active phytoconstituent [49].

Terminalia serica bark extract was reported for antidiabetic activity in vero cells (lineage of kidney epithelial cells of African green monkeys). Further, acetone extract was studied by bioassay-guided fractionation and it was confirmed that the active phytoconstituent of the extract is lupeol. The extract showed inhibitory activity on α-glucosidase and α-amylase activity at 66.5 µM [50].

Seong and group reported antidiabetic activity of *Pueraria lobata.* Ethanolic extract of the root of *Pueraria lobata* was studied by molecular docking simulation for α-glucosidase and protein tyrosine phosphatase 1B (PTP1B) inhibitory activities. The potential inhibitory activities were studied by *in silico* molecular docking and enzyme kinetics using the Lineweaver-Burk and Dixon plots of extract. Further, the extract was studied for the presence of lupeol and lupenone. Both of the compounds were reported for potent PTP1B inhibition with IC_{50} values of 38.89±0.17 and 15.11±1.23µM, respectively. Lupeol and lupenone exhibited potent α-glucosidase inhibitory activity [51].

In 2016, Ramu reported the *in vivo* antihyperglycemic activity of ethanol extract of banana flower in an alloxan-induced diabetic rat model. are the active phytoconstituents of banana flower. 4-week oral treatment of umbelliferone (100 mg/kg body weight) and lupeol (200 mg/kg body weight) showed a reversal of urine and serum biochemical levels and fasting hyperglycemia. To study the antidiabetic activity, diabetic animals were fed with banana flower 100 mg/kg body weight daily for 28 days. This treatment has shown significant improvement in body weight, polyphagia, polyuria polydipsia and urine sugar levels. The histopathological study has shown the regeneration of β-cells in the liver [52].

In 2019, researchers documented that Lupeol has the ability to stimulate fibroblast proliferation and angiogenesis *via* regulating the expressions of growth factors and cytokines involved in wound healing. The wound healing study was carried out in STZ-induced diabetic rats. The posterior dorsal region of rats was extended through the *panniculus carnosus* using a 2 cm diameter punch. Further diabetic rats treated with 0.2 w/w lupeol-based cream and animals were observed for cutaneous wound healing. Histopathological results showed decreased inflammatory cell infiltration and increased proliferation of fibroblasts. Lupeol treatment also showed an increase in vascularization of collagen fibers. ELISA assay showed decreased levels of pro-inflammatory mediators. These results indicated that lupeol has wound healing potential in diabetic rats [53].

Lupeol has antioxidant, anti-inflammatory, anti-dyslipidemic, anti-hyperglycemic, and anti-mutagenic in various disease-targeted animal models. These reports indicated that lupeol has great antidiabetic under various routes of administration. This antidiabetic activity is due to potential targeting proteins such as α-amylase, α-glucosidase and PTP1B and targeting Bcl-2 family, IL-1 receptor-associated kinase-mediated toll-like receptor 4 (IRAK-TLR4),phosphatidylinositol-3-kinase (PI3-K)/Akt, nuclear factor kappa B (NF-kB) and Wnt/β-catenin signaling pathways [54].

Lupeol in Cardiovascular Diseases

Seven weeks of oral lupeol supplementation at a dose of 670 mg/kg in male rats of SHRSP/Izumo strain (stroke-prone spontaneously hypertensive rats) has shown a significant reduction in blood pressure and urinary 8-hydroxy--0-deoxyguanosine as compared with the normal control group. Antihypertensive activity of lupeol is due to down-regulation of hepatic mRNA expressions of genes involved in cholesterol and triglyceride synthesis [55].

Yin and group reported the anticoagulant activity of flowers of *Malus pumila*. The phytoconstituents of *Malus pumila* flowers were isolated by using column chromatography and identified for the presence of lupeol and other eight phytoconstituents. The *in vitro* anticoagulant activity was evaluated by prothrombin time, activated partial thromboplastin time, fibrinogen and thrombin time. The compounds showed a reduction in prothrombin time, activated partial thromboplastin time, and thrombin time. This anticoagulant activity of flowers of *Malus pumilaha* has a great application in CVDs [56].

Crataeva nurvala stem bark is well known for a rich source of terpene and its ester namely lupeol and lupeol linoleate. Sudharsan and group reported the hypocholesterolemic activity of lupeol and lupeol linoleate in the cyclophosphamide-induced lipidaemic model in male albino wistar rats. These phytoconstituents were dissolved in olive oil. Lipidaemic animals were treated with lupeol and lupeol linoleate for 10 days by oral gavage. The study showed that lupeol and lupeol linoleate has great potential to reverse the cyclophosphamide-induced abnormal changes in lipid fractions and serum lipoproteins in serum and cardiac tissue. A study concluded that lupeol linoleate has great cardioprotective activity compared to lupeol [57].

Another study of lupeol and lupeol linoleate was done in hypercholesterolemic male wistar albino rats by Sudhahar and group in 2007. The animals were fed with a high-cholesterol diet containing 4% cholesterol and 1% cholic acid for 30 days. Lupeol and lupeol linoleate treatment has reduced triglycerides, total cholesterol, and phospholipids along with decreased activities of aspartate aminotransferase, lactate dehydrogenase, alkaline phosphatase and alanine aminotransferase in the heart tissue of hypercholesterolemic rats. This study concluded that lupeol and lupeol linoleate minimized the abnormal biochemical changes and lipid abnormalities in hypercholesterolemic rats. These cardioprotective effects of lupeol and lupeol linoleate are beneficial in the treatment of the hypercholesterolemic condition [58].

2. Limonene

It is a colorless, liquid and classified as a cyclic monoterpene. It is majorly present in the oil of citrus fruit peels and plants like *A. marmelos* and *Lavandula stoechas.*

Limonene in Diabetes

Panaskar and group studied the antidiabetic, antioxidant and antiglycation activity of chloroform leaf extract of plant *A. marmelos* in STZ-induced diabetic rats. 60 days oral treatment of chloroform extract of *A. marmelos* has been inhibited protein glycation, protein carbonyl and pentoside formation and in diabetic animals. The chloroform extract was further studied to confirm the active phytoconstituent responsible for bioactivity by gas chromatography and mass spectroscopy (GC-MS). The bio-guided fraction of chloroform extract *A. marmelos* revealed as limonene is an active principle, which is responsible for the antidiabetic, antioxidant and antiglycation activity. Limonene also prevented kidney damage and other secondary complications of diabetes [59].

Murali *et al.* evaluated the antidiabetic and antioxidant effect of limonene in STZ-induced diabetes in rats. 45 days oral treatment of limonene has significantly increased enzyme activity namely catalase, glutathione peroxidase, superoxide dismutase, and glutathione-S-transferase. In the same study, limonene treatment also reduced the formation of lipid peroxidation by-products level, when compared with the diabetic group. Limonene showed antioxidant as well as antidiabetic potential in diabetic rats [60].

Mechanism of antidiabetic activity of limonene was studied in STZ-induced diabetic wistar albino rats by Bacanli in 2017. The study reported that the antidiabetic potential of limonene is due to significant inhibition of DNA damage, malondialdehyde (MDA) and glutathione peroxidase enzyme activities. It also significantly increased total glutathione, superoxide dismutase, catalase and glutathione peroxidase activities. Limonene has shown a reduction in liver enzymes and lipid parameters in diabetic rats [61].

Sebai and group studied the phytochemical profile of *Lavandula stoechas* essential oils in alloxan-induced diabetes rats. Diabetic rats were treated for 15 days with 50 mg/kg intraperitoneal injection of essential oils from *Lavandula stoechas.* The essential oils from the plant were isolated by hydrodistillation and analyzed by GC-MS. The principle compound limonene was detected. The study showed a reduction in blood glucose, lipoperoxidation and antioxidant enzyme activities in diabetic rats. This study concluded that *Lavandula stoechas* has great potential in diabetes and oxidative stress in diabetic rats [62].

Conforti and group studied *in vitro* hypoglycaemic, antioxidant and anticholinesterase activity of n-hexane extract of the diamante citron peel. The extract analysed and confirmed the presence of limonene. The study showed that the n-hexane extract of diamante citron peel has great plasma sugar lowering (hypoglycemic) and antioxidant activity in the beta-carotene bleaching test, 2,2-diphenyl-2-picrylhydrazyl hydrate (DPPH) and bovine brain peroxidation assay [63]. Tan and group studied the hypoglycemic and antioxidant activity of monoterpenes including limonene. Limonene has shown radical scavenging activity in DPPH and 3-ethylbenzothiazoline-6-sulfonic acid assay. Also, it inhibited α-glucosidase, α-amylase enzyme activity and upregulated mRNA expression of glucose transporter in 3T3-L1 adipocytes [64]. This antioxidant activity can be a protective approach for the treatment of oxidative stress and damage caused by free radicals in chronic diseases like diabetes.

Limonene is not only effective in diabetes but also it has a great potential in the management of diabetic complication *via* inhibiting polyol and formation of AGEs. Limonene inhibited aldose reductase associated glucose flux, which is responsible for protein glycation involved in diabetic complications in STZ-induced diabetic rats [65]. Joglekar and group studied antiglycative properties of limonene in 2013. In this study, limonene was evaluated using bovine serum albumin (BSA) as a protein model. The study showed that limonene has a great potential to inhibit protein glycation at 50 μM concentration. This glycation inhibition due to limonene is confirmed through LC-MS analysis. PatchDock was carried out to find out the glycation specificity of limonene. The study revealed that limonene has a major specificity to bind IB, IIA and IIB sub-domains of BSA. These results showed that limonene is a potent protein glycation inhibitor and hence used in the management of diabetic complications [66].

Limonene in Cardiovascular Diseases

Antihypertensive activity of limonene has been studied in monocrotaline-induced pulmonary hypertension, lung injury and right ventricular hypertrophy in male Wistar rats. 21 days of daily oral treatment of limonene at a dose of 400 mg/kg has significantly reduced monocrotaline-induced hypertension and related complications. Histopathology study revealed that limonene treatment reduced the increases in pulmonary arterial media thickness and interstitial fibrosis. It also increased macrophage number in intra-alveolar spaces and lymphocytes around pulmonary veins [67].

3. Arjunolic Acid

Arjunolic acid is triterpenoid saponin mainly found in *Terminalia arjuna, Combretum nelsonii, Combretum dolichopetalum, Lagerstroemia speciosa* and *Leandra chaeton*. It has multifunctional therapeutic applications in Ayurveda for oxidative stress, diabetes and cardiac problems. It has great potential in the prevention of platelet aggregation, coagulation, lowering blood pressure and myocardial necrosis [68].

Arjunolic Acid in Diabetes

Manna and group extensively studied the antidiabetic activity of arjunolic acid. 28 days oral treatment of arjunolic acid in STZ-induced rats showed inhibition of various signaling pathways like phospho-p38, phospho-ERK1/2 and NF-κB involved in diabetes. It has also shown improvement in the release of cytochrome c and mitochondrial transmembrane potential by inhibiting the formation of reactive oxygen species in STZ-induced diabetes [69].

Uzor and Osadebehas reported the antidiabetic potential of the root of *Combretum dolichopetalum* in alloxan-induced diabetic Swiss albino mice. Diabetic animals were treated with 20 mg/kg dose of arjunolic acid for 28 days. Arjunolic acid has shown a synergistic effect with other phytoconstituents present in *Combretum dolichopetalum*. Antidiabetic activity of arjunolic acid is due to inhibition of α-glucosidase in yeast α-glucosidase enzyme with IC_{50} value 18.63 ± 0.32 µg/mL [70].

Hou and group reported *in vitro* antidiabetic activity of arjunolic acid from ethyl acetate extract of leaves of *Lagerstroemia speciosa* by α-glucosidase and α-amylase inhibitory activity. In this study, ethyl acetate extract of leaves of *Lagerstroemia speciosa* was analyzed and confirmed the presence of arjunolic acid and other bioactive principles. Oral treatment of arjunolic acid revealed that inhibition of α-glucosidase and α-amylase inhibitory activity [32]. The mechanism of action of antidiabetic activity of arjunolic acid was reported by Manna and Sil in 2012. Antidiabetic activity of arjunolic acid is due to the prevention of the production of ROS, advanced glycation end product and 8OHdG/2dG ratio. Arjunolic acid also prevented the signal transduction for the activation of NF-κB, protein kinase C and mitogen-activated protein kinases in diabetes. Hence, arjunolic acid may be used in the treatment of diabetes and the prevention of its complications [71].

Arjunolic Acid in Cardiovascular Diseases

Manna and group reported cardioprotective activity of arjunolic acid in arsenic-induced cardiac oxidative damage mice. Arsenic toxicity induced with oral administration of sodium arsenite at a dose of 10 mg/kg body weight for 2 days. This led to the accumulation of arsenic in the cardiac tissue and reduced cardiac antioxidant enzymes like catalase, superoxide dismutase, glutathione reductase, glutathione-S-transferase and glutathione peroxidase. Treatment of arjunolic acid prior to induction at a dose of 20 mg/kg body weight for 4 days has shown free radical scavenging activity in DPPH and ferric reducing/antioxidant power assay. Hence, arjunolic acid has a potential application in the protection of cardiac tissue from arsenic toxicity [72].

Arjunolic acid was reported for antihypertensive and cardioprotective activities in buthionine sulfoximine induced oxidative stress in rats. Hypertension was induced in rats by *i.p.* administration of 2 mmol/kg body weight. Hypertensive rats were treated with arjunolic acid for 28 days. Arjunolic acid recovered systolic blood pressure, glutathione hydroxylase level as compared to standard ascorbic acid group systolic blood pressure. Limonene has an antihypertensive effect similar to ascorbic acid. This study concluded that arjunolic acid has potential in the regulation of hypertension. Furthermore, arjunolic acid has also been reported to reduce AGEs and activate the intracellular antioxidant mechanism. Hence, it can be the lead compound for the development of cardioprotective agent [73].

Type 1 diabetes is associated with increases in vascular inflammation and cardiovascular complications. Manna and group studied the cardioprotective role of arjunolic acid in STZ-induced diabetic rats. Hyperglycemia caused alterations in oxidative stress-related biomarkers and reduced intracellular ATP and nicotinamide adenine dinucleotide concentrations. Arjunolic acid at the dose of 20 mg/kg body weight reduced hyperglycemia, oxidative stress, vascular inflammation and membrane disintegration and blood pressure in diabetic rats. This study concluded that arjunolic acid will be a beneficial phytoconstituent in the treatment of diabetes and cardiac complications [71].

The cardioprotective mechanism of arjunolic acid was studied by Bansal in 2017. This study reported that the cardioprotective activity of arjunolic acid is due to the downregulation of collagen expressions. Arjunolic acid has a capacity to bind and stabilize the ligand-binding site of peroxisome proliferator-activated receptor α (PPARα). Further, the study confirmed with PPARα knockdown rats for increased expressions of PPARα in cardiac fibroblast, renal artery and the ligated heart. Activated PPARα inhibits the TGF-β-activated kinase1 (TAK1) phosphorylation, ultimately resulting in improvement in excess collagen synthesis in cardiac hypertrophy. This study concluded thatarjunolic acid has PPARα agonistic activity and hence showed improvement in hypertrophy-associated cardiac fibrosis [74].

4. Ursolic Acid

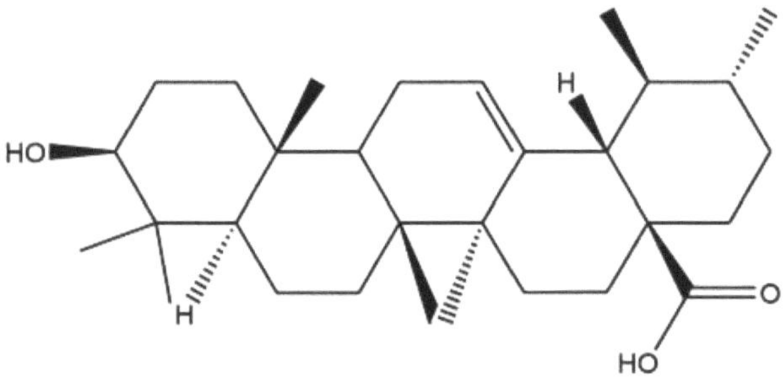

Ursolic acid is a pentacyclic triterpenoid, present in plant *Mirabilis jalapa, Punica granatum, Cornus officinalis,* apples, bilberries, basils, peppermint, cranberries, rosemary, and thyme.

Ursolic Acid in Diabetes

Glucose metabolism is regulated by endogenous Takeda G-protein-coupled receptor 5 (TGR5) and G-protein-coupled bile acid receptor (GPBAR1). Activation of TGR5 causes an increase in the secretion of incretin and reduces blood glucose levels. The role of ursolic acid on TGR5 was studied by Lo and group in transfected cultured Chinese hamster ovary (CHO-K1) cells with the TGR5 gene. The functional activity of transfected cells has been confirmed by glucose uptake using a fluorescent indicator, incretin levels secreted by NCI-H716 cells and glucagon-like peptide (GLP-1) levels were estimated by using ELISA assay. *In vitro* study of ursolic acid has shown a dose-dependent increase in glucose uptake in CHO-K1 cells, induced GLP-1 secretion in NCI-H716 cells. *In vivo* effect of ursolic acid has been studied in STZ-induced diabetic rats, revealed that activation of TGR5 and increased plasma GLP-1 levels. *In vitro* and *in vivo* study of ursolic acid confirmed that it has great potential to activate TGR5 and increase GLP-1 secretion [75].

Ding and group reported α-glucosidase inhibitory activity of ursolic acid in 2018. This study revealed the kinetics and inhibitory mechanism of ursolic acid on α-glucosidase. Ursolic acid has shown potent α-glucosidase inhibitory activities with IC_{50} value (1.69±0.03) ×10^{-5} mol/L. Ursolic acid has the capacity to bind to α-glucosidase induced conformational change and fluorescence quenching. The binding constants of ursolic acid with α-glucosidase at 298K was found to be (1.87±0.02) ×10^3 mol/L. Further, a molecular docking study reported that ursolic acid has great binding specificity at cavity 4 on α-glucosidase. This binding was associated with a reduction in the catalytic activity of α-glucosidase. Hence, ursolic acid can be developed as a potential antidiabetic compound [76, 77]. He and group reported hypoglycemic activity of fruits of *Cornus officinalis* in STZ-induced diabetic mice. Oral treatment of ursolic acid inhibited α-glucosidase and also exhibited free radical scavenging activity in diabetic mice [78].

Literature showed that antidiabetic activity of ursolic acid is mainly due to reduced glucose absorption, endogenous glucose production and improvement in lipid homeostasis and insulin sensitivity. Ursolic acid has also shown antioxidant, anti-inflammatory and antiatherogenic activity, which is relevant for the prevention of diabetes and its complications [79].

Ursolic Acid in Cardiovascular Diseases

Cardioprotective activity of ursolic acid was carried out in Dahl salt-sensitive and insulin-resistant rat model of genetic hypertension by Somova and group in 2003. Rats were administered ursolic acid 60 mg/kg body weight *i.p.* daily for 6 weeks. Plasma biochemical analysis of treated animals revealed that ursolic acid has a potent diuretic, natriuretic-saluretic activity, and direct cardiac effect by decreasing heart rate, hypoglycemic activity, antihyperlipidemic activity and antioxidant activity in Dahl salt-sensitive rats. This study confirmed that ursolic acid has great potential to prevent the development of hypertension and antidiabetic agent [80].

Ursolic acid was reported as a cardioprotective agent in diabetes-induced cardiac disease in male Sprague-Dawley rat rats by Wang in 2018. 8-week oral treatment of ursolic acid at the dose of 35 mg/kg body weight in diabetic rats showed downregulation of TGF-β1, TNF-α and MCP-1. It is also upregulated MMP-2 in the myocardium. The histopathology of the heart has shown an improvement in cardiac structure and function in diabetic rats [81]. In another study, the mechanism of action of ursolic acid in type 2 diabetes was studied by Yang and group in 2018. The male diabetic mice were treated with 100 mg/kg ursolic acid for 8 weeks. This study reported that the cardioprotective action of ursolic acid is due to inhibition of NLRP3 inflammasome activation and reducing myocardial inflammatory injury in diabetic rats [82].

5. Glycyrrhetinic Acid

Glycyrrhetinic acid is an important phytochemical present in *Glycyrrhiza glabra.*

Glycyrrhetinic Acid in Diabetes

Antidiabetic activity of glycyrrhetinic acid has been studied in the STZ-induced diabetic model in wistar adult male albino rats. Diabetic animals were treated orally with glycyrrhetinic acid at a dose of 50, 100 and 200 mg/kg body weight for 45 days. Plasma biochemistry analysis of treatment groups showed a decrease in blood glucose and glycated hemoglobin level, an increase in plasma insulin and hemoglobin level. It also improved gluconeogenic enzyme activity. Glycyrrhetinic acid reduced levels of glucose-6-phosphate and fructose--phosphate and activated glucokinase and glucose-6-phosphate dehydrogenase in the liver along with glycogen. Glycyrrhetinic acid at 100 mg/kg dose showed the potential to reduce blood glucose levels in diabetic rats compared to the standard glibenclamide group [83].

Glycyrrhetinic Acid in Cardiovascular Diseases

Glycyrrhetinic acid has been also reported for hypolipidemic activity by stimulation of plasma glucose and lipid profile in STZ-induced diabetic rats. Diabetic rats were randomized into seven groups such as normal control, diabetic control, glycyrrhetinic acid control, 3 groups of treatment group (50,100 and 200 mg/kg body weight) and one standard glibenclamide group. 28 days oral treatment of glycyrrhetinic acid has been shown that increased levels of plasma total cholesterol, free fatty acid, triglyceride and phospholipid while significantly decreased levels of high-density lipoprotein (HDL)-cholesterol in diabetic rats. The study concluded that glycyrrhetinic acid has the potential to normalize lipid profile and control blood glucose levels in diabetic rats [84].

Parisella and group reported cardiotonic activity of root extract of liquorice in an *in vitro* study by Langendorff for perfused rat heart. In this study, glycyrrhetinic acid improved cardiac contractility, relaxation and increased heart rate. This mechanism is further confirmed by western blotting. Glycyrrhetinic acid acts on cardiac tissue *via* signal transduction of endothelin receptor type B/Akt/nitric oxide synthase/nitric oxide axis [85].

Jiang and group reported *in vitro* and *in vivo* anticoagulant activity of glycyrrhetinic acid in 2014. The *in vitro* analysis was done by using enzyme activities of plasmin, trypsin, Factor Xa (FXa), thrombin and enzyme kinetic activities. *In vivo* analysis was done by using a rat venous stasis model and tail-bleeding model for evaluation of thrombus formation and bleeding time, respectively. This study reported that glycyrrhetinic acid has inhibited FXa with IC_{50} value 32.6 ± 1.24 µM/L and a dose-dependent increase in plasma clotting time. Intragastric Administration of glycyrrhetinic acid at the dose of 50 mg/kg resulted in a decrease in 34.8% of venous thrombus weight compared to the control in the rat venous stasis model. The moderate haemorrhagic effect was recorded at a dose of 200, 300 and 400 mg/kg in the rat tail-bleeding model along with an increase in bleeding time 1, 1.5, 2 fold, respectively. This study has concluded that glycyrrhetinic acid has a potent FXa inhibitory activity and hence, it can be used for the treatment of coagulation disorders such as deep venous thrombosis [86].

Wu and group reported the cardioprotective activity of glycyrrhetinic acid in ischemia-reperfusion induced cardiac arrhythmias in rat hearts. Rats were treated intravenous administration (15 min prior to occlusion of a left anterior descending artery) of glycyrrhetinic acid. 5, 10 and 20 mg/kg dose treatment of glycyrrhetinic acid showed a significant decrease in ventricular tachycardia score at 20 mg/kg dose and prolonged action potential durations. This cardioprotective activity of glycyrrhetinic acid is due to blockade of transient outward potassium current and L-type calcium current. Hence, glycyrrhetinic acid can be a great choice for the treatment of arrhythmia, ischemia and other CVDs [87].

In vitro cardioprotective study of glycyrrhetinic acid was carried out in H9c2 (multinucleated myoblast cells) cells under oxygen and glucose deprivation by Wang and group in 2017. Glycyrrhetinic acid treatment showed significant improvement in morphology and pathology of H9c2 cells studied by Hoechst 33342 staining and transmission electron microscopy. Glycyrrhetinic acid also inhibited secretion of lactate dehydrogenase, aspartate transaminase and creatine kinase-myocardialisoenzyme from H9c2 cells in enzyme-linked immune sorbent assay. Protein expression analysis revealed that the cardioprotective activity of glycyrrhetinic acid is due to the modulation of phosphatidylinositol 3-kinase/Akt signaling pathway [88].

Literature also reported that glycyrrhetinic acid has the potential to inhibit the DNA binding capacity of mechanosensitive transcription factor activation protein. This study has been carried out in pressure-induced increase in biochemical stress for the formation of superficial veins in mice. Glycyrrhetinic acid inhibited the angiogenic sprouting of human venous endothelial cells and smooth muscle cells. Mouse veins have been subjected to biomechanical stress and treated with glycyrrhetinic acid. Glycyrrhetinic acid has a potential of venous remodeling in the mouse auricle [89].

6. Ginsenoside

Ginsenosides are steroidal saponin and triterpene glycosides extremely found in the roots of plants from genus *Panax* namely *P.ginseng, P. notoginseng* and *P. quinquefolius.* Ginsenosides Rg1, Rb1 and Re are reported for antidiabetic and cardioprotective activity.

Ginseosides in Diabetes

Antidiabetic activity of ginsenoside Rg1 was studied by Liu and group in high-fat-diet fed mice and C57BL/6J (glucagon challenged) diabetic mice. Oral treatment of 50 mg/kg Rg1 dose of ginsenoside Rg1 showed a decrease in glucose 6-phosphatase, transcription of phosphoenolpyruvate carboxykinase enzymes and increased binding of Akt to FoxO1 *via* phosphorylation. The molecular mechanism of antidiabetic activity of ginsenoside Rg1 was studied by gene silencing. This study showed that ginsenoside Rg1 treatment may responsible for Akt phosphorylation at Ser473 for a reduction in gluconeogenesis in diabetic mice [90].

Song and group reported the molecular mechanism involved in the antidiabetic activity of ginsenoside Rb1 in high-fat diet-induced type 2 diabetes in Mice. 28 days oral administration of 10 mg/kg dose of ginsenoside Rb1 has reduced 11β-Hydroxysteroid dehydrogenase type I levels in adipose tissue and liver. Ginsenoside Rb1 treatment also increased insulin sensitivity *via* suppressing 11β-Hydroxysteroid dehydrogenase type I in type 2 diabetic mice [91].

Yu and group studied antidiabetic and cardioprotective activities of ginsenoside

Rg1 in endoplasmic reticulum stress-induced apoptosis in wistar rats. 84 days oral administration of 10, 15 and 20 mg/kg/day showed a dose-dependent decrease in plasma blood glucose levels. The serum samples also significantly decreased cardiac troponin-1 at 10 and 15 mg/kg dose. Ginsenoside Rg1 treatment significantly increased cardiac function parameters and reduced apoptotic myocardial cells. This study concluded that ginsenoside Rg1 has a potential cardioprotective role in endoplasmic reticulum stress-induced apoptosis in diabetic rats [92].

Shi and group reported anti-angiopathy activity of ginsenoside Re in early, Type 1 and Type 2 diabetic wistar rats. Early diabetes was induced by high-sucrose-hih-fat diet, type 1 by alloxan and type 2 by high fat and STZ. 56 days intragastric administration of 20 mg/kg of ginsenoside Re efficiently reduced plasma levels of blood glucose, triglycerides, total cholesterol, vascular endothelial growth factor, interleukin-6 and phosphorylation of p38 and c-Jun N-terminal kinase. Ginsenoside Re also increased plasma levels of high-density lipoprotein and insulin in diabetic mice. The antidiabetic and anti-angiopathy activity of ginsenoside Re may due to activation of p38, c-Jun N-terminal kinase, mitogen activated protein kinase signaling [93].

Ginsenosides in Cardiovascular Diseases

Yu and group reported cardioprotective activity of ginsenoside Rg1in STZ induced diabetic rat model. 84 days intraperitoneal treatment of ginsenoside Rg1 showed a dose-dependent reduction in serum creatinine kinase, malondialdehyde and cardiac troponin I. It also showed an increase in serum and cardiac superoxide dismutase, glutathione peroxidase and catalase. These results revealed that ginsenoside Rg1 has great potential in cardiovascular injury in diabetics [94].

7. Corosolic Acid

It is pentacyclic triterpene present in *Lagerstroemia speciosa, Weigela subsessilis* and leaves of *Eriobotrya japonica.*

Corosolic Acid in Diabetes

Miura and group reported antidiabetic activity of corosolic acid in 2004. Corosolic acid at the single dose of 10 mg/kg reduced blood glucose level in KK-Ay mice (cross between diabetic KK and lethal yellow mice) in type 2 diabetes animal model compared to the normal control group. The mechanism of antidiabetic activity of corosolic acid is due to a significant increase in translocation of glucose transporter isoform 4 (GLUT4) from the low-density microsomal membrane to plasma membrane compared with normal control. Hence, corosolicacid has the great potential to develop as an antidiabetic agent in type 2 diabetes [95].

Miura and group reported the antidiabetic activity of corosolic acid in KK-Ay (Type 2 diabetes model) diabetic mice. Single oral administration of corosolic acid at a dose of 2 mg/kg body weight for 2 weeks significantly reduced plasma insulin, insulin tolerance test and plasma glucose levels. The study concluded that corosolic acid has the potential to reduce insulin resistance in KK-Ay mice. This study revealed that corosolic acid will be a future drug for the treatment of Type 2 diabetes [96].

Cellular mechanisms and signaling pathway of corosolic acid as an antidiabetic agent were studied by Shi and group in 2008. *In vitro* analysis of corosolic acid in L6 myotubes and Chinese hamster ovary cells overexpressing human insulin receptor (CHO/hIR) cells. This study showed that corosolic acid enhances glucose uptake and facilitates glucose transporter isoform 4 translocation in L6 myotubes and CHO/hIR cells, respectively. Corosolic acid mediated these actions *via* activation of the insulin pathway and these activities can be blocked by phosphatidylinositol 3-kinase. Treatment of corosolic acid also inhibited several diabetes-related enzymatic activities like tyrosine phosphatases, src homology phosphatase- 1 and 2 [97].

Ethyl acetate extract of *Weigela subsessilis* leaves has rich triterpenoid content including corosolic acid. Ethyl acetate extract was studied for antidiabetic activity in insulin- and basal- stimulated L6 muscle cell lines. This study reported that corosolic acid at 25 and 50 μm concentration has shown potent glucose uptake activity without cytotoxicity in cell lines. This antidiabetic activity of ethyl acetate extract of *Weigela subsessilis* leaves may be due to insulin mimicking the activity of corosolic acid [98].

In vitro analysis of corosolic acid as antidiabetic activity was studied by Zhang and group in 2017. The antidiabetic activity was evaluated by α-glucosidase and α-amylase assay. The IC_{50} value for α-amylase and α-glucosidase inhibitory activity of corosolic acid was 31.2±3.4 μM and 17.2±0.9μM, respectively.

Further, the kinetic study revealed non-competitive inhibition against α-amylase. This study concluded that corosolic acid can be a potential therapeutic agent for diabetes [99].

Recently, in 2019, kinetics, molecular simulation and interactions involved in the α-glucosidase inhibitory activity of corosolic acid were studied by Ni and group. The study was done by using circular dichroism spectra and three-dimensional fluorescence spectra. The results showed that corosolic acid inhibited α-glucosidase in a non-competitive manner with IC_{50} value 1.35×10^{-5} mol/L. This inhibitory activity was confirmed with intrinsic fluorescence of α-glucosidase quenching during the binding of corosolic acid at 298 K and binding constant was found to be 3.47×10^3 mol/L. The binding was mainly driven by hydrophobic forces. This resulted in the extension and loss of the α-helix content of protein polypeptide. The molecular simulation study showed that corosolic acid has great specificity towards amino acid residues Arg315, Arg442, Ser157, Phe303, Gln353 and Tyr158 of the α-glucosidase enzyme. This interaction hinders the release of substrate and product and hence inhibits the catalytic activity of α-glucosidase. This study concluded that corosolic has a potential application in the treatment of diabetes [100].

Corosolic acid has shown dose-dependent gluconeogenesis in the perfused liver and isolated hepatocytes of rats at the dose of 20-100 μM. This activity is due to the stimulation of the production of gluconeogenic intermediate, fructose-2,--bisphosphate. This is the key intermediate for the measurement of hepatic glucose output and glycolysis in the liver. An increase in fructose-2,--bisphosphate is due to a decrease in intracellular cyclic adenosine monophosphate in isolated rat hepatocytes. Corosolic acid also stimulated glucokinase activity without affecting glucose-6-phosphate activity in isolated hepatocytes. This report provides a strong mechanism of corosolic acid as an antidiabetic agent [101].

Corosolic Acid in Cardiovascular Diseases

Yamaguchi and group studied the effects of corosolic acid in obesity, hyperinsulinemia, hypertension, hyperglycemia and hyperlipidemia together with inflammation and oxidative stress in SHR/NDmcr-cp (cp/cp) (SHR-cp) (metabolic syndrome rat model) rats. SHR-cp rats (6 weeks old) fed with a high-fat diet containing corosolic acid (0.072%) for 14 days. Treatment of corosolic acid reduced serum free fatty acid (after 2 weeks of treatment) and blood pressure (after 8 weeks of treatment). Corosolic acid also inhibited oxidative stress markers namely 8-hydroxydeoxyguanosine (59%) and thiobarbituric acid-reactive substances (27%), after 2 weeks of treatment. This study concluded that corosolic acid has the potential to prevent abnormal lipid metabolism, hypertension, inflammation and oxidative stress in SHR-cp rats. This study also suggested that corosolic acid can be used to prevent atherosclerosis-related diseases [102].

Chen and group studied the molecular mechanism of anti-atherosclerotic activity of corosolic acid in apolipoprotein E-deficient mice by targeting NF- κB and MCP-1 pathway. Apolipoprotein E-deficient mice fed 0.15% cholesterol and 21% fat (western-type diet) and treatment group supplemented with corosolic acid (0.3 mg/day/ mice) for 12 weeks. The anti-inflammatory activity of corosolic acid was evaluated in the LPS-induced inflammation model. Atherosclerosis lesions were evaluated by serum profiles, histological lesions and gene expressions. This study reported that corosolic acid has significantly decreased monocyte chemoattractant protein expressions, NF-κB signaling pathway and atherosclerotic lesion area in apolipoprotein E-deficient mice [103].

The vasodilatory effect of corosolic acid was studied by Vazquez and group in 2018 in isolated rat aorta assay. This study reported that the EC_{50} value is 108.9 ± 6.7 µM and Emax value is 96.4 ± 4.2%. The vasodilatory effect of corosolic acid is due to the activation of H_2S/ATP- sensitive potassium channel (K_{ATP}) and NO/cyclic guanosine monophosphate pathway [104].

Recently, Vasodilatory activity of corosolic acid from flowers of the Mexican *Crataegus gracilior* was studied by Torres and group in 2019. *In vitro* analysis of extract containing 1% corosolic acid produced vasodilatory activity on isolated rat aortic rings with EC_{50} 1.83 ± 1.39 µg/mL and Emax = 100 ± 3.4%. This vasodilatory activity corosolic acid can be used to prevent the hypotensive effect in CVDs [105].

8. Pomolic Acid

It is present in leaves of *Licania pittieri* and *Weigela subsessilis*. It is also reported in fruit pulp of *Rhamnus davurica* and roots of *Sanguisorba officinalis*.

Pomolic Acid in Diabetes

Pomolic acid is a ursane triterpenoid that was isolated from ethyl acetate extract of *Weigela subsessilis* leaves. Pomolic acid has been studied for glucose uptake activity and enhancement of basal and insulin- stimulates L6 muscle cells. The Pomolic acid exhibited to 1.6-2.8 fold increase in glucose uptake activity and also reduced cell viability at doses of 25 and 50 µM by 19% and 21.8% at 24 h treatment, respectively. This study reported pomolic acid as insulin mimicking and insulin-sensitizing activity for the treatment of diabetes [106].

Pomolic Acid in Cardiovascular Diseases

Methanolic extract of *Licania pittieri* leaves has been reported for hypotensive activity in rats. The Bioactivity-guided fractionation of methanol extract has been done by measuring changes in heart rate and mean arterial blood pressure in normal rats. This study has led to the isolation of Pomolic acid. Pomolic acid at the dose of 0.4 mg/kg *i.v.* decreased heart rate by 38.7% and mean arterial blood pressure by 24.1% for more than 45 minutes. Additionally, Pomolic acid also reported for hemostasis activity in nose bleeding study. Pomolic acid has been proved as a potent inhibitor of platelets in humans induced by Epinephrine and adenosine diphosphate. The IC_{50} value was found to be 60 nM. This study of pomolic acid was reported for the first time as a hypotensive and platelet anti-aggregating agent and also suggested as a potential phytoconstituents for the treatment of CVDs [107].

CONCLUDING REMARKS

As per the WHO, diabetes and CVDs are the main leading causes of mortality and morbidity throughout the world. Many synthetic drugs are in the market and widely used for the treatment and management of diabetes and cardiovascular diseases. These medications have side effects and toxicity on other vital organs. In this regard, natural product research has been gained importance due to its safety profiles. Mentioned terpenoids have been reported for antidiabetic and cardiovascular protective activity. Terpenoids have exhibited antidiabetic activity *via* a reduction in glucose absorption, an increase in insulin secretion, glucose uptake and formation of AGEs. Terpenoids have also exhibited cardioprotective activity *via* normalizing blood pressure, vasorelaxation, and increasing heart rate. Thus, terpenoids are important phytochemicals that need to be developed as drugs for diabetes and cardiovascular diseases by systemic, pre-clinical and clinical studies.

CONSENT FOR PUBLICATION

Not applicable.

CONFLICT OF INTEREST

There is no conflict of interest declared.

ACKNOWLEDGEMENTS

Declared none.

REFERENCES

[1]   World Health Organization [Internet]. Classification of diabetes 2019; [cited 2019 Sep 5].1-40.https://apps.who.int/iris/handle/10665/325182

[2]   World Health Organization Library. Global report on diabetes [Internet]. Cataloguing-in-publication data global report on diabetes; [cited 2019 Sep 5]. 2016; 1-88. Available from: http://www.who.int/about/licensing/copyright_form/ index.html

[3]   Adam F. Cardiovascular disease: types, symptoms, prevention, and causes [Internet] [cited 2019 Aug 14]. 2019. Available from: https://www.medicalnewstoday.com/articles/257484.php

[4]   Kulkarni YA, Garud MS, Oza MJ, Barve KH, Gaikwad AB. Diabetes, diabetic complications, and flavonoids Fruits, Vegetables, and Herbs. Elsevier 2016; pp. 77-104. http://linkinghub.elsevier.com/ retrieve/pii/B9780128029725000056 Internet [cited 2018 May 16] [http://dx.doi.org/10.1016/B978-0-12-802972-5.00005-6]

[5]   Garud MS, Kulkarni YA. Hyperglycemia to nephropathy via transforming growth factor beta 2014. http://www.ncbi.nlm.nih.gov/pubmed/24919657 [http://dx.doi.org/10.2174/1573399810666140606103645]

[6]   Suryavanshi SV, Kulkarni YA. NF-κβ: A potential target in the management of vascular complications of diabetes. [cited 2019 May 14] Frontiers in Pharmacology. Frontiers Media, SA 2017; Vol. 8: p. 798. Available from: http://www.ncbi.nlm.nih.gov/pubmed/29163178

[7]   Jensen J, Omar M, Kistorp C, Poulsen MK, Tuxen C, Gustafsson I, *et al.* Empagliflozin in heart failure patients with reduced ejection fraction: a randomized clinical trial (Empire HF). Trials [Internet] 2019; 20(1): 374.2019; Available from: https://trialsjournal. biomedcentral.com/articles/10.1186/s13063-019-3474-5

[8]   International Diabetes Federation - What is diabetes [Internet]. [cited 2019 Aug 14]. Available from: https://www.idf.org/aboutdiabetes/what-is-diabetes.html

[9]   Dei Cas A, Khan SS, Butler J, Mentz RJ, Bonow RO, Avogaro A, *et al.* Impact of diabetes on epidemiology, treatment, and outcomes of patients with heart failure. JACC Hear Fail [Internet] 2015; 3(2): 136-45. Available from: https://linkinghub.elsevier. com/retrieve/pii/S221317791400451X [http://dx.doi.org/10.1016/j.jchf.2014.08.004]

[10]   Kasznicki J, Drzewoski J. Heart failure in the diabetic population - pathophysiology, diagnosis and management. Arch Med Sci 2014; 10(3): 546-6. Available from: http://www.ncbi.nlm.nih.gov/ pubmed/25097587

[11]   Brunstrom M, Carlberg B. Effect of antihypertensive treatment at different blood pressure levels in patients with diabetes mellitus: systematic review and meta-analyses. BMJ 2016; 335: i717. Available from: http://www.ncbi.nlm.nih. gov/pubmed/2692033310.1136/bmj.i717

[12]   Putta S, Yarla NS, Kilari EK, Surekha C, Aliev G, Divakara MB, *et al.* Therapeutic potentials of

triterpenes in diabetes and its associated complications. Curr Top Med Chem 2016; 16(23): 2532-42. Available from: http://www.ncbi.nlm.nih.gov/pubmed/27086788

[13]   Ludwiczuk A, Skalicka WK, Georgiev MI. Terpenoids. Pharmacognosy [Internet]. 2017; 233-66. Available from: https://www.sciencedirect.com/science/article/pii/ B9780128021040000111

[14]   Bian G, Ma T, Liu T. *In vivo* platforms for terpenoid overproduction and the generation of chemical diversity.   Methods   Enzymol   2018;   608:   97-129.   Available   from: https://www.sciencedirect.com/science/article/ pii/S0076687918301769

[15]   Dev S. Terpenoids Natural products of woody plants I. Berlin, Heidelberg: Springer 1989; pp. 691-807. http://www.springerlink.com/index/10.1007/978-3-642-74075-6_19 Internet [cited 2019 Aug 19] [http://dx.doi.org/10.1007/978-3-642-74075-6_19]

[16]   Connolly JD, Hill RA. Dictionary of terpenoids. Flavour Fragr J [Internet] 1992; 7(4): 242-3. Available from: http://doi.wiley.com/10.1002/ffj.2730070418

[17]   Gershenzon J, Dudareva N. The function of terpene natural products in the natural world. Nat Chem Biol [Internet] 2007; 3: 408-14. Available from: http://agri.ckcest.cn/ass/NK003-20151109011.pdf [http://dx.doi.org/10.1038/nchembio.2007.5]

[18]   Shagufta P. Introductory chapter: terpenes and terpenoids. IntechOpen 2018; pp. 1-12. https://kopernio.com/viewer?doi=10.5772/intechopen.79683&route=6 [Internet]

[19]   Nam B, So Y, Kim HY, Kim JB, Jin C, Han AR, *et al.* A new monoterpene from the leaves of a radiation mutant cultivar of *perilla frutescens* var. crispa with inhibitory activity on LPS induced NO production. Molecules [Internet] 2017; 22(9): 1471. Available from: http://www.mdpi.com/ 1420-3049/22/9/1471

[20]   Tian SH, Chai XY, Zan K, Zeng KW, Tu PF. Three new eudesmane sesquiterpenes from Artemisia vestita. Chinese Chem Lett [Internet]. 2013 Sep 1 [cited 2019 Aug 10]; 24(9): 797–800. Available from: https://www.sciencedirect.com/science/article/pii/ S1001841713002817

[21]   Arias HR, Feuerbach D, Schmidt B, Heydenreich M, Paz C, Ortells MO. Drimane sesquiterpenoids noncompetitively inhibit human α4β2 nicotinic acetylcholine receptors with higher potency compared to human α3β4 and α7 subtypes. J Nat Prod [Internet]. 2018 Apr 27 [cited 2019 Aug 10]; 81(4): 811–7. Available from: http://pubs.acs.org/doi/ 10.1021/acs.jnatprod.7b00893

[22]   Li SF, Jiao YY, Zhang ZQ, Chao JB, Jia J, Shi XL, *et al.* Diterpenes from buds of Wikstroemia chamaedaphne showing anti-hepatitis B virus activities. Phytochemistry [Internet]. 2018 Jul 1 [cited 2019   Aug   10];   151:17–25.   Available   from: https://www.sciencedirect.com/ science/article/pii/S0031942218300311

[23]   Krstic G, Jadranin M, Todorovic NM, Pesic M, Stankovic T, Aljancic IS, *et al.* Jatrophane diterpenoids with multidrug-resistance modulating activity from the latex of Euphorbia nicaeensis. Phytochemistry [Internet]. 2018 Apr 1 [cited 2019 Aug 10]; 148: 104–12. Available from: https://www.sciencedirect.com/ science/article/pii/S0031942218300232

[24]   Cabanillas AH, Tena Perez V, Maderuelo Corral S, Rosero Valencia DF, Martel QA, Ortega Domenech M, *et al.* Cybastacines A and B: antibiotic sesterterpenes from a Nostoc sp. Cyanobacterium. J Nat Prod [Internet]. 2018 Feb 23 [cited 2019 Aug 10]; 81(2): 410–3. Available from: http://pubs.acs.org/doi/ 10.1021/acs.jnatprod.7b00638

[25]   Annang F, Perez Victoria I, Appiah T, Perez MG, Domingo E, Martin J, *et al.* Antiprotozoan sesterterpenes and triterpenes isolated from two Ghanaian mushrooms. Fitoterapia [Internet]. 2018 Jun 1   [cited   2019   Aug   10];   127:341–8.   Available   from: https://www.sciencedirect.com/ science/article/pii/S0367326X18302958 [http://dx.doi.org/10.1016/j.fitote.2018.03.016]

[26]   Zhu N, Sun Z, Hu M, Li Y, Zhang D, Wu H, *et al.* Cucurbitane-type triterpenes from the tubers of Hemsleya penxianensis and their bioactive activity. Phytochemistry [Internet]. 2018 Mar 1 [cited 2019 Aug 10]; 147:49–56. Available from: https://www.sciencedirect.com/science/article/pii/S00319422

17304089

[27]   Chen Y, Na L, Fan J, Zhao J, Hussain N, Jian Y, *et al.* Seco-dammarane triterpenoids from the leaves of Cyclocarya paliurus. Phytochemistry [Internet]. 2018 Jan 1 [cited 2019 Aug 10]; 145:85–92. Available from: https://www.sciencedirect.com/ science/article/pii/S0031942217303394

[28]   Chen S, Ding M, Liu W, Huang X, Liu Z, Lu Y, *et al.* Anti-inflammatory meroterpenoids from the mangrove endophytic fungus Talaromyces amestolkiae. Phytochemistry [Internet]. 2018 Feb 1 [cited 2019 Aug 10]; 146:8–15. Available from: https://www.sciencedirect.com/science/ article/pii/S0031942217303606

[29]   Wood KW, Lad L, Luo L, Qian X, Knight SD, Nevins N, *et al.* Antitumor activity of an allosteric inhibitor of centromere-associated protein-E. Proc Natl Acad Sci U S A [Internet]. 2010 Mar 30 [cited 2017 Nov 23]; 107(13): 5839–44. Available from: http://www.ncbi.nlm.nih.gov/pubmed/20167 803 [http://dx.doi.org/10.1073/pnas.0915068107]

[30]   Xu S, Wang G, Peng W, *et al.* Corosolic acid isolated from *Eriobotrya japonica* leaves reduces glucose level in human hepatocellular carcinoma cells, zebrafish and rats. Sci Rep 2019; 9(1): 4388. [http://dx.doi.org/10.1038/s41598-019-40934-7] [PMID: 30867526]

[31]   Liu X, Zhu L, Tan J, Zhou X, Xiao L, Yang X, *et al.* Glucosidase inhibitory activity and antioxidant activity of flavonoid compound and triterpenoid compound from Agrimonia Pilosa Ledeb. BMC Complement Altern Med [Internet]. 2014 Jan 10 [cited 2020 Feb 19]; 14:12. Available from: http://www.ncbi.nlm.nih.gov/ pubmed/24410924

[32]   Hou W, Li Y, Zhang Q, Wei X, Peng A, Chen L, *et al.* Triterpene acids isolated from Lagerstroemia speciosa leaves as alpha glucosidase inhibitors. Phyther Res [Internet]. 2009 May [cited 2019 Aug 30]; 23(5): 614–8. Available from: http://www.ncbi.nlm.nih.gov/ pubmed/19107840

[33]   Hamid K, Alqahtani A, Kim MS, *et al.* Tetracyclic triterpenoids in herbal medicines and their activities in diabetes and its complications. Curr Top Med Chem 2015; 15(23): 2406-30. [http://dx.doi.org/10.2174/1568026615666150619141940] [PMID: 26088353]

[34]   Yu SJ, Yu JH, Yu ZP, *et al.* Bioactive terpenoid constituents from *Eclipta prostrata.* Phytochemistry 2020; 170112192 [http://dx.doi.org/10.1016/j.phytochem.2019.112192] [PMID: 31726325]

[35]   Badole SL, Chaudhari SM, Jangam GB, Kandhare AD, Bodhankar SL. Cardioprotective activity of pongamia pinnata in streptozotocin-nicotinamide induced diabetic rats. Biomed Res Int. 2015.

[36]   Mnonopi N, Levendal RA, Davies-Coleman MT, Frost CL. The cardioprotective effects of marrubiin, a diterpenoid found in *Leonotis leonurus* extracts. J Ethnopharmacol 2011; 138(1): 67-75. [http://dx.doi.org/10.1016/j.jep.2011.08.041] [PMID: 21893184]

[37]   Pietri S, Maurelli E, Drieu K, Culcasi M. Cardioprotective and anti-oxidant effects of the terpenoid constituents of *Ginkgo biloba* extract (EGb 761). J Mol Cell Cardiol 1997; 29(2): 733-42. [http://dx.doi.org/10.1006/jmcc.1996.0316] [PMID: 9140830]

[38]   Dudareva N, Pichersky E, Gershenzon J. Biochemistry of plant volatiles. Plant Physiol [Internet]. 2004 [cited 2019 Aug 8]; 135:1893–902. Available from: www.plantphysiol. org/cgi/doi/10.1104/pp.104.049981

[39]   Lichtenthaler HK. The 1-deoxy-d-xylulose-5-phosphate pathway of isoprenoid biosynthesis in plants. Annu Rev Plant Physiol Plant Mol Biol [Internet]. 1999 Jun 28 [cited 2019 Aug 8]; 50(1): 47–65. Available from: http://www.annualreviews.org/doi/10.1146/annurev.arplant.50.1.47

[40]   Schuhr CA, Radykewicz T, Sagner S, Latzel C, Zenk MH, Arigoni D, *et al.* Quantitative assessment of crosstalk between the two isoprenoid biosynthesis pathways in plants by NMR spectroscopy [Internet]. Vol. 2, Phytochemistry Reviews. 2003 [cited 2019 Aug 8]. Available from: https://search.proquest.com/docview/ 2259410705?pq-origsite=gscholar

[41]   Grochowski LL, Xu H, White RH. Methanocaldococcus jannaschii uses a modified mevalonate pathway for biosynthesis of isopentenyl diphosphate. J Bacteriol [Internet]. 2006 [cited 2019 Aug 10];

188(9): 3192–8. Available from: http://jb.asm.org/

[42]   Withers ST, Keasling JD. Biosynthesis and engineering of isoprenoid small molecules. Appl Microbiol Biotechnol [Internet]. 2006 Dec 18 [cited 2019 Aug 10]; 73(5): 980–90. Available from: http://link.springer.com/10.1007/s00253-006-0593-1

[43]   Munne BS, Alegre L. The function of tocopherols and tocotrienols in plants. CRC Crit Rev Plant Sci [Internet]. 2002 Jan 24 [cited 2019 Aug 10]; 21(1): 31–57. Available from: https://www.tandfonline.com/doi/full/10.1080/0735-260291044179

[44]   Kamalakkanan N, Rajadurai M, Prince PSM. Effect of *Aegle marmelos* fruits on normal and streptozotocin-diabetic wistar rats. J Med Food [Internet]. 2003 Jul 7 [cited 2019 Aug 13]; 6(2): 93–8. Available from: http://www.liebertpub.com/doi/10.1089/ 109662003322233486

[45]   Ghazanfar K, Mubashir K, Dar SA, Nazir T, Hameed I, Ganai BA, *et al.* Gentiana kurroo Royle attenuates the metabolic aberrations in diabetic rats; swertiamarin, swertisin and lupeol being the possible bioactive principles. J Complement Integr Med [Internet]. 2017 Jan 28 [cited 2019 Aug 19]; 14(3). Available from: http://www.degruyter. com/view/j/jcim.2017.14.issue-3/jcim-2017-0002/j-im-2017-0002.xml

[46]   Soni LK, Dobhal MP, Arya D, Bhagour K, Parasher P, Gupta RS. *In vitro* and *in vivo* antidiabetic activity of isolated fraction of Prosopis cineraria against streptozotocin-induced experimental diabetes: a mechanistic study. Biomed Pharmacother [Internet]. 2018 Dec [cited 2019 Aug 19]; 108:1015–21. Available from: http://www.ncbi.nlm. nih.gov/pubmed/30372801

[47]   Khan MF, Maurya CK, Dev K, Arha D, Rai AK, Tamrakar AK, *et al.* Design and synthesis of lupeol analogues and their glucose uptake stimulatory effect in L6 skeletal muscle cells 2014. http://www.ncbi.nlm.nih. gov/pubmed/24813738
        [http://dx.doi.org/10.1016/j.bmcl.2014.04.059]

[48]   Papi RK, Singh AB, Puri A, Srivastava AK, Narender T. Synthesis of novel triterpenoid (lupeol) derivatives and their in vivo antihyperglycemic and antidyslipidemic activity. Bioorg Med Chem Lett [Internet]. 2009 Aug 1 [cited 2019 Aug 29]; 19(15): 4463–6. Available from: http://www.ncbi.nlm.nih.gov/pubmed/ 19515563

[49]   Ighodaro OM, Akinloye OA. Antidiabetic potential of Sapium ellipticum (Hochst) pax leaf extract in streptozotocin (STZ)-induced diabetic wistar rats. BMC Complement Altern Med [Internet]. 2017 Dec 8 [cited 2019 Aug 29]; 17(1): 525. Available from: http://www.ncbi.nlm.nih.gov/pubmed/29216879

[50]   Nkobole N, Houghton PJ, Hussein A, Lall N. Antidiabetic activity of Terminalia sericea constituents. Nat Prod Commun [Internet]. 2011 Nov [cited 2019 Aug 29]; 6(11): 1585–8. Available from: http://www.ncbi.nlm.nih.gov/pubmed/22224265

[51]   Seong SH, Roy A, Jung HA, Jung HJ, Choi JS. Protein tyrosine phosphatase 1B and α-glucosidase inhibitory activities of *Pueraria lobata* root and its constituents. J Ethnopharmacol [Internet]. 2016 Dec 24 [cited 2019 Aug 29]; 194:706–16. Available from: http://www.ncbi.nlm.nih.gov/pubmed/27769948

[52]   Ramu R. Assessment of in vivo antidiabetic properties of umbelliferone and lupeol constituents of banana (musa sp. var. nanjangud rasa bale) flower in hyperglycaemic rodent model. Essop MF, editor. PLoS One [Internet]. 2016 Mar 22 [cited 2019 Aug 29]; 11(3): e0151135. Available from: http://www.ncbi.nlm.nih.gov/pubmed/27003006

[53]   Beserra FP, Vieira AJ, Gushiken LFS, de Souza EO, Hussni MF, Hussni CA, *et al.* Lupeol, a dietary triterpene, enhances wound healing in streptozotocin-induced hyperglycemic rats with modulatory effects on inflammation, oxidative stress, and angiogenesis 2019.
        [http://dx.doi.org/10.1155/2019/3182627]

[54]   Tsai FS, Lin LW, Wu CR. Lupeol and its role in chronic diseases 2016. http://link.springer.com/ 10.1007/978-3-319-41342-6_7
        [http://dx.doi.org/10.1007/978-3-319-41342-6_7]

[55]   Ardiansyah YE. Shirakawa H, Hata K, Hiwatashi K, Ohinata K, Goto T KM. Lupeol supplementation improves blood pressure and lipid metabolism parameters in stroke-prone spontaneously hypertensive rats. Biosci Biotechnol Biochem [Internet]. 2012 Jan 23 [cited 2019 Aug 19]; 76(1): 183–5. Available from: http://www.ncbi.nlm.nih.gov/pubmed/22232260

[56]   Yin Z, Zhang Y, Zhang J, Wang J, Kang W. Coagulatory active constituents of *Malus pumila* Mill. flowers. Chem Cent J [Internet]. 2018 Dec 3 [cited 2019 Aug 30]; 12(1): 126. Available from: http://www.ncbi.nlm.nih.gov/pubmed/30506434

[57]   Sudharsan PT, Mythili Y, Sudhahar V, Varalakshmi P. Role of lupeol and its ester on cyclophosphamide-induced hyperlipidaemic cardiomyopathy in rats. J Pharm Pharmacol [Internet]. 2005 Nov [cited 2019 Aug 30]; 57(11): 1437–44. Available from: http://www.ncbi.nlm.nih.gov/pubmed/ 16259776

[58]   Sudhahar V, Kumar SA, Sudharsan PT, Varalakshmi P. Protective effect of lupeol and its ester on cardiac abnormalities in experimental hypercholesterolemia. Vascul Pharmacol [Internet]. 2007 Jun [cited 2019 Aug 30]; 46(6): 412–8. Available from: http://www.ncbi.nlm.nih.gov/ pubmed/1733616410.1016/j.vph.2006.12.005

[59]   Panaskar SN, Joglekar MM, Taklikar SS, Haldavnekar VS, Arvindekar AU. *Aegle marmelos* correa leaf extract prevents secondary complications in streptozotocin-induced diabetic rats and demonstration of limonene as a potent antiglycating agent. J Pharm Pharmacol [Internet]. 2013 Jun [cited 2018 Jun 13]; 65(6): 884–94. Available from: http://www.ncbi. nlm.nih.gov/pubmed/23647682

[60]   Murali R, Karthikeyan A, Saravanan R. Protective Effects of d -Limonene on lipid peroxidation and antioxidant enzymes in streptozotocin-induced diabetic rats. Basic Clin Pharmacol Toxicol [Internet]. 2013 Mar [cited 2019 Aug 19]; 112(3): 175–81. Available from: http://www.ncbi.nlm.nih.gov/pubmed/22998493

[61]   Bacanlı M, Anlar HG, Aydın S, Cal T, Arı N, Undeger BU, *et al.* d-Limonene ameliorates diabetes and its complications in streptozotocin-induced diabetic rats. Food Chem Toxicol [Internet]. 2017 Dec [cited 2019 Aug 19]; 110: 434–42. Available from: http://www.ncbi.nlm.nih. gov/pubmed/28923438

[62]   Sebai H, Selmi S, Rtibi K, Souli A, Gharbi N, Sakly M. Lavender (*Lavandula stoechas* L.) essential oils attenuate hyperglycemia and protect against oxidative stress in alloxan-induced diabetic rats. Lipids Health Dis [Internet]. 2013 Dec 28 [cited 2019 Aug 30];12(1):189. Available from: http://www.ncbi.nlm.nih. gov/pubmed/24373672

[63]   Conforti F, Statti GA, Tundis R, Loizzo MR, Menichini F. *In vitro* activities of *Citrus medica* L. cv. Diamante (Diamante citron) relevant to treatment of diabetes and Alzheimer's disease. Phyther Res [Internet]. 2007 May [cited 2019 Aug 30]; 21(5): 427–33. Available from: http://www.ncbi.nlm.nih. gov/pubmed/17236166

[64]   Tan XC, Chua KH, Ravishankar RM, Kuppusamy UR. Monoterpenes: Novel insights into their biological effects and roles on glucose uptake and lipid metabolism in 3T3-L1 adipocytes. Food Chem [Internet]. 2016 Apr 1 [cited 2019 Aug 30];196:242–50. Available from: http://www.ncbi.nlm.nih. gov/pubmed/26593489

[65]   Jagdale AD, Bavkar LN, More TA, Joglekar MM, Arvindekar AU. Strong inhibition of the polyol pathway diverts glucose flux to protein glycation leading to rapid establishment of secondary complications in diabetes mellitus. J Diabetes Complications [Internet]. 2016 Apr [cited 2019 Aug 30]; 30(3): 398–405. Available from: http://www.ncbi.nlm.nih. gov/pubmed/26896333

[66]   Joglekar MM, Panaskar SN, Chougale AD, Kulkarni MJ, Arvindekar AU. A novel mechanism for antiglycative action of limonene through stabilization of protein conformation 2013. http://www.ncbi.nlm. nih.gov/pubmed/23872839
[http://dx.doi.org/10.1039/c3mb00020f]

[67]   Touvay C, Vilain B, Carre C, Mencia JM, Braquet P. Effect of limonene and sobrerol on monocrotaline-lnduced lung alterations and pulmonary hypertension 1995. http://www.ncbi.nlm.nih. gov/pubmed/7542078

[http://dx.doi.org/10.1159/000237000]

[68] Hemalatha T, Pulavendran S, Balachandran C, Manohar BM, Puvanakrishnan R. Arjunolic acid: a novel phytomedicine with multifunctional therapeutic applications 2010. http://www.ncbi.nlm.nih.gov/pubmed/21046976

[69] Manna P, Sinha M, Sil PC. Protective role of arjunolic acid in response to streptozotocin-induced type-I diabetes via the mitochondrial dependent and independent pathways 2009. http://www.ncbi.nlm.nih.gov/ pubmed/19133311 [http://dx.doi.org/10.1016/j.tox.2008.12.008]

[70] Uzor PF, Osadebe PO. Antidiabetic activity of the chemical constituents of *Combretum dolichopetalum* root in mice. EXCLI J [Internet]. 2016 [cited 2019 Aug 30]; 15: 290–6. Available from: http://www.ncbi.nlm.nih.gov/pubmed/27298614

[71] Manna P, Sil PC. Arjunolic acid: beneficial role in type 1 diabetes and its associated organ pathophysiology. Free Radic Res [Internet]. 2012 Jul 3 [cited 2019 Aug 17]; 46(7): 815–30. Available from: http://www.tandfonline.com/doi/full/10.3109/10715762.2012.683431 [http://dx.doi.org/10.3109/10715762.2012.683431]

[72] Manna P, Sinha M, Sil PC. Arsenic-induced oxidative myocardial injury: protective role of arjunolic acid. Arch Toxicol [Internet]. 2008 Mar 16 [cited 2019 Aug 30]; 82(3): 137–49. Available from: http://www.ncbi.nlm.nih.gov/pubmed/1819739910.1007/s00204-007-0272-8

[73] Khatkar S, Nanda A, Ansari SH. Comparative evaluation of conventional and novel extracts of stem bark of *Terminalia arjuna* for antihypertensive activity in bso induced oxidative stress based rat model. Curr Pharm Biotechnol [Internet]. 2019 Apr 16 [cited 2019 Aug 17]; 20(2): 157–67. Available from: http://www.ncbi.nlm.nih.gov/pubmed/30806310

[74] Bansal T, Chatterjee E, Singh J, Ray A, Kundu B, Thankamani V, *et al.* Arjunolic acid, a peroxisome proliferator-activated receptor α agonist, regresses cardiac fibrosis by inhibiting non-canonical TGF-β signaling. J Biol Chem [Internet]. 2017 Oct 6 [cited 2019 Aug 30]; 292(40): 16440–62. Available from: http://www.ncbi.nlm.nih.gov/ pubmed/28821620

[75] Lo SH, Li Y, Cheng KC, Niu CS, Cheng J-T, Niu HS. Ursolic acid activates the TGR5 receptor to enhance GLP-1 secretion in type 1-like diabetic rats. Naunyn Schmiedebergs Arch Pharmacol [Internet]. 2017 Nov 30 [cited 2019 Aug 17]; 390(11): 1097–104. Available from: http://www.ncbi.nlm.nih. gov/pubmed/28756460

[76] Ding H, Hu X, Xu X, Zhang G, Gong D. Inhibitory mechanism of two allosteric inhibitors, oleanolic acid and ursolic acid on α-glucosidase 2018. https://linkinghub.elsevier.com/retrieve/pii/S0141813017336255

[77] Kalaycıoglu Z, Uzascı S, Dirmenci T, Erim FB. α-Glucosidase enzyme inhibitory effects and ursolic and oleanolic acid contents of fourteen *Anatolian Salvia* species. J Pharm Biomed Anal [Internet]. 2018 Jun 5 [cited 2019 Aug 30]; 155: 284–7. Available from: http://www.ncbi.nlm.nih.gov/pubmed/29677678

[78] He K, Song S, Zou Z, Feng M, Wang D, Wang Y, *et al.* The hypoglycemic and synergistic effect of loganin, morroniside, and ursolic acid isolated from the fruits of Cornus officinalis. Phyther Res [Internet]. 2016 Feb [cited 2019 Aug 30]; 30(2): 283–91. Available from: http://www.ncbi.nlm.nih.gov/pubmed/26619955

[79] Silva FG, Oliveira PJ, Duarte MF. Oleanolic, ursolic, and betulinic acids as food supplements or pharmaceutical agents for type 2 diabetes: Promise or illusion? J Agric Food Chem [Internet]. 2016 Apr 20 [cited 2019 Aug 30]; 64(15): 2991–3008. Available from: http://www.ncbi.nlm.nih.gov/ pubmed/27012451

[80] Somova LO, Nadar A, Rammanan P, Shode FO. Cardiovascular, antihyperlipidemic and antioxidant effects of oleanolic and ursolic acids in experimental hypertension 2003. http://www.ncbi.nlm.nih.gov/ pubmed/12725563 [http://dx.doi.org/10.1078/094471103321659807]

[81] Wang X, Gong Y, Zhou B, Yang J, Cheng Y, Zhao J, *et al.* Ursolic acid ameliorates oxidative stress, inflammation and fibrosis in diabetic cardiomyopathy rats 2018. http://www.ncbi.nlm.nih.gov/pubmed/29156537
[http://dx.doi.org/10.1016/j.biopha.2017.11.032]

[82] Yang ZL, Xu HL, Cheng Y, Zhao JG, Zhou YJ, Weng YJ, *et al.* Effect of ursolic acid on cardiomyopathy of mice with diabetes and its mechanism. Zhongguo Ying Yong Sheng Li Xue Za Zhi [Internet]. 2018 Apr 8 [cited 2019 Aug 30]; 34(4): 309-312 339. Available from: http://www.ncbi.nlm.nih.gov/ pubmed/30788937

[83] Kalaiarasi P, Pugalendi KV. Antihyperglycemic effect of 18β-glycyrrhetinic acid, aglycone of glycyrrhizin, on streptozotocin-diabetic rats. Eur J Pharmacol [Internet]. 2009 Mar 15 [cited 2019 Aug 17]; 606(1–3): 269–73. Available from: http://www.ncbi.nlm.nih.gov/pubmed/19374864

[84] Kalaiarasi P, Kaviarasan K, Pugalendi KV. Hypolipidemic activity of 18β-glycyrrhetinic acid on streptozotocin-induced diabetic rats. Eur J Pharmacol [Internet]. 2009 Jun 10 [cited 2019 Aug 17]; 612(1–3): 93–7. Available from: http://www.ncbi.nlm.nih.gov/pubmed/19361497

[85] Parisella ML, Angelone T, Gattuso A, Cerra MC, Pellegrino D. Glycyrrhizin and glycyrrhetinic acid directly modulate rat cardiac performance. J Nutr Biochem [Internet]. 2012 Jan [cited 2019 Aug 31]; 23(1): 69–75. Available from: http://www.ncbi.nlm.nih. gov/pubmed/21414764

[86] Jiang L, Wang Q, Shen S, Xiao T, Li Y. Discovery of glycyrrhetinic acid as an orally active, direct inhibitor of blood coagulation factor xa. Thromb Res [Internet]. 2014 Mar [cited 2019 Aug 31]; 133(3):   501–6.   Available   from: http://www.ncbi.nlm.nih.gov/pubmed/2441202910.1016/j.thromres.2013.12.025

[87] Wu HJ, Yang JY, Jin M, Wang SQ, Wu DL, Liu YN, *et al.* Glycyrrhetinic acid protects the heart from ischemia/reperfusion injury by attenuating the susceptibility and incidence of fatal ventricular arrhythmia during the reperfusion period in the rat hearts. Cell Physiol Biochem [Internet]. 2015 [cited 2019 Aug 31]; 36(2): 741–52. Available from: http://www.ncbi.nlm.nih.gov/ pubmed/26021262

[88] Wang L, He Y, Wan H, Zhou H, Yang J, Wan H. Protective mechanisms of hypaconitine and glycyrrhetinic acid compatibility in oxygen and glucose deprivation injury. J Zhejiang Univ B [Internet]. 2017 Jul 18 [cited 2019 Aug 31]; 18(7): 586–96. Available from: http://www.ncbi.nlm.nih.gov/ pubmed/28681583

[89] Kuk H, Arnold C, Wagner AH, Hecker M, Sticht C, Korff T. Glycyrrhetinic acid antagonizes pressure-induced venous remodeling in mice 2018. http://www.ncbi.nlm.nih.gov/pubmed/29670539
[http://dx.doi.org/10.3389/fphys.2018.00320]

[90] Liu Q, Zhang FG, Zhang WS, Pan A, Yang YL, Liu JF, *et al.* Ginsenoside Rg1 inhibits glucagon-induced hepatic gluconeogenesis through Akt-FoxO1 interaction 2017. http://www.thno.org/v07p4001.htm
[http://dx.doi.org/10.7150/thno.18788]

[91] Song B, Ding L, Zhang H, *et al.* Ginsenoside Rb1 increases insulin sensitivity through suppressing 11β-hydroxysteroid dehydrogenase type I. Am J Transl Res 2017; 9(3): 1049-57. https://www.ncbi.nlm.nih.gov/pubmed/28386332 [Internet].
[PMID: 28386332]

[92] Yu H, Zhen J, Yang Y, Gu J, Wu S, Liu Q. Ginsenoside Rg1 ameliorates diabetic cardiomyopathy by inhibiting endoplasmic reticulum stress-induced apoptosis in a streptozotocin-induced diabetes rat model. J Cell Mol Med [Internet]. 2016 Apr [cited 2019 Sep 5]; 20(4): 623–31. Available from: http://doi.wiley.com/10.1111/jcmm.12739

[93] Shi Y, Wan X, Shao N, Ye R, Zhang N, Zhang Y. Protective and anti-angiopathy effects of ginsenoside Re against diabetes mellitus via the activation of p38 MAPK, ERK1/2 and JNK signaling. Mol Med Rep [Internet]. 2016 Nov [cited 2019 Sep 5]; 14(5): 4849–56. Available from: https://www.spandidos-publications.com/10.3892/mmr.2016.5821

[94]   Yu H, Zhen J, Pang B, Gu J, Wu S. Ginsenoside Rg1 ameliorates oxidative stress and myocardial apoptosis in streptozotocin-induced diabetic rats. J Zhejiang Univ B [Internet]. 2015 May 12 [cited 2019 Sep 5]; 16(5): 344–54. Available from: http://link.springer.com/10.1631/jzus.B1400204

[95]   Miura T, Itoh Y, Kaneko T, Ueda N, Ishida T, Fukushima M, *et al.* Corosolic acid induces GLUT4 translocation in genetically type 2 diabetic mice. Biol Pharm Bull [Internet]. 2004 Jul [cited 2019 Aug 16]; 27(7): 1103–5. Available from: http://www.ncbi.nlm.nih.gov/pubmed/15256748

[96]   Miura T, Ueda N, Yamada K, Fukushima M, Ishida T, Kaneko T, *et al.* Antidiabetic effects of corosolic acid in KK-Ay diabetic mice. Biol Pharm Bull [Internet]. 2006 Mar [cited 2019 Aug 31]; 29(3): 585–7. Available from: http://www.ncbi.nlm.nih.gov/pubmed/16508174 http://www.ncbi.nlm.nih.gov/ pubmed/16508174

[97]   Shi L, Zhang W, Zhou YY, Zhang YN, Li JY, Hu LH, *et al.* Corosolic acid stimulates glucose uptake via enhancing insulin receptor phosphorylation. Eur J Pharmacol [Internet]. 2008 Apr 14 [cited 2019 Aug 31]; 584(1): 21–9. Available from: http://www.ncbi.nlm.nih.gov/pubmed/18348886

[98]   Lee MS, Thuong PT. Stimulation of glucose uptake by triterpenoids from *Weigela subsessilis*. Phyther Res [Internet]. 2010 Jan [cited 2019 Aug 31]; 24(1): 49–53. Available from: http://www.ncbi.nlm.nih.gov/pubmed/19548274

[99]   Zhang B, Xing Y, Wen C, Yu X, Sun W, Xiu Z, *et al.* Pentacyclic triterpenes as α-glucosidase and α-amylase inhibitors: Structure-activity relationships and the synergism with acarbose. Bioorg Med Chem Lett [Internet]. 2017 Nov 15 [cited 2019 Aug 31]; 27(22): 5065–70. Available from: http://www.ncbi.nlm.nih.gov/ pubmed/28964635

[100]   Ni M, Pan J, Hu X, Gong D, Zhang G. Inhibitory effect of corosolic acid on α □glucosidase: kinetics, interaction mechanism, and molecular simulation. J Sci Food Agric [Internet]. 2019 Jul 10 [cited 2019 Aug 31];jsfa.9862. Available from: http://www.ncbi.nlm.nih.gov/pubmed/31206698

[101]   Yamada K, Hosokawa M, Fujimoto S, Fujiwara H, Fujita Y, Harada N, *et al.* Effect of corosolic acid on gluconeogenesis in rat liver. Diabetes Res Clin Pract [Internet]. 2008 Apr [cited 2019 Aug 16]; 80(1): 48–55. Available from: http://www.ncbi.nlm.nih.gov/ pubmed/18177973

[102]   Yamaguchi Y, Yamada K, Yoshikawa N, Nakamura K, Haginaka J, Kunitomo M. Corosolic acid prevents oxidative stress, inflammation and hypertension in SHR/NDmcr-cp rats, a model of metabolic syndrome. Life Sci [Internet]. 2006 Nov [cited 2019 Aug 31]; 79(26): 2474–9. Available from: https://linkinghub.elsevier.com/retrieve/pii/S0024320506006400

[103]   Chen H, Yang J, Zhang Q, Chen LH, Wang Q. Corosolic acid ameliorates atherosclerosis in apolipoprotein E-deficient mice by regulating the nuclear factor-κB signaling pathway and inhibiting monocyte chemoattractant protein-1 expression. Circ J [Internet]. 2012 [cited 2019 Aug 31]; 76(4): 995–1003. Available from: http://joi.jlc.jst.go.jp/JST.JSTAGE/circj/CJ-11- 0344?from=CrossRef

[104]   Luna VF, Ibarra AC, Camacho CM, Rojas MA, Rojas MJ, Garcia A, *et al.* Vasodilator activity of compounds isolated from plants used in mexican traditional medicine. Molecules [Internet]. 2018 Jun 18 [cited 2019 Aug 17]; 23(6): 1474. Available from: http://www.ncbi.nlm.nih.gov/pubmed/ 29912156

[105]   Torres DA, Eloy R, Moustapha B, Cesar IA, Edmundo MS, Jesus CR, *et al.* Vasorelaxing effect and possible chemical markers of the flowers of the Mexican Crataegus gracilior. Nat Prod Res [Internet]. 2019 Mar 13 [cited 2019 Aug 31]; 1–4. Available from: http://www.ncbi.nlm.nih.gov/pubmed/ 30864868

[106]   Lee MS, Thuong PT. Stimulation of glucose uptake by triterpenoids from *Weigela subsessilis*. Phyther Res [Internet]. 2010 Jan 1 [cited 2019 Aug 16]; 24(1): 49-53. Available from: http://doi.wiley.com/ 10.1002/ptr.2865

[107] Estrada O, Alvarado CC, Fernandez A, Lopez M, Romero VE, Vasquez J, *et al.* Pomolic Acid isolated from the leaves of *Licania pittieri* inhibits ADP- and epinephrine-induced platelet aggregation and has hypotensive effect on rats. Curr Bioact Compd [Internet]. 2009 Sep 1 [cited 2019 Aug 16]; 5(3): 219–25. Available from: http://www.eurekaselect.com/openurl/content.php?genre=article& issn=1573-4072&volume=5&issue=3&spage=219

Antidiabetic and Antihypertensive Medicinal Plants of Asia: Active Ingredients, Safety, Pharmacology, and Traditional Uses

Subrata Das[1], Anupam Das Talukdar[1], Manabendra Dutta Choudhury[1] and Sanjoy Singh Ningthoujam[2,*]

[1] *Department of Life Science and Bioinformatics, Assam University, Silchar, India*

[2] *Department of Botany, Ghanapriya Women's College, Dhanamanjuri University, Imphal, India*

Abstract: Diabetes mellitus and hypertension are the two most common diseases in modern civilized countries. It is suggested that hypertension is more likely to be associated with type II diabetes as the patient acquires both diseases at old age. Though several therapeutic approaches were developed to treat the complications, plant-based therapeutics remains one of the most promising approaches. Moreover, traditional medicine remains as a primary health care system in the resource constraint societies. The use of medicinal plants for therapeutic uses has a long tradition in Asia in the form of Ayurveda, Traditional Chinese Medicine, Unani, Jamu, *etc*. In recent years, the scientific community has focused on natural products derived from ethnomedicinal plants for their wide therapeutic potentials, including diabetes mellitus and hypertension. Phenformin, metformin, repaglinide (Prandin), nateglinide (Starlix), pioglitazone, rosiglitazone, acarbose, miglitol are some of the antidiabetic marketed drugs of plant origin. Lignans, cinnamaldehyde, and protodioscin are newly isolated anti-diabetic drugs from plant sources. This chapter attempts to highlight the medicinal plants of Asia used for antidiabetic and antihypertensive purposes with regard to their phytochemical potentials, biosafety, and scientific evaluation of their traditional uses.

Keywords: Antidiabetic, Antihypertensive, Asia, Medicinal plants, Plant-based therapeutics, Traditional medicine.

INTRODUCTION

Diabetes

Diabetes mellitus (DM) is an important chronic disease triggered by an inappropriate balance of glucose homeostasis [1]. DM is a severe chronic

* **Corresponding author Sanjoy Singh Ningthoujam:** Department of Botany, Ghanapriya Women's College, Dhanamanjuri University, Imphal, India; Email: ningthouja@hotmail.com

M. Eddouks (Ed.)

metabolic disorder that affects health, quality of life, and life expectancy of patients, as well as the health care system. According to the World Health Organization (WHO), 171 million people worldwide suffer from diabetes; this number is expected to be more than double by 2030 and around 3.2 million deaths every year are attributable due to diabetes; six deaths every single minute [2]. Reports of the WHO showed that the diabetes epidemic is more pronounced in India than in other parts of the world. 32 million people had diabetes in the year 2000 [3]. The International Diabetes Federation (IDF) estimates the total number of diabetic condition subjects to be around 40.9 million in India, and this is further set to increase to 69.9 million by the year 2025. Reports of WHO have also shown that non-insulin-dependent diabetes mellitus (NIDDM) and its complications are increasing in sub-Saharan Africa. and the incidence of the disease is growing annually [4]. Diabetes is the most heterogeneous challenging disease. It can merely be categorized into type 1 diabetes mellitus and type 2 diabetes mellitus [5]. The distinction between type 1 and type 2 diabetes mellitus solely depends on the clinical appearance, such as age at disease commencement, the incidence of ketosis, and insulin dependence. Type 1 diabetes mellitus, occurring mainly in childhood or young adulthood, is earmarked by T cell-mediated autoimmune destruction of beta cells, absolute insulin dependence, and the need for insulin treatment. Type 2 diabetes mellitus, mainly occurring in adulthood, is the outcome of insulin resistance and relative insulin deficit [6]. Diabetes or hyperglycaemic condition can be caused through the inhibition of key enzymes α-glucosidase and α-amylase for starch digestion. Drugs that are in use now, such as miglitol, acarbose, nojirimycin, voglibose, and 1-deoxynojirimycin possess unbearable toxicity, which triggers the finding of natural inhibitors of glucosidase and amylase from the plant sources [7].

Hypertension

High blood pressure or hypertension (HTN) is a common cardiovascular complication, which has become a global problem. 15–20% of all adults with ailments, such as arteriosclerosis, stroke, myocardial infarction, and end-stage renal diseases are due to hypertension [8]. It is stated that NIDDM is the result of prolonged hypertension complications. These two diseases (NIDDM and hypertension) are interconnected metabolic syndromes. Prolonged persistent hypertension serves as a risk factor for stroke and chronic renal failure [9]. Angiotensin-I converting enzyme (ACE) is a key enzyme that controls the regulation of blood pressure. It translates angiotensin I to angiotensin II, which is an effective vasoconstrictor. The inhibition of ACE activity provides an antihypertensive potential by simultaneously lowering blood pressure in non-diabetic and diabetic patients [10]. Lisinopril, captopril, and enalapril are drugs currently used as ACE inhibitors and have been reported to be harmless and effective. Search for non-toxic ACE inhibitors provides a direction towards the use of dietary phenolic phytochemicals and is shown to have promising effectiveness [11]. In recent decades, the consumption of vegetables for antihypertensive and antidiabetic phytochemicals has attracted growing interest. Many experimental and epidemiological studies have reliably verified a positive connection between the intake of these natural foodstuffs and reduced risks of several degenerative diseases, including NIDDM [7]. Phytochemical rich foods consist of several antioxidants, especially antioxidative vitamins, including ascorbic acid (vitamin C), α-tocopherol (vitamin E), and β-carotene (provitamin A), which may provide a defensive role against these complications. Studies indicated that polyphenolic compounds are the main phytochemicals, with greater antioxidant properties found in plants [7]. Phenolics in plant products are present in free or aglycone and bound or glycoside forms [12]. The free phenolics are more easily absorbed and thus provide helpful bioactivities in food assimilation. However, the number of different bound phenolics are assimilated and absorbed at several sites of the gastrointestinal tract where they do their duty for the benefit of health [7]. Type 2 diabetes mellitus and hypertension are two highly predominant diseases among the aged that make them vulnerable to vascular disease. The occurrence of type 2 diabetes in the age group of 65 years and older is approximately between 15% and 25% [13], whereas, for hypertension, the range is between 50% and 70% [14].

Diabetes and Hypertension

Diabetes and hypertension are interconnected in most diabetic people and the prevalence of getting hypertension is two folds that of the non-diabetic person [15, 16]. Prolonged diabetes damages arteries and causes a condition called atherosclerosis. This condition leads to the development of high blood pressure along with other circulatory hindrance. In type 2 diabetes due to insulin resistance, hyperinsulinemia develops, which regulates the Angiotensin-I converting enzyme to convert Angiotensin-I to Angiotensin-II. As a result, Angiotensin-II regulates the vasoconstriction and develops hypertension in diabetic condition [10]. Below mentioned Fig. (**1**) demonstrates the connection link between diabetes and hypertension.

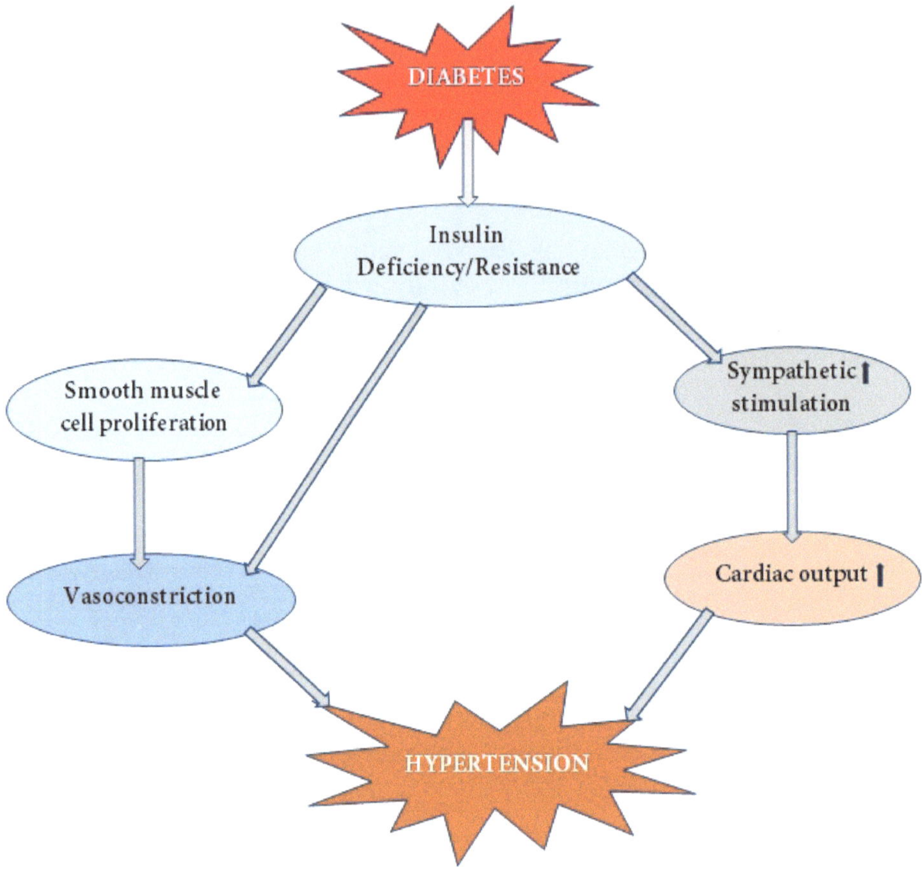

Fig. (1). Relation between Diabetes and Hypertension.

ANTIDIABETIC MEDICINAL PLANTS OF ASIA AND THEIR ACTIVE INGREDIENTS IN TRADITIONAL USES

Brassica juncea (L.) Czern

This plant is usually used as a spice in food preparation and belongs to the Brassicaceae family. The seed extract of the plant is used as a potent hypoglycemic agent which was examined in streptozotocin(STZ)-induced diabetic male albino rat [17]. The bioactive phytochemical compounds found in the plant include flavonoids, phenolic acids, carotenoids (lutein, zeaxanthin, β-carotene), polyphenols, alkaloids, saponins, tannins, phytosterols chlorophyll, anthocyanins, phytosterols, glucosinolates, glycosides, terpenoids, Vitamin E, vitamin C, aliphatic and aromatic amines [18].

Syzygium cumini (L.) Skeels

S. cumini, the native Indian tree, belongs to the Myrtaceae family and popularly known as Indian blackberry or Jamun. The ancient system of Indian medicine Ayurveda indicated the use of its fruits in diabetes. This plant is found in the Asian sub-continent and tropical regions of the world. Ripened fruits are deep purple berries similar in appearance to the purple grape. The pulp of the Jamun berry contains the delphinidin, malvidin glucosides, anthocyanins, and petunidin, which produce its bright purple colour. The seed and fruit pulp extracts of the Jamun have been known to possess antidiabetic properties [19].

Coccinia grandis (L.) Voigt

It is a perennial climbing herb that spread vegetatively or by seed. It belongs to the Cucurbitaceae family and commonly known as scarlet gourd, Ivy gourd, Tindora. It is native to India, Asia, and Central Africa. The leaves show antidiabetic, hypoglycemic, and antioxidant activities [20]. The bioactive compounds include secondary metabolites like glycoside, bamyrine, alkaloids, saponin, lupeol, cephalandrine, cephalandrol, cucurbitacin, and flavonoids [21].

Alangium salviifolium (L.f.) Wangerin

A. salvifolium is a small deciduous tree of 10–15 m height, it flowers between February and June. It is widely distributed in South East Asia, *i.e.,* India to China, Thailand, Philippines, Indonesia, and Papua New Guinea. It belongs to the Alangiaceae family. In Indian traditional medicine, it is widely used as an antidiabetic, antiulcer, analgesic, anti-inflammatory agent [22]. Preliminary phytochemical study reveals the presence of various compounds like tubulosine, psychotrine, cephaeline, isotobulosine, and alangiside in roots, alangicine, marckidine, dimethyl psychotrine, marckine, land amarckinine in root bark, alangimarkine, deoxytobulosine, ankorine, alangine, sterols and three triterpenoids, N-methylcephaeline, cepheline, deoxytobulosine in fruits and alamanine, alangimarine, emetine, alangimaridine, psychotrine, and cephaeline in seeds [23].

Albizia odoratissima (L.f.) Benth

A. odoratissima belongs to the Mimosaceae family and is usually known as 'Black Siris'. The bark is acrid, astringent, depurative, cooling, expectorant, and useful against bronchitis, cough, diabetes & burning sensation [24]. Bark and leaf extract of the plant revealed the presence of carbohydrates, flavonoids, glycosides, steroids, phenolic compounds, tannins, and saponin, such as echinocystic acid, oleanolic acid, acacic acid, lactone or machaerinic acid γ-lacton [25, 26].

Axonopus compressus (Sw.) P.Beauv

It is commonly known as broadleaf carpet grass. It is an invasive weed in the paddy field but a grass that is generally used as permanent pasture, ground cover, and turf in moist low fertility soils, particularly in shaded situations. A perennial graminoid or grass-like plant is widely naturalized in the humid tropics and subtropics especially West tropical Africa, South Africa, India, the Philippines, Indonesia, Australia, and the Pacific Islands. The methanolic leaf extract of the plant possesses antidiabetic activity in alloxan-induced diabetic rats [27]. The phytochemicals in the extracts are alkaloid, saponin, inulin, β-sitosterol, and tannin respectively which exert antidiabetic activity [28].

Berberis vulgaris L.

B. vulgaris belongs to the Berberidaceae family. It is a well-known cultivated medicinal plant in Asia and Europe. The phytochemical screening of genus Berberis has led to the isolation of phenolic compounds, alkaloids, sterols, tannins, and triterpenes [29]. In *B. vulgaris* berberine is the major compound isolated and this component is responsible for the antidiabetic activity [30]. Berberine is an isoquinoline alkaloid produced by the plants [31, 32].

Caesalpinia digyna Rottler

*C. digyna*belongs to the Fabaceae family and is a scandent, large, prickly shrub or climber, growing wild in the scrub forests of the Himalayas. The root extract of *C. digyna* is used as antidiabetic, antitubercular, and radioprotective agents [33]. Chemicals profiling of the extract revealed the presence of cellallocinnine, caesalpinine A, gallic acid, bergenin, pipecolic acid, ellagic acid, friedelin, hexacosanoic acid, β-sitosterol, and stigmasterol [34].

Catharanthus roseus (L.) G.Don

C. roseus is an evergreen shrub or herbaceous plant, which is less than 1 m in height. It belongs to the Apocynaceae family. It consists of several important alkaloids which are useful in diabetes, asthma, constipation, blood pressure, cancer, and menstrual problem [35]. Commonly *C. roseus* is known as Periwinkle or Rosy Periwinkle in Southern Asia. The Phytochemical evaluation shows the presence of alkaloids like vinblastin, vincristine, vindeline, vindesine, actineoplastidemeric, and tabersonine in aerial parts whereas vinceine, ajmalicine, raubasin, vineamine, catharanthine, reserpine are present in roots and basal stem. An anthocyanin pigment rosindin is found in the flower of *C. roseus* [36].

Centaurium erythraea Rafn

C. erythraea is a flowering plant belonging to the family Gentianaceae. It is a biennial herb that grows up to half a meter. It is commonly known as a common centaury. It is reported to have antidiabetic activity in STZ-induced diabetes mice [37]. Phytochemical investigation of the plant revealed several plant secondary metabolites, including centapiricin, centauroside, flavonoids, gentiopicroside, gentiopicrin, isocumarin, phenolic acids, and their derivatives, swertiamarin, terpenoids, and xanthones. Among these Swertiamarin is the key compound found in the plant along with others such as p-coumaric, ferulic, O-hydroxyphenyl acetic, eustomin, protocatechuic, vanillic, sinapic, syringic, hydroxyterephthalic, oleanolic acid, 2,5-dihydroxy-terephthalic acids, β-sitosterol, campesterol, and stigmasterol [38].

Aeglemarmelos (L.) Correa

This plant belongs to the family Rutaceae. The plant is very common in the Indian sub-continent and grows in the deciduous forest. The fruits of this plant play an important role in Indian ayurvedic medicine for curing diabetes mellitus [39]. The plant is commonly known as a wood apple or Bel or Holy fruit tree. The root bark extract of the plant showed hypoglycemic activity, leaf extract produced insulin-like activity in diabetic rats [40]. Fruit extract possesses antidiabetic, anti-hyperlipidemic, and antioxidant activity in STZ diabetic rats [41]. The phyto-chemical profiling of the bel obtained many compounds such as Isoamyl acetate, Hexanal, β-phellandrene, Limonene, Acetoin, p-cymenne, (E)-2-octenal, dehydro-p-cymene, Linalool oxide, α-cubebene, trans-p-mentha-2,8-dienol, 3,5-Octadiene-2-one, β-cubebene, Citronellal, β-caryophyllene, Pulegone, Hexadecane, α-humulene, Carvone, Verbenone, dihydro-β-ionone, Carvyl acetate, E-6,10-dimethyl-5,9-undecadien-2-one, Caryophyllene oxide, β-ionone, Hexadecanoic acid and humulene oxide [42].

Allium cepa L.

It is a widely cultivated plant throughout India. It belongs to the family Liliaceae and it is commonly known as onion. The leaves and bulb of onion play an important part in the diet. The bulb of onion is utilized as a food component to provide flavour and fragrance to a great variety of dishes. It is observed that ether extracts of onion, lower the blood sugar level in normal rabbits [43]. Prolonged treatment with onion containing diet produced a hypoglycemic effect in diabetic rats [44]. Onions are a significant source of phytonutrients as flavonoids, fructooligosaccharides, and thiosulfonates, which play a vital role in the Mediterranean diet [45]. Quercetins are the most abundant flavonoids found in onions which consist of high levels of phenolic compounds and a rich source of anthocyanins with antidiabetic and antioxidant activities [45].

Allium sativum **L.**

A. sativum is commonly called as garlic and is used as a flavoring substance in food. It belongs to the family Amaryllidaceae. From ancient times the plant is known for its ethnomedicinal properties. It is now cultivated worldwide for food and medicine. Allicin, a compound isolated from garlic, showed hypoglycemia in mild diabetic rabbits [46]. In an experiment, alloxan-induced diabetic rats fed with *A. sativum* for 15 days could reduce the blood glucose level as compared to the control group [47]. Allicin, Diallyltrisulphide, and Bis(allixinato)oxovanadium are three important compounds in the garlic for its antidiabetic activity [48].

Aloe vera **(L.) Burm. F.**

It is commonly known as Aloe and it belongs to the family Liliaceae. In Indian Ayurveda, it is widely used for its medicinal properties and cultivated throughout Indian states. The extract of the plant has a prominent anti-hyperglycemic activity in type 2 diabetes [49]. Leaf pulp extract of *A. vera* exhibited hypoglycemic activity on type 1 and type 2 diabetic rats, the effect becomes enhanced in type 2 diabetes as related to glibenclamide [50]. Important phytosterols of *A. vera* are lophenol, 24-ethyl-lophenol, 24-methyl-lophenol, cycloartenol and 24-methylene-cycloartenol [51].

Andrographispaniculata **(Burm. F.) Nees**

It is an annual herb belonging to the family of Acanthaceae and in Indian Ayurveda, it is known as *Kalamegha* meaning dark cloud. Commonly, it is known as chireta or king of bitterness. Plant extract efficiently produced anti-hyperglycemic and hypoglycemic activity in normal rats [52]. In the alloxan-induced diabetic rat, the estrous cycle was restored due to the antidiabetic potentials of the plant extract [53]. Andrographolide, labdane, lactone, 14-deoxyandrographolide, neoandrographolide, andrograpanin, isoandrographolide, 14-deoxy-11, 12-didehydroandrographolide, and 14-deoxy-14,15-didehydro-andrographolide are some of the phytochemicals isolated from the plant [54].

Annona squamosa **L.**

A squamosa is a semi-deciduous tree, with a broad, open crown or spreading branches, widely available in India. It is under the family Annonaceae. It is commonly known as the custard apple or sugar apple tree. The plant is known for its medicinal and nutraceuticals properties. In Northern India, the plant is used for its anti-diabetic properties and aqueous leaf extract showed hypoglycemic activity in diabetic rats [55]. The fruit pulp extract of the plant has been shown to recover the glucose tolerance of alloxan-diabetic rats [56]. Bioactive phytochemicals isolated from the plant are squamocenin, reticulatain-2, annotemoyin-2, squamocin-B, motrilin, squamostatin-D, squamocin, squamocin-I, squamostatin-E, cherimolin-1 and cherimolin-2 [57].

Azadirachtaindica A. Juss

A. indica is commonly known as Neem or Indian lilac tree. It is an evergreen tree of the Indian subcontinent. It is under the family Meliaceae of the Angiosperm. From ancient time neem tree has been used for various medicinal purposes. Aqueous extract of leaf showed hypoglycemic activity in normal rats [58]. Crude ethanol extract of the leaf has the potential to lower the blood sugar level of alloxan-diabetic rats [59]. The important constituents for the medicinal property of the plants are azadirachtin, nimbin, nimbolinin, salannin, nimbidol, nimbidin, gedunin, sodium nimbinate, quercetin, ascorbic acid, nimbanene, 6-desacetylnimbinene, n-hexacosanol, nimbandiol, nimbolide, nimbiol amino acid, 7-desacetyl-7-benzoylgedunin, ß-sitosterol, 7-desacetyl-7-benzoylazadiradione, 17-hydroxyazadiradione, and polyphenolic flavonoids [60].

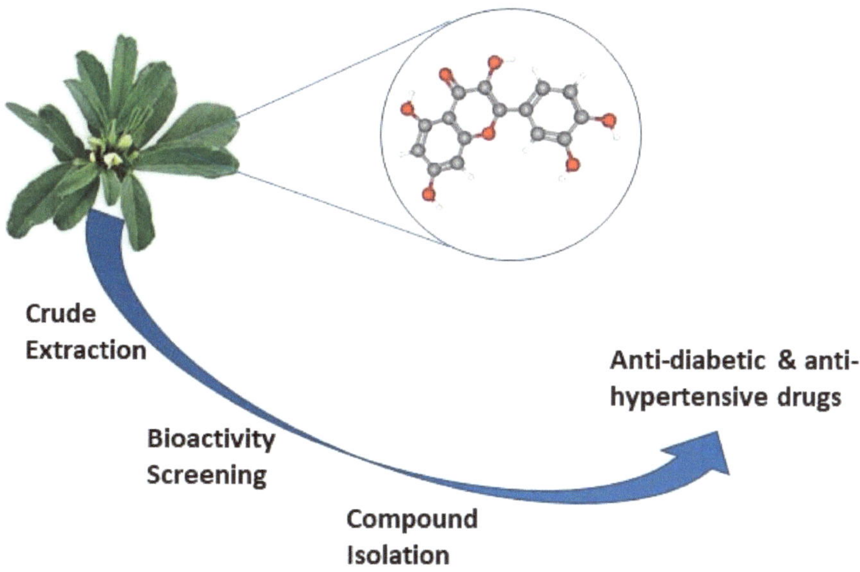

Fig. (2). Schematic representation of anti-diabetic & anti-hypertensive drug development from natural product.

Cinnamomumtamala (Buch. -Ham.) T. Nees & Eberm

It is commonly known as Indian bay leaf or tejapatta and belongs to the family Lauraceae. The leaf of the plant is used as a spice and it is cultivated in different parts of India [61]. Powdered leaf extract of the plant is known to possess antidiabetic activity [62]. Isolated major bioactive compounds of the plant are eugenol, methyl eugenol, Beta-Caryophyllene, trans-cinnamyl acetate, cinnamaldehyde, Tans-cinnamyl acetate, and ascabin [63].

Table 1. Some other antidiabetic plant and their traditional uses.

S. No.	Plant Name	Traditional Uses
1	*Swertia chirayita* (Roxb.) Buch. -Ham. ex C.B.Clarke	antidiabetic, antimicrobial, anticholinergic and chemopreventive [64]
2	*Solanum melongena* L.	antidiabetic [2], Analgesic activity [65], Anti-inflammatory activity [66]
3	*Momordica dioica* Roxb.ex Willd.	antidiabetic, hepatoprotective, antihypertensive, anti-inflammatory, antiasthmatic, antipyretic, antileprosy [67]
4	*Momordica charantia* L.	Antidiabetic [68], anti-inflammatory, anti-tumor, antimicrobial [69]
5	*Coriandrum sativum* L.	antidiabetic [70], antibacterial, antifungal and anti-oxidative [71]
6	*Olea europaea* L.	antidiabetic [70], antidiabetic, anticonvulsant, antioxidant, anti-inflammatory, immunomodulatory, analgesic, antimicrobial, antiviral, antihypertensive, anticancer, antihyperglycemic, antinociceptive, gastroprotective [72]
7	*Ferula assa-foetida* L.	antidiabetic [70], anticancer, anti-inflammatory, antimicrobial [73]
8	*Trigonella foenum-graecum* L.	antidiabetic [68, 70], anticholesterolemic, anti-inflammatory, antitumor, carminative [74]
9	*Citrus macroptera* Montr.	antidiabetic [75], antimicrobial [76]
10	*Linumus itatissimum* L.	antidiabetic, atherosclerosis, hypertension [77, 78]
11	*Anacardium occidentale* L.	antidiabetic, anti-inflammatory, antimicrobial and analgesic [79]
12	*Annona muricata* L.	antidiabetic, anti-inflammatory, antihypertension, anticancer [57, 80]
13	*Dichrostachys cinerea* (L.) Wight & Arn.	antidiabetic [81], antibacterial [82]
14	*Phaseolus vulgaris* L.	antidiabetic, cardiovascular disease [83]
15	*Ocimum gratissimum* L.	antidiabetic, anti-inflammatory [84]

(Table 1) cont.....

S. No.	Plant Name	Traditional Uses
16	*Moringa oleifera* Lam.	antidiabetic, hypercholesterolemia, high blood pressure, insulin resistance, non-alcoholic liver disease, cancer and inflammation [85]
17	*Psidiumguajava* L.	diabetes, diarrhea, dysentery, gastroenteritis, hypertension [86]
18	*Cymbopogon citratus* (DC.) Stapf	diabetes, cancer, obesity, cardiovascular diseases [87]
19	*Parkia timoriana* (DC.) Merr	antibacterial, antidiabetic, antiproliferative [88]
20	*Oxalis corniculata* L.	antidiabetic, anti-inflammatory, antifungal, antiulcer, antinociceptive, anticancer, hepatoprotective [89]

ANTIHYPERTENSIVE MEDICINAL PLANTS OF ASIA AND THEIR ACTIVE INGREDIENTS IN TRADITIONAL USES

Apiumgraveolens L.

A. graveolens is commonly known as Celery and it belongs to the family Apiaceae. The plant is cultivated for vegetables all around the world and its seeds are also useful for spices. The plant is known for its antihypertensive activity in Chinese medicine. It has been stated the extract of the plant lowers systolic and diastolic blood pressure [90]. The phytochemicals responsible for the HTN activity are celerin, apiumetin, bergapten, osthenol, apiumoside, isopimpinellin, apigravrin, isoimperatorin, 8-hydroxy methoxypsoralen, graveobioside A and B, apigenin, isoquercitrin, apiin, phytic acid and celereoside [91].

Aristolochia manshuriensis Kom

In China, it is commonly known as Guan Mu Tong, and it belongs to the family Aristolochiaceae. In Chinese traditional medicine, the extract of the plant is used for its hypotensive properties. The bioactive components responsible for the activity are magnoflorine, aristolochic acid, hederagenin, aristoloside, oleanolic acid, and tannins [92].

Avena sativa L.

A. sativa belongs to the family Poaceae. It is commonly known as green oat and is now cultivated worldwide. The cereal grains are consumed for their high dietary fiber and antioxidants. A diet rich in soluble fiber in whole oats significantly lower the blood pressure in hypertensive conditions and improve blood pressure control. It is an effective dietary therapy for the prevention of HTN [93]. Oat grains are the rich source of protein, important minerals, a mixed-linkage polysaccharide, lipids, β-glucan, which form an important part of dietary oat fiber, and also contains other phyto-elements like avenanthramides, flavonoids, flavonolignans, an indole alkaloid-gramine, triterpenoid, sterols, saponins, and tocols [94].

Plantagoovata **Forssk**

It is commonly known as blond psyllium or isabgol and falls under the family Plantaginaceae. The psyllium is very rich in dietary fiber and is useful in Indian traditional medicine. A study shows that taking *P. ovata* supplements daily can lower blood pressure. Plantagin, anvrtyn, aucubin, diastase, hetrozeid, plantenolic acid, succinic acid, and aeocoeine are some of the phytoconstituents found in the plant [95].

Camellia sinensis **(L.) Kuntze**

It is an evergreen perennial shrub or small tree that belongs to the family Theaceae. It is commonly known as the Tea plant as tea is obtained from the leaf of the plant. Tea possesses many types of medicinal properties and is a common beverage taken in worldwide. Population research shows that consumption of green tea and oolong tea decreased the risk of developing HTN [96]. Bioactive phytochemicals of tea revealed the presence of caffeine, gallic acid, (-) - epicatechin, (+)-catechin, (-)-epiafzelechin, theobromine,(+)-afzelechin-3-O-gallate, (-) -epicatechin-3-O-gallate, ampelopsin, quemefin-3-O-alpha-L- arabino pyranosid, (+)-catechin-3-O-gallate, (-)-epiafzelechin-3-O-gallate, and (-)-epica techin-3-O-p-hydroxybenzoate [97].

Trachyspermumammi **(L.) Sprague**

T. ammi is commonly known as Ajwain. It falls under the family Umbelliferae. The seed or fruit of the plant is mostly used in the cuisine of India, Pakistan, Afghanistan. In an experiment, it was found that the crude extract of the plant shows a fall in blood pressure and heart rate of anesthetized normotensive rats [98]. 3-methyl-2-butenyl- γ –glucoside, P-hydroxy benzoic acid,γ -sitosteryl-glucoside-6'- octadecanoate, bis(5-formylfurfuryl) ether 5- (hydroxymethyl) furfural; daucosterol; uracil; α-D-fructofuranosides methyl; cappariside (4-hydroxy-5- methylfuran-3-carboxylic acid), stachydrine, corchoionoside C ((6S,9S)-roseoside), (6S)-hydroxy-3-oxo-a-ionol glucosides and prenylglucoside are some of the phytochemicals of the plant [99].

Chamaecristaabsus (L.) H.S.Irwin & Barne by

C. absus is commonly known as Chaksu and belongs to family Fabaceae. It is dispersed throughout India and Sri Lanka. In the Indian traditional system of Ayurveda, the plant has been used from long ancient times. A study shows that an intravenous administration of the crude extract of the plant reduces blood pressure in a dose-dependent manner and also decreases heart rate at higher doses [100]. Isochaksine, Luteolin, Allelochemical, Galactomannan, Linoleic acid, Raffinose, and Beta-sitosterol are isolated from the seed of the plant [101].

Sennaoccidentalis (L.) Link

It is commonly called as Coffee weed and belongs to the family Fabaceae. It is an annual herb or shrub and a common weed throughout India. The leaf of the plant is used as an antihypertensive principle in the ethnic medicine system. A study showed that crude extract of leaf reduced blood pressure by relaxing the smooth muscle and inhibiting Ca^{2+} influx channel [102]. Chrysophanol, jaceidin-7-rhamnoside, emodin, metteucinol-7-rhamnoside,physcion, 4, 4, 5, 5-tetrahydroxy-2,2- dimethyl-1,1-bianthraquinone, pinselin (cassiallin), aloe-emodin,rhein, islandicin, xanthorin, helminthosporin, sitosterol, campesterol, stigmasterol, 1,8-dihydroxyanthraquinone; α-hydroxyanthraquinone, 1,7- dihydroxy-3-methoxy-xanthone quercetin, germichrysone, questin, singueanol-I,methylgermitorosone, pinselin; bis(tetrahydro)anthracene derivatives; occidentalol-1,occidentalol-II, C-glycosidic flavonoids, cassiaoccidentalins A, B and C flavonoids, anthraquinones, 1,8-dihydroxy-2- methylanthraquinone; 1,4,5-trihydroxy-7-methoxy-3- methyl-anthraquinone, and N-methyl- morpholine are some of the phytoconstituents of the plant isolated [103].

Coleus forskohlii (Willd.) Briq

C. forskohlii belongs to the family Lamiaceae and it is commonly known as Karpurvali. In Indian Ayurveda, the plant is used to treat heart diseases. Coleonol, a diterpene isolated from the plant, has been shown to reduce the blood pressure of anesthetized cats and rats [104]. The phytochemicals isolated from the plant are oleanolic acid, chamaecydin, forskolin G, betulinic acid, 6 alpha-hydroxydeme-thylcryptojaponol, alpha-cedrene, forskolin H, forskolin A, forskolin J, 6-acetyl-1-deoxyforskolin, and beta-sitosterol [105].

Cuscuta reflexa Roxb

C. reflexa occurs throughout India. It is commonly known as dodder and belongs to the family Convolvulaceae. The plant is very important in terms of ethnomedicinal perspective. The extract of the plant is known to possess antihypertensive activity. It has been found to reduce systolic and diastolic blood pressure in anesthetized rats [106]. The bioactive phytoconstituents isolated from the plant are lauric acid, palmitic acid, myristic acid, palmitoleic acid, stearic acid, diterpene, Phenol, 3,5-bis (1,1- dimethylethyl), squalene, and oleic acid [107].

Table 2. Some other antihypertensive plant and their traditional uses.

S. No.	Plant Name	Traditional Uses
1	*Zea mays* L.	Antihypertensive, anticancer, hypoglycemic and hypotensive [70]
2	*Allium cepa* L.	Antihypertensive [70], hypoglycemic [44]
3	*Olea europaea* L.	Antihypertensive [70], antidiabetic, anticonvulsant, antioxidant, anti-inflammatory, immunomodulatory [72]
4	*Allium sativum* L.	Antihypertensive [108], antidiabetic [47]
5	*Echinodorus grandiflorus* (Cham. & Schltdl.) Micheli	Antihypertensive [109], anti-inflammatory, diuretic, cardioprotective [110]
6	*Centaurea bruguierana* (DC.) Hand. - Mazz.	Antihypertensive [109], antidiabetic [111]
7	*Eruca vesicaria* (L.) Cav.	Antihypertensive [109], antigenotoxic, antidiuretic [112]
8	*Sechium edule* (Jacq.) Sw.	Antihypertensive [109], antidiabetic [113]
9	*Marrubium vulgare* L.	Antihypertensive [109], antispasmodic, antidiabetic, gastroprotective, anti-inflammatory, antimicrobial, anticancer [114]
10	*Moringa oleifera* Lam.	Antihypertensive [109], antidiabetic, hypercholesterolemia, insulin resistance, non-alcoholic liver disease, cancer and inflammation [85]
11	*Myristica fragrans* Houtt.	Antihypertensive [109], hypolipidemic, hypocholesterolemic, antimicrobial, antidepressant, aphrodisiac, memory enhancing, antioxidant and hepatoprotective [115]
12	*Coix lacryma-jobi* L.	Antihypertensive [109], anti-inflammatory, antioxidant, hypolipidemic, anticancer [116]
13	*Rubus brasiliensis* Mart.	Antihypertensive [109], antidiabetic, gastroprotective, anti-inflammatory, rheumatism, sore throat, antihemorrhoid [117]
14	*Solanum paniculatum* L.	Antihypertensive [109]
15	*Hedychium coronarium* J. Koenig	Antihypertensive [109]
16	*Lumnitzera racemosa* Willd.	Antihypertensive [118]
17	*Lycopersicon esculentum* Mill.	Antihypertensive [119]
18	*Ocimum basilicum* L.	Antihypertensive [120]

(Table 2) cont.....

S. No.	Plant Name	Traditional Uses
19	*Peganum harmala* L.	Antihypertensive [121]
20	*Phyllanthus amarus* Schumach. & Thonn.	Antihypertensive [92]
21	*Hibiscus sabdariffa* L.	Antihypertensive [122]
22	*Daucus carota* L.	Antihypertensive [123]

CONCLUSION

In the present scenario diabetes and hypertension are the two most common complications worldwide. Modernization of human culture and the use of techniques play a role in increasing obesity, diabetes, and hypertension. There is an urgent requirement of effective and nontoxic remediation for maintaining diabetes and hypertension worldwide. Natural compounds are believed to be a safe and non-toxic therapeutic agent for the development of the drug. Bioactivity analysis and toxicity screening of phytochemical compounds play an important role in the development of a drug for a particular ailment (Fig. **2**). Drugs from natural sources are safer than synthetic origin as these compounds show lesser or negligible toxicity. So, in recent times natural compounds are the best source of therapeutic drugs. In this context, the above illustration showed several antidiabetic and antihypertensive plants and their role in traditional medication. However, their sustainable use and proper validation of phytoconstituents with bioactivity analysis will play a major role in the management of the complication. And also, this will increase the chance of developing a novel compound for other such complications like anticancer, antitumor, anti-inflammatory, immunomodulatory conditions.

CONSENT FOR PUBLICATION

Not applicable.

CONFLICT OF INTEREST

There is no conflict of interest declared.

ACKNOWLEDGEMENTS

Declared none.

REFERENCES

[1]   Rossetti L, Giaccari A, DeFronzo RA. Glucose toxicity. Diabetes Care 1990; 13(6): 610-30.
[http://dx.doi.org/10.2337/diacare.13.6.610] [PMID: 2192847]

[2]   Kwon Y-I, Apostolidis E, Shetty K. *In vitro* studies of eggplant (*Solanum melongena*) phenolics as inhibitors of key enzymes relevant for type 2 diabetes and hypertension. Bioresour Technol 2008; 99(8): 2981-8.
[http://dx.doi.org/10.1016/j.biortech.2007.06.035] [PMID: 17706416]

[3]   Wild S, Roglic G, Green A, Sicree R, King H. Global prevalence of diabetes: estimates for the year 2000 and projections for 2030. Diabetes Care 2004; 27(5): 1047-53.
[http://dx.doi.org/10.2337/diacare.27.5.1047] [PMID: 15111519]

[4]   Choukem SP, Kengne AP, Dehayem YM, Simo NL, Mbanya JC. Hypertension in people with diabetes in sub-Saharan Africa: revealing the hidden face of the iceberg. Diabetes Res Clin Pract 2007; 77(2): 293-9.
[http://dx.doi.org/10.1016/j.diabres.2006.11.007] [PMID: 17184871]

[5]   Tuomi T, Santoro N, Caprio S, Cai M, Weng J, Groop L. The many faces of diabetes: a disease with increasing heterogeneity. Lancet 2014; 383(9922): 1084-94.
[http://dx.doi.org/10.1016/S0140-6736(13)62219-9] [PMID: 24315621]

[6]   Yi B, Huang G, Zhou Z. Different role of zinc transporter 8 between type 1 diabetes mellitus and type 2 diabetes mellitus. J Diabetes Investig 2016; 7(4): 459-65.
[http://dx.doi.org/10.1111/jdi.12441] [PMID: 27181765]

[7]   Adefegha SA, Oboh G. Antioxidant and inhibitory properties of Clerodendrumvolubile leaf extracts on key enzymes relevant to non-insulin-dependent diabetes mellitus and hypertension. J Taibah Uni Sci 2016; 10: 521-33.
[http://dx.doi.org/10.1016/j.jtusci.2015.10.008]

[8]   Je J-Y, Park P-J, Kim E-K, Ahn C-B. Antioxidant and angiotensin I converting enzyme inhibitory activity of Bambusae caulis in Liquamen. Food Chem 2009; 113: 932-5.
[http://dx.doi.org/10.1016/j.foodchem.2008.08.022]

[9]   Bakris GL, Williams M, Dworkin L, *et al.* Preserving renal function in adults with hypertension and diabetes: a consensus approach. Am J Kidney Dis 2000; 36(3): 646-61.
[http://dx.doi.org/10.1053/ajkd.2000.16225] [PMID: 10977801]

[10]   Pahor M, Psaty BM, Alderman MH, Applegate WB, Williamson JD, Furberg CD. Therapeutic benefits of ACE inhibitors and other antihypertensive drugs in patients with type 2 diabetes. Diabetes Care 2000; 23(7): 888-92.
[http://dx.doi.org/10.2337/diacare.23.7.888] [PMID: 10895836]

[11]   Li Q-L, Li B-G, Zhang Y, Gao X-P, Li C-Q, Zhang G-L. Three angiotensin-converting enzyme inhibitors from Rabdosia coetsa. Phytomedicine 2008; 15(5): 386-8.
[http://dx.doi.org/10.1016/j.phymed.2007.09.013] [PMID: 17977703]

[12]   Oboh G, Ademiluyi AO, Akinyemi AJ, Henle T, Saliu JA, Schwarzenbolz U. Inhibitory effect of polyphenol-rich extracts of jute leaf (Corchorusolitorius) on key enzyme linked to type 2 diabetes (α-amylase and α-glucosidase) and hypertension (angiotensin I converting) *in vitro*. J Funct Foods 2012; 4: 450-8.
[http://dx.doi.org/10.1016/j.jff.2012.02.003]

[13]   Fillenbaum GG, Pieper CF, Cohen HJ, Cornoni-Huntley JC, Guralnik JM. Comorbidity of five chronic health conditions in elderly community residents: determinants and impact on mortality. J Gerontol A Biol Sci Med Sci 2000; 55(2): M84-9.
[http://dx.doi.org/10.1093/gerona/55.2.M84] [PMID: 10737690]

[14]   Wolz M, Cutler J, Roccella EJ, Rohde F, Thom T, Burt V. Statement from the national high blood pressure education program: prevalence of hypertension. Am J Hypertens 2000; 13(1 Pt 1): 103-4.
[http://dx.doi.org/10.1016/S0895-7061(99)00241-1] [PMID: 10678279]

[15]   Epstein M, Sowers JR. Diabetes mellitus and hypertension. Hypertension 1992; 19(5): 403-18.
[http://dx.doi.org/10.1161/01.HYP.19.5.403] [PMID: 1568757]

[16]   Arayne MS, Sultana N, Mirza AZ, Siddiqui FA. Simultaneous determination of gliquidone, fexofenadine, buclizine, and levocetirizine in dosage formulation and human serum by RP-HPLC. J Chromatogr Sci 2010; 48(5): 382-5.
[http://dx.doi.org/10.1093/chromsci/48.5.382] [PMID: 20515533]

[17]   Thirumalai T, Therasa SV, Elumalai EK, David E. Hypoglycemic effect of Brassica juncea (seeds) on streptozotocin induced diabetic male albino rat. Asian Pac J Trop Biomed 2011; 1(4): 323-5.
[http://dx.doi.org/10.1016/S2221-1691(11)60052-X] [PMID: 23569784]

[18]   Danlami U, Orishadipe Abayomi T, Lawal DR. Phytochemical, nutritional, and antimicrobial evaluations of the aqueous extract of Brassica Nigra (Brassicaceae) seeds. American J Appl Chem 2016; 4: 161-3.
[http://dx.doi.org/10.11648/j.ajac.20160404.17]

[19]   Veigas JM, Narayan MS, Laxman PM, Neelwarne B. Chemical nature, stability, and bioefficacies of anthocyanins from the fruit peel of SyzygiumcuminiSkeels. Food Chem 2007; 105: 619-27.
[http://dx.doi.org/10.1016/j.foodchem.2007.04.022]

[20]   Hossain S A, Uddin S N, Salim A, Haque R. Phytochemical and Pharmacological screening of Cocciniagrandis Linn. Journal of scientific and innovative research 2014; 3: 65-71.

[21]   Dewanjee S, Kundu M, Maiti A, Majumdar R, Majumdar A, Mandel S. *In vitro* evaluation of the antimicrobial activity of crude extract from plants Diospyrosperegrina, Cocciniagrandis, and Swieteniamacrophylla. Trop J Pharm Res 2007; 6: 773-8.
[http://dx.doi.org/10.4314/tjpr.v6i3.14658]

[22]   Venkateshwarlu R, Raju AB, Yerragunta VG. Phytochemistry and pharmacology of Alangiumsalvifolium: A review. J Pharm Res 2011; 4: 1423-5.

[23]   Jain S, Sinha A, Bhakuni DS. The biosynthesis of β-carboline and quinolizidine alkaloids of Alangium lamarckii. Phytochemistry 2002; 60(8): 853-9.
[http://dx.doi.org/10.1016/S0031-9422(02)00057-2] [PMID: 12150812]

[24]   Kumar D, Kumar S, Kohli S, Arya R, Gupta J. Antidiabetic activity of methanolic bark extract of Albizia odoratissima Benth. in alloxan induced diabetic albino mice. Asian Pac J Trop Med 2011; 4(11): 900-3.
[http://dx.doi.org/10.1016/S1995-7645(11)60215-0] [PMID: 22078953]

[25]   Rajan M, Kumar VK, Kumar PS, Venkatachalam T, Anbarasan V. Pharmacognostical and phytochemical studies of the leaves of AlbiziaOdoratissima (LF) Benth. Int J Pharmacognosy Phytochem Res 2011; 3: 47-55.

[26]   Singab A, Bahgat D, Al-Sayed E, Eldahshan O. Saponins from genus Albizia: phytochemical and biological review. Med Aromat Plants S 2015; 3: 2167-0412.

[27]   Ibeh BO, Ezeaja MI. Preliminary study of antidiabetic activity of the methanolic leaf extract of Axonopus compressus (P. Beauv) in alloxan-induced diabetic rats. J Ethnopharmacol 2011; 138(3): 713-6.
[http://dx.doi.org/10.1016/j.jep.2011.10.009] [PMID: 22032842]

[28]   Ogie-Odia E, Eseigbe D, Ilechie M, Erhabor J, Ogbebor E. Foliar epidermal and phytochemical studies of the grasses Cymbopogoncitratus (stapf.), Axonopuscompressus (P. Beauv.), and Eragrostistremula (SW Beauv) in Ekpoma, Edo state, Nigeria. ScientificWorldJournal 2010; 5.

[29]   Arayne MS, Sultana N, Bahadur SS. The berberis story: Berberis vulgaris in therapeutics. Pak J Pharm Sci 2007; 20(1): 83-92.
[PMID: 17337435]

[30]   Mohammadzadeh N, Mehri S, Hosseinzadeh H. *Berberis vulgaris* and its constituent berberine as antidotes and protective agents against natural or chemical toxicities. Iran J Basic Med Sci 2017; 20(5): 538-51.
[PMID: 28656089]

[31] Meliani N, Dib MelA, Allali H, Tabti B. Hypoglycaemic effect of Berberis vulgaris L. in normal and streptozotocin-induced diabetic rats. Asian Pac J Trop Biomed 2011; 1(6): 468-71.
[http://dx.doi.org/10.1016/S2221-1691(11)60102-0] [PMID: 23569815]

[32] Imanshahidi M, Hosseinzadeh H. Pharmacological and therapeutic effects of Berberis vulgaris and its active constituent, berberine. Phytother Res 2008; 22(8): 999-1012.
[http://dx.doi.org/10.1002/ptr.2399] [PMID: 18618524]

[33] Singh R, De S, Belkheir A. Avena sativa (Oat), a potential neutraceutical and therapeutic agent: an overview. Crit Rev Food Sci Nutr 2013; 53(2): 126-44.
[http://dx.doi.org/10.1080/10408398.2010.526725] [PMID: 23072529]

[34] Srinivasan R, Chandrasekar M, Nanjan M. Phytochemical investigations of Caesalpiniadigyna root. J Chem 2011; 8: 1843-7.

[35] Kabesh K, Senthilkumar P, Ragunathan R, Kumar RR. Phytochemical analysis of Catharanthusroseus plant extract and its antimicrobial activity. Int J Pure App Biosci 2015; 3: 162-72.

[36] Sain M, Sharma V. Catharanthusroseus (An anti-cancerous drug yielding plant). A Review of Potential Therapeutic Properties. Int J Pure App Biosci 2013; 1: 139-42.

[37] Arumugam G, Manjula P, Paari N. A review: Antidiabetic medicinal plants used for diabetes mellitus. J Acute Dis 2013; 2: 196-200.
[http://dx.doi.org/10.1016/S2221-6189(13)60126-2]

[38] Jerković I, Gašo-Sokač D, Pavlović H, *et al*. Volatile organic compounds from Centaurium erythraea Rafn (Croatia) and the antimicrobial potential of its essential oil. Molecules 2012; 17(2): 2058-72.
[http://dx.doi.org/10.3390/molecules17022058] [PMID: 22349896]

[39] Kamalakkanan N, Rajadurai M, Prince PSM. Effect of Aegle marmelos fruits on normal and streptozotocin-diabetic Wistar rats. J Med Food 2003; 6(2): 93-8.
[http://dx.doi.org/10.1089/109662003322233486] [PMID: 12935319]

[40] Ponnachan PT, Paulose CS, Panikkar KR. Effect of leaf extract of Aegle marmelose in diabetic rats. Indian J Exp Biol 1993; 31(4): 345-7.
[PMID: 8359833]

[41] Kamalakkannan N, Prince PSM. The effect of Aegle marmelos fruit extract in streptozotocin diabetes: a histopathological study. J Herb Pharmacother 2005; 5(3): 87-96.
[http://dx.doi.org/10.1080/J157v05n03_08] [PMID: 16520300]

[42] Charoensiddhi S, Anprung P. Bioactive compounds and volatile compounds of Thai bael fruit (Aeglemarmelos (L.) Correa) as a valuable source for functional food ingredients. Int Food Res J 2008; 15: 287-95.

[43] Augusti KT. Studies on the effects of a hypoglycemic principle from Allium Cepa Linn. Indian J Med Res 1973; 61(7): 1066-71.
[PMID: 4757998]

[44] El-Demerdash FM, Yousef MI, El-Naga NI. Biochemical study on the hypoglycemic effects of onion and garlic in alloxan-induced diabetic rats. Food Chem Toxicol 2005; 43(1): 57-63.
[http://dx.doi.org/10.1016/j.fct.2004.08.012] [PMID: 15582196]

[45] Goldman IL, Kopelberg M, Debaene JE, Schwartz BS. Antiplatelet activity in onion (Allium cepa) is sulfur dependent. Thromb Haemost 1996; 76(3): 450-2.
[http://dx.doi.org/10.1055/s-0038-1650598] [PMID: 8883285]

[46] Mathew PT, Augusti KT. Studies on the effect of allicin (diallyl disulphide-oxide) on alloxan diabetes. I. Hypoglycaemic action and enhancement of serum insulin effect and glycogen synthesis. Indian J Biochem Biophys 1973; 10(3): 209-12.
[PMID: 4792931]

[47] Jelodar GA, Maleki M, Motadayen MH, Sirus S. Effect of fenugreek, onion and garlic on blood

glucose and histopathology of pancreas of alloxan-induced diabetic rats. Indian J Med Sci 2005; 59(2): 64-9.
[http://dx.doi.org/10.4103/0019-5359.13905] [PMID: 15738612]

[48]   Adachi Y, Yoshida J, Kodera Y, Katoh A, Takada J, Sakurai H. Bis(allixinato)oxovanadium(IV) complex is a potent antidiabetic agent: studies on structure-activity relationship for a series of hydroxypyrone-vanadium complexes. J Med Chem 2006; 49(11): 3251-6.
[http://dx.doi.org/10.1021/jm060229a] [PMID: 16722643]

[49]   Ghannam N, Kingston M, Al-Meshaal IA, Tariq M, Parman NS, Woodhouse N. The antidiabetic activity of aloes: preliminary clinical and experimental observations. Horm Res 1986; 24(4): 288-94.
[http://dx.doi.org/10.1159/000180569] [PMID: 3096865]

[50]   Okyar A, Can A, Akev N, Baktir G, Sütlüpinar N. Effect of Aloe vera leaves on blood glucose level in type I and type II diabetic rat models. Phytother Res 2001; 15(2): 157-61.
[http://dx.doi.org/10.1002/ptr.719] [PMID: 11268118]

[51]   Tanaka M, Misawa E, Ito Y, *et al.* Identification of five phytosterols from Aloe vera gel as anti-diabetic compounds. Biol Pharm Bull 2006; 29(7): 1418-22.
[http://dx.doi.org/10.1248/bpb.29.1418] [PMID: 16819181]

[52]   Borhanuddin M, Shamsuzzoha M, Hussain AH. Hypoglycaemic effects of Andrographis paniculata Nees on non-diabetic rabbits. Bangladesh Med Res Counc Bull 1994; 20(1): 24-6.
[PMID: 7880153]

[53]   Reyes BA, Bautista ND, Tanquilut NC, *et al.* Anti-diabetic potentials of Momordica charantia and Andrographis paniculata and their effects on estrous cyclicity of alloxan-induced diabetic rats. J Ethnopharmacol 2006; 105(1-2): 196-200.
[http://dx.doi.org/10.1016/j.jep.2005.10.018] [PMID: 16298503]

[54]   Chao W-W, Lin B-F. Isolation and identification of bioactive compounds in Andrographis paniculata (Chuanxinlian). Chin Med 2010; 5: 17.
[http://dx.doi.org/10.1186/1749-8546-5-17] [PMID: 20465823]

[55]   Shirwaikar A, Rajendran K, Dinesh Kumar C, Bodla R. Antidiabetic activity of aqueous leaf extract of Annona squamosa in streptozotocin-nicotinamide type 2 diabetic rats. J Ethnopharmacol 2004; 91(1): 171-5.
[http://dx.doi.org/10.1016/j.jep.2003.12.017] [PMID: 15036485]

[56]   Gupta RK, Kesari AN, Murthy PS, Chandra R, Tandon V, Watal G. Hypoglycemic and antidiabetic effect of ethanolic extract of leaves of Annona squamosa L. in experimental animals. J Ethnopharmacol 2005; 99(1): 75-81.
[http://dx.doi.org/10.1016/j.jep.2005.01.048] [PMID: 15848023]

[57]   Yu J, Gui H, Luo X, Sun L, Zhu P, Yu Z. Studies on the chemical constituents of Annonamuricata. Yao xuexuebao= ActapharmaceuticaSinica 1997; 32: 431-7.

[58]   Chattopadhyay RR. A comparative evaluation of some blood sugar lowering agents of plant origin. J Ethnopharmacol 1999; 67(3): 367-72.
[http://dx.doi.org/10.1016/S0378-8741(99)00095-1] [PMID: 10617074]

[59]   Kar A, Choudhary BK, Bandyopadhyay NG. Comparative evaluation of hypoglycaemic activity of some Indian medicinal plants in alloxan diabetic rats. J Ethnopharmacol 2003; 84(1): 105-8.
[http://dx.doi.org/10.1016/S0378-8741(02)00144-7] [PMID: 12499084]

[60]   Alzohairy MA. Therapeutics role of Azadirachta Indica (Neem) and their active constituents in disease prevention [88]AL-SNAFI, A. E. 2014. The pharmacology of Apiumgraveolens. -A review. International Journal for Pharmaceutical Research Scholars 2016; 3: 671-7.

[61]   Saxena A, Mukherjee S, Shukla G. Progress of diabetes research in India during the 20th century National Institute of Science and Communication. New Delhi: CSIR 2006; p. 104.

[62]   Gupta R, Bajpai KG, Johri S, Saxena AM. An overview of Indian novel traditional medicinal plants

with anti-diabetic potentials. Afr J Tradit Complement Altern Med 2007; 5(1): 1-17.
[PMID: 20162049]

[63]　Kumar S, Sharma S, Vasudeva N. Chemical compositions of Cinnamomumtamala oil from two different regions of India. Asian Pac J Trop Dis 2012; 2: S761-4.
[http://dx.doi.org/10.1016/S2222-1808(12)60260-6]

[64]　Suryawanshi S, Mehrotra N, Asthana RK, Gupta RC. Liquid chromatography/tandem mass spectrometric study and analysis of xanthone and secoiridoid glycoside composition of Swertia chirata, a potent antidiabetic. Rapid Commun Mass Spectrom 2006; 20(24): 3761-8.
[http://dx.doi.org/10.1002/rcm.2795] [PMID: 17120271]

[65]　Vohora SB, Kumar I, Khan MS. Effect of alkaloids of *Solanum melongena* on the central nervous system. J Ethnopharmacol 1984; 11(3): 331-6.
[http://dx.doi.org/10.1016/0378-8741(84)90078-3] [PMID: 6482482]

[66]　Han S-W, Tae J, Kim J-A, *et al.* The aqueous extract of *Solanum melongena* inhibits PAR2 agonist-induced inflammation. Clin Chim Acta 2003; 328(1-2): 39-44.
[http://dx.doi.org/10.1016/S0009-8981(02)00377-7] [PMID: 12559597]

[67]　Talukdar SN, Hossain MN. Phytochemical, phytotherapeutical and pharmacological study of Momordicadioica. Evid Based Complement Alternat Med 2014; 2014806082
[http://dx.doi.org/10.1155/2014/806082] [PMID: 25197312]

[68]　Arayne MS, Sultana N, Mirza AZ, Zuberi MH, Siddiqui FA. *In vitro* hypoglycemic activity of methanolic extract of some indigenous plants. Pak J Pharm Sci 2007; 20(4): 268-73.
[PMID: 17604247]

[69]　Jia S, Shen M, Zhang F, Xie J. Recent advances in Momordicacharantia: functional components and biological activities. Int J Mol Sci 2017; 18: 2555.
[http://dx.doi.org/10.3390/ijms18122555]

[70]　Alzweiri M, Sarhan AA, Mansi K, Hudaib M, Aburjai T. Ethnopharmacological survey of medicinal herbs in Jordan, the Northern Badia region. J Ethnopharmacol 2011; 137(1): 27-35.
[http://dx.doi.org/10.1016/j.jep.2011.02.007] [PMID: 21335083]

[71]　Mandal S, Mandal M. Coriander (Coriandrum sativum L.) essential oil: Chemistry and biological activity. Asian Pac J Trop Biomed 2015; 5: 421-8.
[http://dx.doi.org/10.1016/j.apjtb.2015.04.001]

[72]　Hashmi MA, Khan A, Hanif M, Farooq U, Perveen S. Traditional uses, phytochemistry, and pharmacology of Oleaeuropaea (olive). Evid Based Complement Alternat Med 2015; 2015541591
[http://dx.doi.org/10.1155/2015/541591] [PMID: 25802541]

[73]　Mahendra P, Bisht S. Ferula asafoetida: Traditional uses and pharmacological activity. Pharmacogn Rev 2012; 6(12): 141-6.
[http://dx.doi.org/10.4103/0973-7847.99948] [PMID: 23055640]

[74]　Sheikhlar A. Trigonellafoenuin-graecum L.(Fenugreek) as a Medicinal Herb in Animals Growth and Health. Science International 2013; 1: 194-1198.

[75]　Uddin N, Hasan MR, Hossain MM, *et al. In vitro* α-amylase inhibitory activity and *in vivo* hypoglycemic effect of methanol extract of Citrus macroptera Montr. fruit. Asian Pac J Trop Biomed 2014; 4(6): 473-9.
[http://dx.doi.org/10.12980/APJTB.4.2014C1173] [PMID: 25182949]

[76]　Waikedre J, Dugay A, Barrachina I, Herrenknecht C, Cabalion P, Fournet A. Chemical composition and antimicrobial activity of the essential oils from New Caledonian Citrus macroptera and Citrus hystrix. Chem Biodivers 2010; 7(4): 871-7.
[http://dx.doi.org/10.1002/cbdv.200900196] [PMID: 20397222]

[77]　Sun J, Deng A, Li Z, Qin H. Studies on chemical constituents of roots of Linum usitatissimum. Zhongguo Zhong Yao Za Zhi 2009; 34(6): 718-20.

[PMID: 19624013]

[78] Tursunova M. Lipids from Seeds of Linumhumile. Chem Nat Compd 2015; 51: 228-31.
[http://dx.doi.org/10.1007/s10600-015-1249-0]

[79] Fadeyi O, Olatunji G, Ogundele V. Isolation and characterization of the chemical constituents of Anacardiumoccidentale cracked bark. Nat Prod Chem Res 2015; 3: 192.

[80] Coria-Téllez AV, Montalvo-Gónzalez E, Yahia EM, Obledo-Vázquez EN. Annonamuricata: A comprehensive review of its traditional medicinal uses, phytochemicals, pharmacological activities, mechanisms of action, and toxicity. Arab J Chem 2018; 11: 662-91.
[http://dx.doi.org/10.1016/j.arabjc.2016.01.004]

[81] Karou SD, Tchacondo T, Djikpo Tchibozo MA, *et al.* Ethnobotanical study of medicinal plants used in the management of diabetes mellitus and hypertension in the Central Region of Togo. Pharm Biol 2011; 49(12): 1286-97.
[http://dx.doi.org/10.3109/13880209.2011.621959] [PMID: 22077164]

[82] Fotie J, Nkengfack A, Peter MG, Heydenreich M, Fomum Z. Chemical constituents of the ethyl acetate extract of the stem bark and fruits of Dichrostachyscinerea and the roots of Parkia bicolor. Bull Chem Soc Ethiop 2004; 18.

[83] Reynoso-Camacho R, Ramos-Gomez M, Loarca-Pina G. Bioactive components in common beans (Phaseolus vulgaris L.). Advances in Agricultural and Food Biotechnology 2006; 217.

[84] Joshi RK. Chemical composition, *in vitro* antimicrobial and antioxidant activities of the essential oils of Ocimumgratissimum, O. sanctum, and their major constituents. Indian J Pharm Sci 2013; 75(4): 457-62.
[http://dx.doi.org/10.4103/0250-474X.119834] [PMID: 24302801]

[85] Vergara-Jimenez M, Almatrafi MM, Fernandez ML. Bioactive components in Moringa Oleifera leaves to protect against chronic disease. Antioxidants 2017; 6(4): 91.
[http://dx.doi.org/10.3390/antiox6040091] [PMID: 29144438]

[86] Naseer S, Hussain S, Naeem N, Pervaiz M, Rahman M. The phytochemistry and medicinal value of Psidiumguajava (guava). Clinical Phytoscience 2018; 4: 32.
[http://dx.doi.org/10.1186/s40816-018-0093-8]

[87] Uraku A. Leaves by Gas Chromatography-Mass Spectrometry (GC-MS) Method. Res J Phytochem 2015; 9: 175-87.
[http://dx.doi.org/10.3923/rjphyto.2015.175.187]

[88] Angami T, Bhagawati R, Touthang L, *et al.* Traditional uses, phytochemistry and biological activities of Parkiatimoriana (DC.) Merr., an underutilized multipurpose tree bean: a review. Genet Resour Crop Evol 2018; 65: 679-92.
[http://dx.doi.org/10.1007/s10722-017-0595-0]

[89] Srikanth M, Swetha T, Veeresh B. Phytochemistry and pharmacology of Oxalis corniculata Linn.: A review. Int J Pharm Sci Res 2012; 3: 4077.

[90] Gharouni M, Sarkarati A. Application of Apiumgraveolens in treatment of hypertension. and treatment. Evid Based Complement Alternat Med 2000; 2016.

[91] Al-Snafi AE. The Pharmacology of *Apiumgraveolens.* - A review. International Journal for Pharmaceutical Research Scholars 2014; 3(1-1): 671-7.

[92] Tabassum N, Ahmad F. Role of natural herbs in the treatment of hypertension. Pharmacogn Rev 2011; 5(9): 30-40.
[http://dx.doi.org/10.4103/0973-7847.79097] [PMID: 22096316]

[93] Keenan JM, Pins JJ, Frazel C, Moran A, Turnquist L. Oat ingestion reduces systolic and diastolic blood pressure in patients with mild or borderline hypertension: a pilot trial. J Fam Pract 2002; 51(4): 369.

[PMID: 11978262]

[94]   Singh U, Kunwar A, Srinivasan R, Nanjan MJ, Priyadarsini KI. Differential free radical scavenging activity and radioprotection of caesalpinia digyna extracts and its active constituent. J Radiat Res (Tokyo) 2009; 50(5): 425-33.
[http://dx.doi.org/10.1269/jrr.08123] [PMID: 19652457]

[95]   Haddadian K, Haddadian K, Zahmatkash M. A review of Plantago plant. Indian J Tradit Know 2004; 13(4): 681-5.

[96]   Yang Y-C, Lu F-H, Wu J-S, Wu C-H, Chang C-J. The protective effect of habitual tea consumption on hypertension. Arch Intern Med 2004; 164(14): 1534-40.
[http://dx.doi.org/10.1001/archinte.164.14.1534] [PMID: 15277285]

[97]   Zhu H-B, Li B-M, Liu C, Chen R-Y. [Chemical constituents of Camellia sinensis var. assamica]. Zhongguo Zhongyao Zazhi 2013; 38(9): 1386-9.
[PMID: 23944074]

[98]   Gilani AH, Jabeen Q, Ghayur MN, Janbaz KH, Akhtar MS. Studies on the antihypertensive, antispasmodic, bronchodilator and hepatoprotective activities of the Carum copticum seed extract. J Ethnopharmacol 2005; 98(1-2): 127-35.
[http://dx.doi.org/10.1016/j.jep.2005.01.017] [PMID: 15763373]

[99]   Yang T, Wang C, Liu H, Chou G, Cheng X, Wang Z. A new antioxidant compound from Capparis spinosa. Pharm Biol 2010; 48(5): 589-94.
[http://dx.doi.org/10.3109/13880200903214231] [PMID: 20645804]

[100] Cheema MA, Priddle OD. Pharmacological investigations of isochaksine, an alkaloid isolated from the seeds of Cassia absus Linn. (Chaksu). Arch Int Pharmacodyn Ther 1965; 158(2): 307-13.
[PMID: 5868585]

[101] Nancy P, Ashlesha V. Pharmacognostic and phytochemical studies of Cassia absus seeds extract. Int J Pharm Pharm Sci 2015; 8: 325-32.

[102] Ajagbonna O, Mojiminiyi F, Sofola O. Relaxant effects of the aqueous leaf extract of cassia occidentailis on rat aortic rings. Afr J Biomed Res 2001; 4.

[103] Kaur I, Ahmad S, Harikumar S. Pharmacognosy, phytochemistry, and pharmacology of Cassia occidentalis Linn. International Journal of Pharmacognosy and Phytochemical Research 2014; 6: 151-5.

[104] Dubey MP, Srimal RC, Nityanand S, Dhawan BN. Pharmacological studies on coleonol, a hypotensive diterpene from Coleus forskohlii. J Ethnopharmacol 1981; 3(1): 1-13.
[http://dx.doi.org/10.1016/0378-8741(81)90010-6] [PMID: 7193263]

[105] Wang YQ, Ma JP, Pan SL, Hou AJ, Huang JM. [Studies on the chemical constituents of Coleus forskohlii]. Zhong Yao Cai 2009; 32(9): 1381-5.
[PMID: 20034210]

[106] Gilani A-U H, Aftab K. Pharmacological actions of Cuscutareflexa. International journal of pharmacognosy 1992; 30: 296-302.

[107] Rai DK, Sharma V, Pal K, Gupta RK. Comparative phytochemical analysis of CuscutareflexaRoxb. Parasite grown on north India by GC-MS. Tropical Plant Research 2016; 3: 428-33.

[108] Aburjai T, Hudaib M, Tayyem R, Yousef M, Qishawi M. Ethnopharmacological survey of medicinal herbs in Jordan, the Ajloun Heights region. J Ethnopharmacol 2007; 110(2): 294-304.
[http://dx.doi.org/10.1016/j.jep.2006.09.031] [PMID: 17097250]

[109] Tahseen MA, Mishra G. Ethnobotany and diuretic activity of some selected Indian medicinal plants: a scientific review. Pharma Innovation 2013; 2: 109.

[110] Marques AM, Provance DW Jr, Kaplan MAC, Figueiredo MR. Echinodorus grandiflorus: Ethnobotanical, phytochemical and pharmacological overview of a medicinal plant used in Brazil.

Food Chem Toxicol 2017; 109(Pt 2): 1032-47.
[http://dx.doi.org/10.1016/j.fct.2017.03.026] [PMID: 28322968]

[111]   Twaij HA, Kery A, Al-Khazraji NK. Some pharmacological, toxicological and phytochemical investigations on Centaurea phyllocephala. J Ethnopharmacol 1983; 9(2-3): 299-314.
[http://dx.doi.org/10.1016/0378-8741(83)90037-5] [PMID: 6677820]

[112]   Barazani O, Ziffer-Berger J. Eruca sativa, a Tasty Salad Herb with Health-Promoting Properties Medicinal and Aromatic Plants of the Middle-East. Springer 2014.

[113]   Coronel O, León-García E, Vela-Gutiérrez G, Medina Jdlc G-V R, García H. Chayote (Sechiumedule (Jacq.) Swartz). Fruit and Vegetable Phytochemicals: Chemistry and Human Health 2017; 979-92.

[114]   Lodhi S, Vadnere GP, Sharma VK, Usman M. Marrubiumvulgare L.: A review on phytochemical and pharmacological aspects. J Intercult Ethnopharmacol 2017; 6: 429-52.
[http://dx.doi.org/10.5455/jice.20170713060840]

[115]   Jaiswal P, Kumar P, Singh V K, Singh D K. Biological Effects of Myristicafragrans. Annual review of biomedical sciences 2009; 11.

[116]   Patel B, Patel G, Shah S, Parmar S. A Review: Coixlacrymajobi L. Research Journal of Pharmacognosy and Phytochemistry 2017; 9: 248-52.
[http://dx.doi.org/10.5958/0975-4385.2017.00046.2]

[117]   Süntar I, Koca U, Keleş H, Akkol EK. Wound healing activity of RubussanctusSchreber (Rosaceae): preclinical study in animal models. Evid Based Complement Alternat Med 2011; 2011816156
[http://dx.doi.org/10.1093/ecam/nep137] [PMID: 19755505]

[118]   Cheng J-T, Lin T-C, Hsu F-L. Antihypertensive effect of corilagin in the rat. Can J Physiol Pharmacol 1995; 73(10): 1425-9.
[http://dx.doi.org/10.1139/y95-198] [PMID: 8748933]

[119]   Engelhard Y N, Gazer B, Paran E. 2006; Natural antioxidants from tomato extract reduce blood pressure in patients with grade-1 hypertension: a double-blind, placebo-controlled pilot study. American heart journal 151: 100. e6-100.
[http://dx.doi.org/10.1016/j.ahj.2005.05.008]

[120]   Azhar I, Aftab K, Usmanghani K. Naturally occurring calcium channel blockers. Hamdard Med 1995; 38: 5-16.

[121]   Gilani AH, Aftab K, Saeed SA, Suria A. Effect of harmalol on blood pressure in anaesthetized rats. Portland Press Limited 1992.
[http://dx.doi.org/10.1042/bst020359s]

[122]   Mojiminiyi FB, Dikko M, Muhammad BY, *et al.* Antihypertensive effect of an aqueous extract of the calyx of Hibiscus sabdariffa. Fitoterapia 2007; 78(4): 292-7.
[http://dx.doi.org/10.1016/j.fitote.2007.02.011] [PMID: 17482378]

[123]   Gilani AH, Shaheen E, Saeed SA, *et al.* Hypotensive action of coumarin glycosides from Daucus carota. Phytomedicine 2000; 7(5): 423-6.
[http://dx.doi.org/10.1016/S0944-7113(00)80064-1] [PMID: 11081994]

CHAPTER 7

Chrysophyllum Cainito L.

A. Sánchez-Recillas[1,*], L. Cerón-Romero[2], R. Ortiz-Andrade[1] and J.C. Sánchez-Salgado[3]

[1] *Laboratorio de Farmacología, Facultad de Química, Universidad Autónoma de Yucatán, Calle 43 No. 613 x Calle 90 Col. Inalámbrica. C.P. 97069, Mérida, Yucatán, Mexico*

[2] *División Académica de Ciencias Básicas, Universidad Juárez Autónoma de Tabasco, Carretera Cunduacán-Jalpa KM. 1. Col. La Esmeralda C.P. 86690, Cunduacán, Tabasco, Mexico*

[3] *Instituto de Inmunología y Enfermedades Complejas. Av. San Jerónimo 819, 106-D, San Jerónimo Lídice, Magdalena Contreras, C.P.10200, Mexico City, Mexico*

Abstract: *Chrysophyllum cainito* L. is part of the family Sapotaceae and native to the Greater Antilles and the West Indies. This specie is a medicinal plant used around the world by many cultures, commonly known as "star apple" or "caimito". Some studies have reported that *C. cainito* possesses many pharmacological properties as antidiabetic, anti-hypersensitivity, antihypertensive, anti-inflammatory, antimicrobial, antinociceptive, antioxidant, gastroprotective and immunosuppressive. Also, phytochemical evidence has revealed that the main secondary metabolites in *C. cainito* are alkaloids, tannins, flavonoids, phenols, sterols, coumarins and triterpenes which are responsible for their pharmacological benefits. *In vitro* and *in vivo* toxicology studies have suggested human consumption of *Chrysophyllum cainito* leaves as safe. This chapter includes scientific information of pharmacology, toxicology and phytochemistry of *C. cainito* seeds, leaves, and fruits with the purpose to contribute valuable scientific information to future research in drug development based on *C. cainito* as a source of raw material.

Keywords: Antidiabetic, Anti-inflammatory, Antimicrobial, Antinociceptive, Antioxidant, *Chrysophyllum cainito* L., Immunosuppressive, Medicinal use, Pharmacology Phytochemicals, Toxicity.

INTRODUCTION

Chrysophyllum cainito is part of the family Sapotaceae and native to the Greater Antilles and the West Indies. It is spread in the lowlands of Central America and now is very common and cultivated throughout the tropics, including Southeast Asia [1]. The fruit is named as star apple, cainito, caimito or cayumito, and its fla-

---

* **Corresponding author Sánchez-Recillas:** Área de Farmacología Experimental, Facultad de Química, Universidad Autónoma de Yucatán (UADY) - Calle 43 No. 613 x Calle 90 Col. Inalámbrica. C.P. 97069. Mérida, Yucatán, México; E-mail: amanda.sanchez@correo.uady.mx

M. Eddouks (Ed.)

vor is a mixture between green grapes and litchi. This specie is used in folk medicine for the treatment of inflammation such as laryngitis, pneumonia, rheumatoid arthritis, and diabetes mellitus [2]. The chemical analysis has described several secondary metabolites including alkaloids, flavonoids, phenols, sterols, and triterpenes which are well known to have pharmacology properties. The biological activity of *C. cainito* has been also investigated comprehensively [1 - 3], and in this chapter, we assemble the information of *C. cainito* describing the ethnomedical, chemical, pharmacological, and toxicological properties providing wide scientific evidence of its medicinal benefits and worthiness as a source of new chemical agents in the drug discovery process.

SYNONYMS

C. cainito L is also known by many other synonyms around the world. The most common synonyms are *Cainito pomiferum* Tusac, *Chrysophyllum bicolor* Poir, *Chrysophyllum bonplandii* Klotzsch ex Miq, *Chrysophyllum monopyrenum* Sw, *Chrysophyllum sericeum* Salisb, *Cynodendron bicolor* (Poir.) Baehni [1], and *Achras caimito* Ruiz & Pavon [2].

BOTANICAL FEATURES [3]

Kingdom: Plantae
Subkingdom: Viridiplantae
Division: Tracheophyta
Class: Magnoliopsida
Superorder: Asteranae
Order: Ericales
Family: Sapotaceae
Genus: *Chrysophyllum* L.
Species: *C. cainito* L.

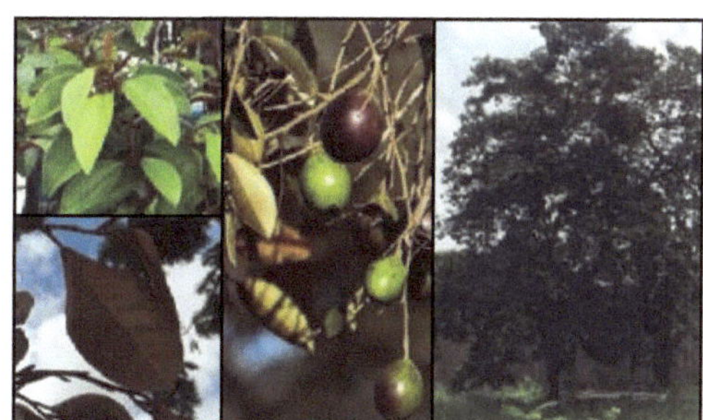

VERNACULAR NAMES

Chrysophyllum cainito is most commonly known as "caimito" or "cayumito". However, many names are reported of this specie (Table **1**).

C. cainito is an evergreen tree with alternate oblong-lanceolate leaves and flowers blooming from May to October, which are small, white to greenish in color. A green to purple fruit with approximately 5-8 cm in diameter is characterized by fleshy and edible pericarp. The epicarp or peel is hard on the external tissues and soft on the internal ones [8]. The fructification is mixed; the first fruits appear in July and are prolonged until the following year [9]. *C. cainito* is propagated by seed and it can germinate to about 60% by mechanical scarification [10 - 13].

Table 1. Reported vernacular names for *Chrysophyllum cainito* L. worldwide.

Geographical Region	Vernacular Name	Reference
AMERICA		
North America		
Mexico	Caimito or Cayumito	[1]
Oaxaca	Canela	[4]
Chiapas	Chicle de monte	[4]
San Luis Potosi	Isi, ocotlan	[4]
United States		
Florida (southern)	Star apple	[6]
Caribbean	Star apple (overall)	[5]
Haiti	Pied caimite or caimitier a feuilles d'or	[2]
French West Indies	Pomme surette, or buis	[2]
Virgin Islands	Cainit	[2]
Trinidad and Tobago	Caimite or kaimit	[2]
Barbados	Star-plum	[2]
Central America	Star apple (overall)	[5]
Belize	Damsel	[2]
El Salvador	Guayabillo	[2]
Nicaragua (eastern)	Apil	[7]
South America	Star apple (overall)	[5]
Colombia	Caimo, caimo morado (purple variety) or caimito madura verde (green variety)	[2]
Bolivia	Caimitero, or murucuja	[2]
Surinam	Sterappel, apra or goudblad boom	[2]
French Guiana	Macoucou	[2]
Argentina	Aguay or olivoa	[2]
EUROPE		
Spain	Caimito or Estrella	[2]
Portugal	Cainito orajara	[2]
France	Caimite or caimitier	[2]
ASIA		
Singapore	Chicle durian	[2]

DISTRIBUTION

C. cainito is native to Caribbean islands and Central America [14, 15]. Pennington (1990) established that this species is native of the Greater Antilles and it is possible that cultivated plants were originated from a reduced population that multiplied it through Antilles and South America in the pre-Columbian era [2, 16]. Historical records of European plant explorers from the 16th and 17th centuries have indicated that *C. cainito* has long been cultivated in neotropics, from Greater and Lesser Antilles to Panama [17]. The species is currently cultivated in Antilles, Mesoamerica, and South America, as well as in some zones of Florida, Hawaii, and south-east Asia [2, 18]. In Mesoamerica and Mexican Caribbean, *C. cainito* might be growing in wild and cultivated settings [1].

CHEMICAL CONSTITUENTS

C. cainito has secondary metabolites such as alkaloids, flavonoids, phenols, sterols, and triterpenes [6, 19], which have been isolated from aerial parts including fresh fruits (Table **2**).

Table 2. Chemical constituents isolated of *Chrysophyllum cainito* L.

No.	Compound Name	Part of the Plant from Where it was Isolated	Chemical Structure	Reference
1	(+)-Catechin	Aerial parts		[6]
2	(-)-Epicatechin	Aerial parts		[6]
3	(+)-Gallocatechin	Aerial parts		[6]

(Table 2) cont.....

No.	Compound Name	Part of the Plant from Where it was Isolated	Chemical Structure	Reference
4	(-)-Epigallocatechin	Aerial parts	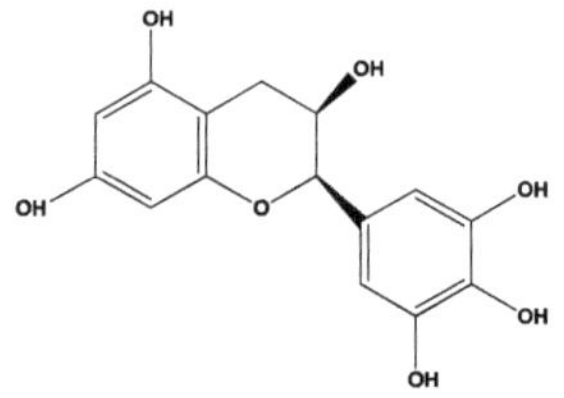	[6]
5	Quercetin	Aerial parts	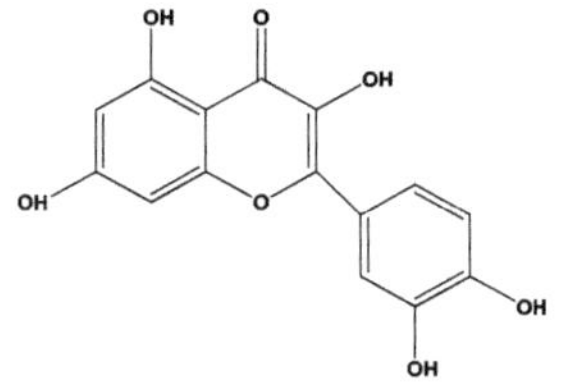	[6]
6	Quercitrin	Aerial parts	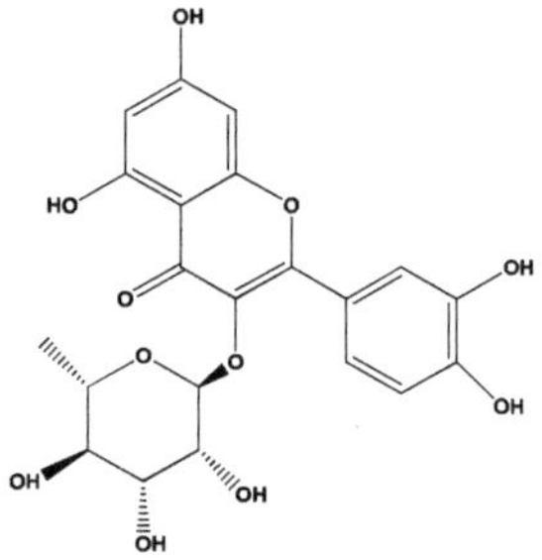	[6]
7	Isoquercitrin	Aerial parts	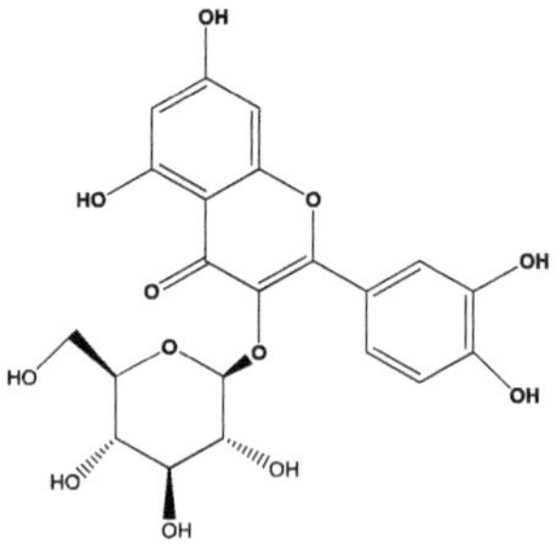	[6]

(Table 2) cont.....

No.	Compound Name	Part of the Plant from Where it was Isolated	Chemical Structure	Reference
8	Myricitrin	Aerial parts	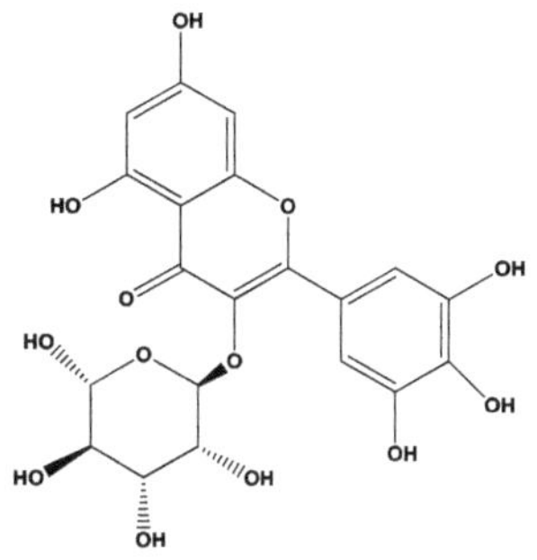	[6]
9	Gallic acid	Fresh fruit	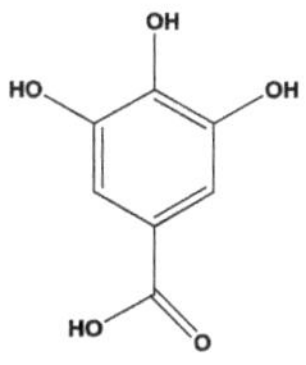	[6]
10	Ursolic acid	Leaves	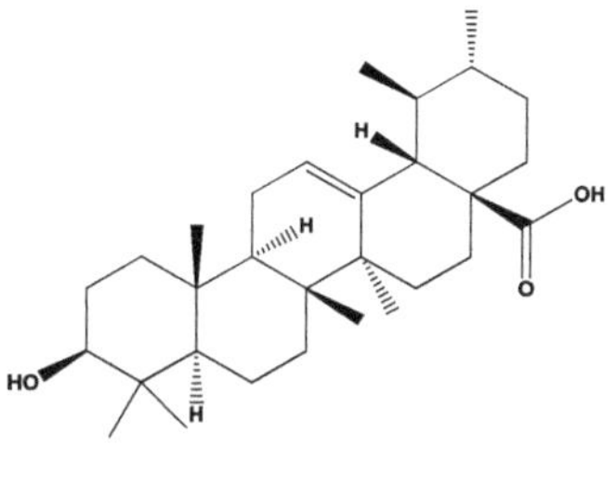	[19]
11	Beta sitosterol	Leaves	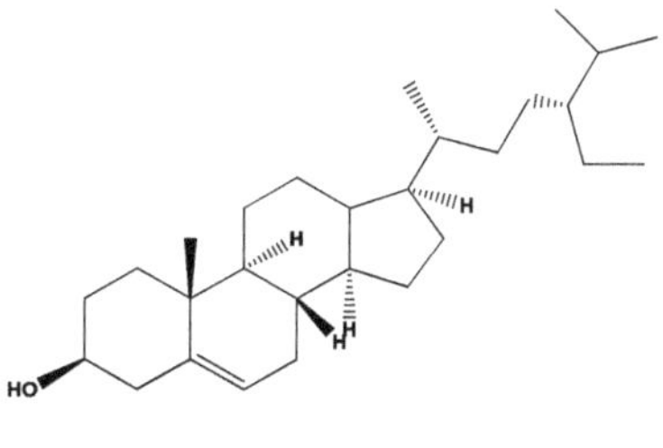	[19]

(Table 2) cont.....

No.	Compound Name	Part of the Plant from Where it was Isolated	Chemical Structure	Reference
12	Lupeol	Leaves	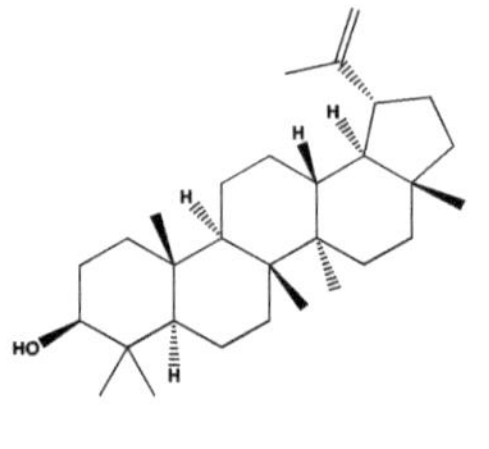	[19]
13	Lupeol acetate	Leaves	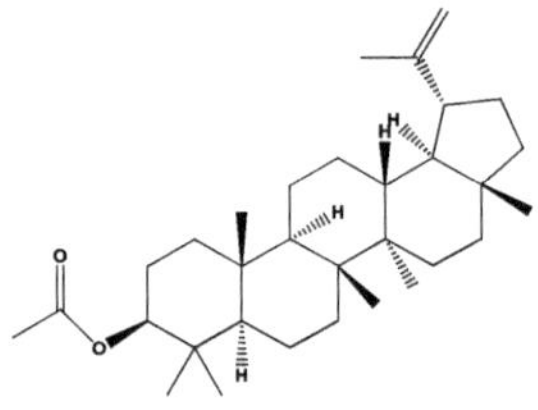	[20]
14	Octocosanoic acid methyl ester	Leaves	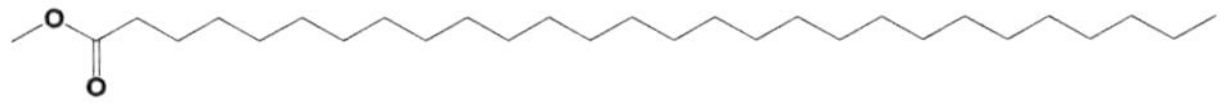	[21]
15	Alpha-amyrin	Leaves	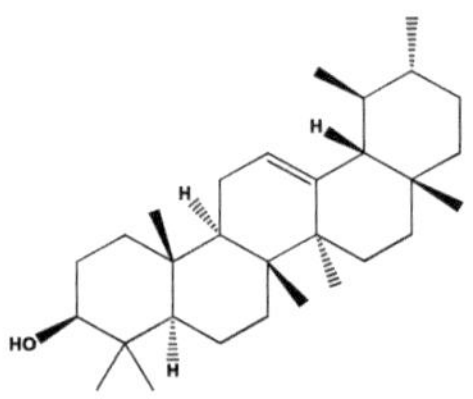	[22]
16	Ascorbic acid	Freeze-dried peel	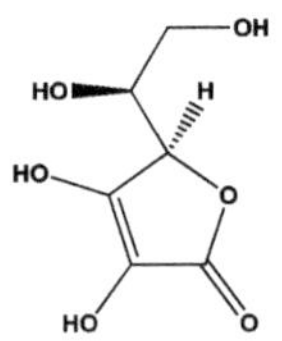	[23]
17	Ferulic acid	Freeze-dried peel	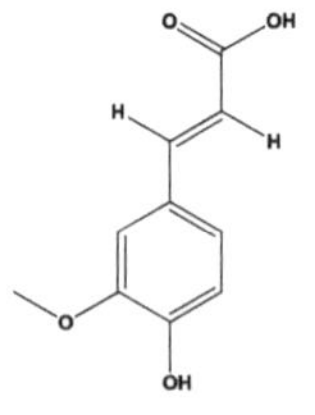	[24]

(Table 2) cont.....

No.	Compound Name	Part of the Plant from Where it was Isolated	Chemical Structure	Reference
18	Ellagic acid	Freeze-dried peel	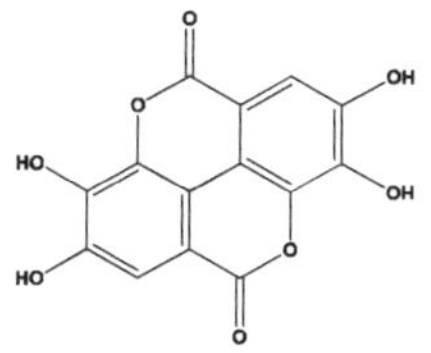	[24]
19	Myricetin	Freeze-dried peel	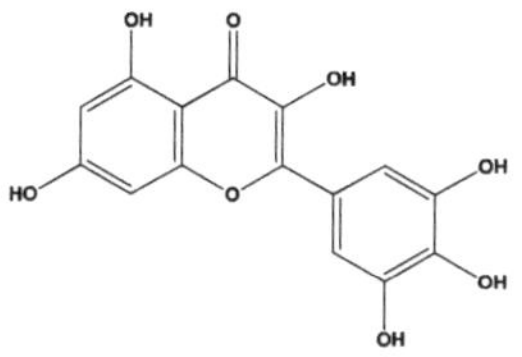	[24]
20	Beta amyrine acetate	Leaves and stems	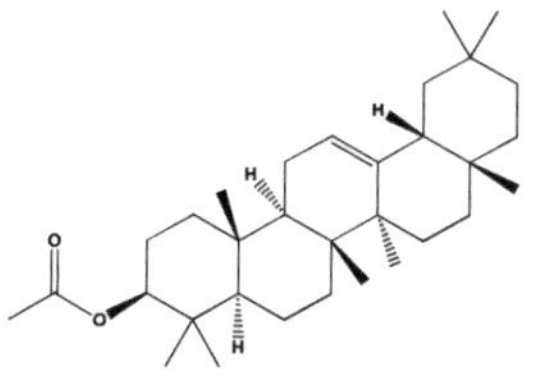	[1]
21	Gentisic acid	Leaves	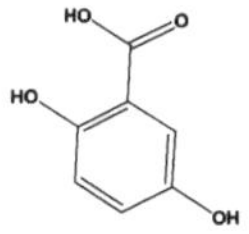	[1]
22	2-hexenal	Aerial parts	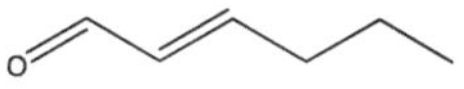	[25]
23	1-hexanol	Aerial parts	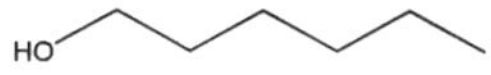	[25]
24	Limonene	Aerial parts	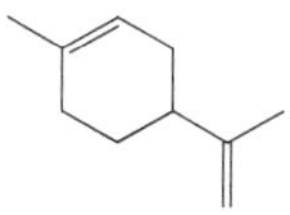	[25]
25	Linalool	Aerial parts	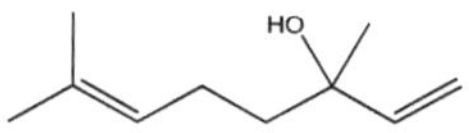	[25]

(Table 2) cont.....

No.	Compound Name	Part of the Plant from Where it was Isolated	Chemical Structure	Reference
26	Copaene	Aerial parts		[25]
27	Hexadecanoic acid	Aerial parts		[25]

PURITY REQUIREMENTS

The physicochemical parameters of the leaves are usually determined by standard pharmacopeia methods and leaves of *C. cainito* showed greater solubility in the polar solvents (Table **3**) [19].

Table 3. Physiochemical properties of *C. cainito*'s leaves.

Parameters	Results
Foreign organic matter	0.214 ± 0.018
Total ash	9.376 ± 0.629
Acid insoluble ash	2.022 ± 0.035
Water soluble ash	7.325 ± 0.143
Ethanol soluble extractive value	8.786 ± 0.012
Water soluble extractive value	9.455 ± 0.135
Ether soluble extractive value	19.268 ± 0.240

Values are (% Mean ± S.D., n=3)

Fruit Composition

C. cainito fruit has the following content per 100 g (Table **4**) [26].

Table 4. Composition of *C. cainito* fruit (100 g of edible portion).

Parameter	Seed	Pulp
Total energy (Kcal/100 g)	474.77±1.09	89.32±0.15
Moisture (%)	56.04±1.64	75.90±4.31

(Table 4) cont.....

Parameter	Seed	Pulp
Proteins (g)	4.63± 0.12	1.96±0.23
Fats (g)	15.81±0.53	0.88±0.31
Total carbohydrates (g)	78.49±0.40	18.39±0.33
Fiber (g)	2.31±0.21	4.19±0.46
Ash (g)	0.84±0.25	0.56±0.10
Calcium (mg/100 mg)	168.0 ± 0.28	37.0 ± 0.25
Magnesium (mg/100 g)	90.0 ± 0.25	5.0 ± 0.24
Phosphorus (mg/100 mg)	18.0 ± 0.31	8.0 ± 0.25
Potassium (mg/100 g)	78.0 ± 0.32	38.0 ± 0.29
Sodium (mg/100 g)	39.0 ± 0.25	21.0 ± 0.32
Ferrous (mg/100 mg)	-	0.8
Vitamin A (mg/100 mg)	0.027 ± 0.44	0.089 ± 0.32
Thiamine (mg/100 mg)	-	0.04
Riboflavin (mg/100 mg)	-	0.03
Niacin (mg/100 mg)	-	1
Vit. C (mg/100mg)	10.0 ± 0.22	43.54 ± 0.57

CHEMICAL ASSAYS

Diverse chemical assays have been developed to easily identify the content of major secondary metabolites. The assays used for these purposes are described below (Table **5**).

Table **5**. Qualitative and quantitative assays for chemical determination of secondary metabolites from *C. cainito*.

Secondary metabolite	Chemical assay	Reference
Saponins	**QL**: Measuring the height of foam formed after vigorous stirring	[27-29]
Alkaloids	**QL**: Silica gel plates eluted with the same mixture used for anthraquinones and exposed to Dragendorff reagent.	[27-29]
Tannins	**QL**: The appearance of a white precipitate after contact with a 1% gelatin solution.	[27-29]
Coumarins	**QL**: A simple test on filter paper exposed to blue fluorescence light could be used to indicate the presence of volatile coumarins.	[27-29]
Phenolic compounds	**QT**: Folin–Ciocalteu colorimetric method using a standard curve prepared with gallic acid is used for determining total phenolic content.	[30-31]

(Table 5) cont.....

Secondary metabolite	Chemical assay	Reference
Flavonoids	**QT**: Total flavonoids are determined by the colorimetric method of aluminum chloride described by Chang *et al.*	[32-33]

QL, qualitative assay; QT, quantitative assay

MEDICINAL USES

C. cainito's fruit is used in folk medicine for the treatment of inflammation processes observed in laryngitis, pneumonia, rheumatoid arthritis, and diabetes mellitus [2, 36 - 38] and has other medicinal properties [6, 20, 39, 40].

In eastern Nicaragua, fruit extract is used to treat diarrhea, fever, and venereal diseases, as well as it might be used as an astringent [7, 36]. The slightly unripe fruits are eaten to overcome gut disturbances in Venezuela. On the other hand, latex is applied on abscesses and it might be a potent vermifuge when administered as dried and powdered preparation in Brazil. Also, it is used as diuretic, febrifuge, and dysentery medicine [2]. In Yucatan (Mexico), *C. cainito* leaves decoction supplemented with *Citrus aurantifolia*, *Annona muricata*, and *Manilkara zapota* is used for weight loss. Some authors have reported that bark decoction has been used locally for abscess and inflammation, orally as dysentery treatment, and the juice as a sexual fortifier [1].

A rind or leaves extract is applied in pectoral, whereas bark decoction is used as a tonic and stimulant as well as to treat diarrhea, dysentery, and hemorrhages, gonorrhea and "catarrh of the bladder". The bitter, pulverized seeds are used as tonic, diuretic, and febrifuge medicine. Cuban population also uses the leaves decoction as a cancer remedy [2].

PHARMACOLOGY

Experimental Pharmacology

Antioxidant activity: The fruit of *C. cainito* is reported to have antioxidant properties. Xiao-dong (2002) reported antioxidant activity (IC$_{50}$= 22 µg/mL) of the fresh fruit evaluated by DPPH assay. Also, nine known polyphenolic antioxidants were identified in fruits, in which epicatechin had the highest concentration (7.3 mg/kg fresh weight). Furthermore, flavonoid quercetin showed the highest antioxidant activity (IC$_{50}$= 40 µM) in the DPPH assay [6].

Moo-Huchin [24] *et al.* evaluated total soluble phenols and flavonoids isolated from the methanolic extract of freeze-dried peels. The antioxidant capacity was determined by DPPH and ABTS assays. Results showed relevant antioxidant activity of the freeze-dried peel extract, which corresponded to 3,310.95 µM Trolox/100 g DW and 1,680.9 µM Trolox/100 g DW, respectively [24]. Besides, Chel-Guerrero *et al.* [27] reported the antioxidant activity of methanol extract of fruit peels by a cupric reducing antioxidant capacity (CUPRAC) assay.

Overall, these bioassay experiments suggested that antioxidant capacity is proportional to the total phenolic content of peel [24, 34]. Sayed *et al.* [21] reported a protective potential of the methanolic extract on gamma radiation-induced damage in rats. Thus, the methanolic extract has a beneficial effect to ameliorate gamma-irradiation-induced alterations *via* improving antioxidant status, decreasing malondialdehyde concentration, as well as improving glutathione level and superoxide dismutase activity. The extract showed a mild increase in the enzyme metallothionein expressed on liver and kidney, and demonstrated improvement of lipid profile, as well as lesser damage in the liver.

Antimicrobial activities: The pulp and seed have shown antimicrobial activities against clinically relevant *Escherichia coli* and some *Salmonella, Staphylococcus, Pseudomonas, Aspergillus, Candida,* and *Penicillium* species. Microbial counts of the fruits ranged from 1.0×10^9 - 2.4×10^{10} for total aerobic plate count, 1.0×10^7 - 2.0×10^7 for the fungal count, and 1.0×10^8 - 1.2×10^9 for the coliform count. The normal flora and spoilage organisms on surfaces and pulp of healthy fruits have *Bacillus, Corynebacterium, Staphylococcus, Micrococcus, Acinetobacter, Enterococcus,* and *Pseudomonas* species. The fungal isolates showed *Rhizopus, Aspergillus, Penicillum,* and *Saccharomyces* species [26].

Immunosuppressive effect: The immune-modulatory effect of leaves of methanol extract was determined in peritoneal murine macrophages isolated from Balb/c mice, which were treated with the extract and stimulated with LPS. The effect on phagocytosis was evaluated by a flow cytometry method. Nitric oxide (NO) and hydrogen peroxide (H_2O_2) production were measured by the Griess reagent and phenol red reaction, respectively. IL-6 and TNF-α levels were measured using an ELISA assay. The methanol extract of *C. cainito* leaves significantly inhibited phagocytosis, and decreased IL-6 and TNF-α production. NO and H_2O_2 released by the macrophages were also diminished in a concentration-dependent sequence [35].

Anti-inflammatory effect: Methanol extract of leaves and its fractions have been evaluated in a carrageenan-induced mechanical hypersensitivity mouse model, using indomethacin as a positive control [20]. The results showed that methanolic extract produced a significant inhibition of general hypersensitivity. Highest inhibition (86.79%) was achieved at 10 mg/kg. A half inhibitory dose (ID_{50}) was calculated as 7.69 mg/kg. An effective chromatographic fraction using chloroform as a solvent carrier was ID_{50} = 14.45 mg/kg. Neutrophil migration assay showed that both methanolic and hexanic fractions significantly reduced the myeloperoxidase activity. However, methanolic extract presented a slight reduction in paw edema compared with the control group. The effect of the methanolic extract seemed to be partially related to the anti-inflammatory activity [20].

Anti-hypersensitivity activity: The mice treated with *C. cainito* methanol extract (leaves) or chloroform fraction showed a decrease in mechanical hypersensitivity suggesting that these substances might reduce inflammatory pains in mice [20].

Meira *et al.* [36] reported similar activity of this extract in acute inflammatory pain models induced by PGE_2, epinephrine, LPS and CFA. Animals treated with the methanolic extract and stimulated with PGE_2, epinephrine, LPS or CFA showed a significantly decreasing mechanical hypersensitivity. In addition, an anti-inflammatory mechanism of action could be elucidated involving production, release or action of some chemical mediators, such as PGE_2, sympathetic amines, and cytokines.

Antidiabetic activity: *C. cainito* fruit or leaf preparations are also used in the treatment of diabetes and its complications. N'guessan *et al.* (2009) formerly described a hypoglycemic effect induced by leave decoction of *C. cainito* in alloxan-induced diabetic rabbits in a dose-dependent manner (10, 20 and 30 g/L). However, rabbits showed toxic adverse events after 8 weeks of treatment [37].

Hedge *et al.* [38] investigated the effects of a hydroalcoholic extract of *C. cainito* fruits in two models of experimental diabetes (streptozotocin and alloxan), observing that *C. cainito* decreased plasma concentrations of glucose, cholesterol, triglycerides, and LDL concentrations in a dose-dependent manner, conversely HDL was increased. In addition, this extract induced a regenerative process in pancreatic β-cells.

On the other hand, Doan *et al.* [39] reported that 500 mg/kg dose of an aqueous extract of *C. cainito* leaves decreased fasting blood glucose levels in alloxan-induced diabetic rodents (from 387.17±29.84 mg/dL to 125.67±62.09 mg/dL after 6 hours' post-administration). Additionally, 50 µg/mL of *C. cainito* aqueous extract significantly increased glucose uptake in the abdominal muscle when stimulated with insulin. Also, it was shown that the extract administration produced a strong inhibition for α-glycosidase activity (IC_{50} = 1.20 ± 0.09 µg/mL) suggesting that *C. cainito* extract works like a metabolic regulator by glucose uptake stimulation and α-glycosidase inhibitory modulation.

Antinociceptive activity: Déciga-Campos *et al.* [40] reported antinociceptive and anti-hyperalgesic effects of *C. cainito* leaves ethanol extract and non-solvent leaves-based herbal preparation. Air-dried leaves of *Citrus limonum, C. cainito, Pouteria campechiana,* and *Annona muricata* were mixed (1:1:1:1 ratio, 500 g each) to obtain a PCCA preparation, which was extracted with ethanol for 90 min. This methodology was used to simulate indications of a traditional Mayan healer (h-men) from the Regional Council of Indigenous Medical Doctors, NACHI COCOM, A.C., from Mérida, Yucatán.

Single extracts of each species were prepared by the same methodology. PCCA and *C. cainito* extracts were evaluated by formalin and capsaicin tests in rats [41]. Systemic administration of PCCA extracts (50–400 mg/kg, p.o.) resulted in a dose-dependent antinociceptive effect in the formalin test (ED_{50} = 197.18 ±14.7 mg/kg). *C. cainito* (46.4%) and PCCA (66%) extracts produced a moderate antinociceptive effect. PCCA extract administered locally (20–160 µg/paw) decreased capsaicin-induced nociception with a maximum effect at 160 mg/paw of 69.5%. The hyperalgesic effect increased in diabetic rats with a lower percentage of formalin (0.5%) with respect to the non-diabetic rats. For the induction of experimental hyperglycemia, Wistar rats were administrated with alloxan (50 mg/kg, i.p.) dissolved in the isotonic saline solution and one-time blood glucose levels (mg/dL) were estimated using a commercial glucometer. Subcutaneous (s.c.) injection of 1% formalin into the right hind paw of non-diabetic rats and 0.5% formalin in diabetic (four weeks) rats produced a typical biphasic pattern of flinching behavior hyperalgesic activity was confirmed with the acetone cold test [42]. The PCCA extract (100–400 mg/kg, p.o.) showed anti-hyperalgesic effects in alloxan diabetic rats [40].

Antihypertensive effects: *C. cainito* contains several phenolic compounds which could have antihypertensive potential. Mao *et al.* [43] reported the evaluation of alcoholic and aqueous extracts of the pulp of plant on *in vitro, ex vivo* and *in vivo* models of hypertension arterial. *C. cainito* fruits were collected from its natural habitat in Hunan province, China, and the dried powder of the fruit of the plant was submitted to the extraction process with soxhlet and ethanol. The extracts were evaluated on *in vitro* inhibition of angiotensin I converting enzyme/ACE [44]; results showed that ethyl acetate fraction from ethanolic extract (ALE-EAF) was more active on ACE inhibition. For *ex vivo* assay of the isolated aortic ring, thoracic aortic of the rat was used; it was kept in the physiological conditions (immersed into organ baths containing 10 mL Krebs solution at 37° C and oxygenated with O_2:CO_2 at 95:5) and changes in basal tension were recorded by BIOPAC system [43]. Stimulation of aortic rings with 120 mM of KCl resulted in a sustained contraction equivalent to 5363 ± 541 mg and was maximum. The additions of the extracts or fractions of *C. cainito* caused the significant relaxant response; in this experiment, also ALE-EAF was more active with 62.82 ± 6.19%

and $46.47 \pm 8.32\%$ of relaxation at 50 μg/mL and 10 μg/mL of gallic acid equivalents, respectively. The ALE-EAF was submitted to *in vivo* experiment. The salt induced hypertensive (SIH) rat model was used to study the antihypertensive activity of active fraction, thus normotensive male albinos Wistar rats were randomly divided into seven groups of six animals each. One group was administrated with tap water intragastrically (i.g): (NT) group; the second group was administrated with 10 mL 18% NaCl kg-per 1 rat body weight day-1 for 30 days (SIH) group; and two positive control groups received 18% NaCl solution and either captopril 10 mg kg-1 day-1 (SI) or 20 mg kg-1 day-1 (SII). The fraction was administrated at 200, 500 and 1000 mg kg-1 day-1 by gavage.

ALE-EAF reduced the elevated arterial pressure of salt induced hypertensive rat significantly to the level of normotensive animal group [43]. On the other hand, Sánchez-Recillas *et al.* [45] reported the vasorelaxant effect in aortic ring tests and hypotensive effect in normotensive Wistar rats of an herbal preparation that included *C. cainito* leaves; this medicinal preparation showed significant vasorelaxation (medium effective concentration: EC_{50}=463.43 μg/mL) in a concentration-dependent manner in aorta's endothelium-intact rings and this effect was partially endothelial-dependent. Acute oral administration of 200 and 300 mg/kg of PCCA (i.g) exhibited a significant decrease in the systolic blood pressure in normotensive rats.

Gastroprotective activity: The methanolic extracts from peels, seeds and pulp of *C. cainito* fruits showed gastroprotective activity in mice using ethanol/HCl- and indomethacin-induced ulcer [46].

Da Rosa *et al.* [46] evaluated the methanol extracts of the peels (0.3 mg/kg), seeds (0.3 mg/kg) and pulp (1 mg/kg) in a model of ethanol/HCl mice. In order to evaluate the systemic activity, the methanol extracts of peels (0.3 mg/kg), seeds (0.3 mg/kg) or pulp (1 mg/kg) were administered intraperitoneally (i.p) and ethanol/HCl was administered after 30 min [47]. In this same model, in another set of experiments, mice (n = 6) received vehicle (VEH, water, 10 mL/kg), omeprazole (OME, 30 mg/kg) or *C. cainito* juice (100 mL/kg) *via* oral gavage, once a day, for 7 days. Another group of animals received feed supplemented with 10% of the methanol extracts and juice from *C. cainito ad libitum* for 7 days. The acidified ethanol was administered 1 h after the last administration of vehicle or juice, or 12 h after the interruption of the supplementation. The mice were weighed during the treatment period. One hour after the ulcerogenic intake, the animals were euthanized [48]. The results showed that the pretreatment with the methanol extract of peels reduced the gastric lesions induced by acidified ethanol at doses of 3 and 10 mg/kg by 72 and 85%, respectively, compared to the ulcerated vehicle-treated group.

The methanol extract of seeds also decreased the gastric lesions by 76 and 72%, at doses of 3 and 10 mg/kg and the methanol extract of pulp reduced the lesions at doses of 10 and 30 mg/kg by 81 and 63%. The administration of the methanol extract of peels (0.3 mg/kg), seeds (0.3 mg/kg) and pulp (1 mg/kg) by intraperitoneal route was able to reduce gastric lesions at 74, 81 and 58%, respectively, compared to the ulcerated group treated with vehicle and the macroscopic and microscopic representative images from the stomachs showed that the methanol extracts of peels, seeds and pulp treatments minimized the loss of gastric epithelial cells from damages and increased mucin levels by 176, 198, and 193% [49].

C. cainito supplementation (10%) for 7 days promoted gastroprotective effects. The four intakes reduced the injured area by 83%, compared to the vehicle group. On the other hand, the daily consumption of fruit juice of C. *cainito* (100 mL/kg) was not able to protect the gastric mucosa against acidified ethanol [50].

Additionally, the methanol extracts of peels, seed and pulp were tested in a model indomethacin-induced gastric ulcer. Briefly, fasted mice were divided into different groups (n= 6) and pretreated with vehicle, water (10 mL/kg), carbenoxolone (200 mg/kg), the methanolic extracts of peels (3 mg/kg), seeds (3 mg/kg) and pulp (3 mg/kg). After 1 h, the animals were orally treated with indomethacin (80 mg/kg) to induce gastric injury. After 6 h, the animals were euthanized in a CO_2 chamber, the stomachs removed and opened along the greater curvature and ulcer was measured. The treatment with the methanol extracts of peels (3 mg/kg, p.o), seeds (3 mg/kg, p.o) and pulp (10 mg/kg, p.o) reduced the ulcer area by 78, 70 and 50%, respectively, compared to the vehicle-treated ulcerated group [51, 52].

Regarding the mode of action [53, 54], the gastroprotective effect of methanolic extract of peels was decreased by the pre-administration of N-ethylmaleimide (NEM, a sulfhydryl group chelator, 10 mg/kg, i.p), glibenclamide (a potassium channel blocker, 10 mg/kg, i.p), yohimbine (10 mg/kg, i.p, an alpha-adrenergic receptor antagonist, 10 mg/kg, i.p) and indomethacin (a cyclooxygenase inhibitor, 10 mg/kg, i.p). The gastroprotective effect of methanolic extract of seeds was reduced by the pre-administration of NEM, glibenclamide, N-Nitro-l-arginine methyl ester (L-NAME, a nitric oxide synthase inhibitor, 70 mg/kg, i.p) and yohimbine, while that methanol extract of pulp had the gastroprotective effect decreased in animals pretreated with NEM and L-NAME. However, the extracts did not reduce gastric acid secretion [55].

TOXICITY

The *C. cainito* seeds contain 1.2% of the bitter, cyanogenic glycoside, lucumin; 0.0037% pouterin; 6.6% of a fixed oil; 0.19% saponin; 2.4% dextrose and 3.75% ash. The leaves possess an alkaloid, resin, resinic acid, and a bitter substance [2]. *In vitro* toxicity of methanol extract from dried peels was evaluated using the brine shrimp lethality (*Artemia salina*) bioassay; this extract exhibited moderate toxicity (LC_{50}= 409.79 – 5.39 µg/mL) while its antiproliferative activity was determined by the sulforhodamine B (SRB) assay against cervical uterine (HeLa), mammary (MCF-7), and colon (HCT-116 and HCT-15) cell lines. The methanol extract of peels increased the susceptibility of MCF-7/Vin+ cells to vinblastine in a manner similar to the one observed in the positive control (IC_{50} vinblastine/IC_{50} vinblastine in the presence of extract) [27]. Also, Coe *et al.* reported that *A. salina* lethality assay of aqueous extract from *C. cainito* leaves did not show relevant cytotoxicity on brine shrimp (LC_{50}= 3435 µg/mL) [7, 27].

Hegde *et al.* [38] reported acute toxicity in rodents of a hydro-alcoholic extract of fruit; their results showed a lethal dose above 2000 mg/kg body weight suggesting it to be safe for oral consumption [38]. Crude methanol extract and bioactive fraction ($CHCl_3$ fraction) of leaves of *C. cainito* were evaluated by motor coordination test on mice using a horizontal rotarod device set to rotate at 22 rpm. The 3, 10 or 30 mg/kg, i.p doses did not affect locomotor activity, motor coordination or body temperature in healthy mice, suggesting it to not produce any change in the mechanical sensitivity [20].

Shailajan *et al.* [56] reported the evaluation of the safety of the standardized ethanol extract of *C. cainito* leaves. Skin irritation study as per OECD guidelines No. 404 was conducted on three female healthy rabbits and ethanol extract of *C. cainito* leaves (20%) was applied on the patch at the right side (test), while the patch on the left side was selected as a control (without application of the extract). Observations for irritation in terms of erythema and edema were recorded after 24 h, 48 h, and 72 h of topical applications. The results obtained were analyzed to determine the primary irritation index. Skin irritation test of the standardized ethanol extract of *C. cainito* leaves (20%) on rabbits showed no signs of dermal irritation after the topical application. In addition, acute oral toxicity study of the same extract was conducted in male albino Wistar rats (n=5/group) as per OECD Test Guidelines No. 420. Oral administration of the standardized extract to rats did not cause any mortality as well as no significant change in the body weight, food and water intake was observed when compared with the animals of the control group [56].

CONTRAINDICATIONS

None reported.

PRECAUTIONS AND WARNINGS

Surgery

Acute oral toxicity studies in animals ensure an adequate safety margin of *C. cainito* leaves for their intended use [56].

CONCLUSION

Chryspohyllum cainito has proven to possess many pharmacological activities, supporting traditional uses and exhibiting new biological functions such as antinociceptive, antimicrobial, and immunosuppressive. Based on the studies reported here, *C. cainito* is considered a medicinal plant with great value due to its secondary metabolites content and its large potential as a source for developing new drugs helpful in the treatment of non-communicable chronic diseases such as cardiovascular diseases, diabetes, and cancer. In this Chapter, an attempt was made to provide valuable scientific information for future research in drug development based on *C. cainito* as a source of raw material.

CONSENT FOR PUBLICATION

Not applicable.

CONFLICT OF INTEREST

There is no conflict of interest declared.

ACKNOWLEDGEMENTS

A. Sánchez-Recillas, L. Cerón-Romero, R. Ortiz-Andrade and JC. Sánchez-Salgado are members of "Red Mexicana de Investigación Preclínica y Desarrollo Farmacéutico" (REMIDEF).

Authors want to thank Dr. Juan Carlos Sánchez-Salgado for his contribution in manuscript and style corrections.

REFERENCES

[1]　Méndez-González M, Durán-García R, Borges-Argáez R, *et al*. Flora medicinal de los Mayas peninsulares.Pronatura, Península de Yucatán, A C. 1st ed. Mérida, Yucatán, México: Centro de Investigación Científica de Yucatán 2012; p. 69.

[2]　Morton JF. Star Apple. In: Miami FL, Ed. Fruits of warm climates. 1987; pp. 408-10.

[3]   http://www.itis.gov

[4]   Martínez M. Catálogo de nombres vulgares y científicos de plantas mexicanas. FCE México 1979; p. 1220.

[5]   Parker IM, López I, Petersen JJ, Anaya N, Cubilla-Rios L, Potter D. Domestication syndrome in Caimito (Chrysophyllum cainito L.): Fruit and seed characteristics. Econ Bot 2010; 64(2): 161-75.
[http://dx.doi.org/10.1007/s12231-010-9121-4] [PMID: 20543881]

[6]   Luo XD, Basile MJ, Kennelly EJ. Polyphenolic antioxidants from the fruits of Chrysophyllum cainito L. (Star Apple). J Agric Food Chem 2002; 50(6): 1379-82.
[http://dx.doi.org/10.1021/jf011178n] [PMID: 11879006]

[7]   Coe FG, Parikh DM, Johnson CA, Anderson GJ. The good and the bad: alkaloid screening and brineshrimp bioassays of aqueous extracts of 31 medicinal plants of eastern Nicaragua. Pharm Biol 2012; 50(3): 384-92.
[http://dx.doi.org/10.3109/13880209.2011.608077] [PMID: 22117166]

[8]   Baudi J. Plantas medicinales existentes en Venezuela y Latino América. Caracas, Venezuela 1987; pp. 95-6.

[9]   Pérez de los SMA Descripción de algunos frutales tropicales subexplotados en el municipio de Paraíso. Tabasco, México: Tesis. CSAT Cárdenas, Tab 1986; p. 133.

[10]   Roig J. Plantas medicinales, aromáticas o venenosas de Cuba. Habana, Cuba: Ministerio de Agricultura de Cuba. Parte I. 1945; p. 189.

[11]   Flores Vindes E M. Editorial Tecnológica. Costa Rica 1999; II: 773-810.

[12]   Rojas-Rodríguez F, Torres-Córdoba G. Árboles del Valle Central de Costa Rica: reproducción Caimito (Chrysophyllum cainito L) Revista Forestal Mesoamericana Kurú (Costa Rica). 2012; 9.(23)

[13]   Álvarez R, Quintero I, Manzano-Méndez J, Gónzalez D. Emergency and seedlings characteristics from Chrysophyllum cainito L. under differents preemergence treatments and sowing seed position. UDO Agric 2009; 9(2): 333-42.

[14]   Geilfus F. El árbol al servicio del agricultor: manual de agroforestería para el desarrollo rural. Turrialba Costa Rica CATIE ENDA CARIBE 1994; p. 778.

[15]   Petersen JJ, Parker IM, Potter D. Domestication of the neotropical tree Chrysophyllum cainito from a geographically limited yet genetically diverse gene pool in Panama. Ecol Evol 2014; 4(5): 539-53.
[http://dx.doi.org/10.1002/ece3.948] [PMID: 25035796]

[16]   León J. Botánica de los cultivos tropicales. San Jose, Instituto interamericano de cooperación para la agricultura (IICA). Editorial Agroamericana. 3 ed.. 2000; No. 84: p. 178.ISBN92-9039-395 5.

[17]   Petersen JJ, Parker IM, Potter D. Origins and close relatives of a semi-domesticated neotropical fruit tree: Chrysophyllum cainito (Sapotaceae). Am J Bot 2012; 99(3): 585-604.
[http://dx.doi.org/10.3732/ajb.1100326] [PMID: 22396333]

[18]   Crane JH. Chrysophyllum cainito star apple.The Encyclopedia of Fruit & Nuts. Wallingford, U.K: CABI 2008; pp. 825-7.

[19]   Shailajan S, Gurjar D. Pharmacognostic and phytochemical evaluation of Chrysophyllum cainito Linn. leaves. Int J Pharm Sci Rev Res 2014; 26(1): 106-11.

[20]   Meira NA, Klein LC Jr, Rocha LW, *et al.* Anti-inflammatory and anti-hypersensitive effects of the crude extract, fractions and triterpenes obtained from Chrysophyllum cainito leaves in mice. J Ethnopharmacol 2014; 151(2): 975-83.
[http://dx.doi.org/10.1016/j.jep.2013.12.014] [PMID: 24342779]

[21]   Sayed DF, Nada AS, Abd El Hameed Mohamed M, Ibrahim MT. Modulatory effects of Chrysophyllum cainito L. extract on gamma radiation induced oxidative stress in rats. Biomed Pharmacother 2019; 111: 613-23.

[http://dx.doi.org/10.1016/j.biopha.2018.12.137] [PMID: 30611985]

[22]   Ajila CM, Naidu KA, Bhat SG, Prasada Rao UJS. Bioactive compounds and antioxidant potential of mango peel extract. Food Chem 2007; 105(3): 982-8.
[http://dx.doi.org/10.1016/j.foodchem.2007.04.052]

[23]   Vieira FG, Borges GdaS, Copetti C, Gonzaga LV, Nunes EdaC, Fett R. Activity and contents of polyphenolic antioxidants in the whole fruit, flesh and peel of three apple cultivars. Arch Latinoam Nutr 2009; 59(1): 101-6.
[PMID: 19480352]

[24]   Moo-Huchin VM, Moo-Huchin MI, Estrada-León RJ, *et al.* Antioxidant compounds, antioxidant activity and phenolic content in peel from three tropical fruits from Yucatan, Mexico. Food Chem 2015; 166: 17-22.
[http://dx.doi.org/10.1016/j.foodchem.2014.05.127] [PMID: 25053022]

[25]   Pino J, Marbot R, Rosado A. Antimicrobial activities and chemical compositions of Chrysophyllum cainito (Star apple) fruit. Microbiol Res Int 2002; 3(3): 41-50.

[26]   Oranusi SU, Braide W, Umeze RU. Antimicrobial activities and chemical compositions of Chrysophyllum cainito (Star apple) fruit. Microbiol Res Int 2015; 3(3): 41-50.

[27]   Chel-Guerrero LD, Sauri-Duch E, Fragoso-Serrano MC, *et al.* Phytochemical Profile, Toxicity, and Pharmacological Potential of Peels from Four Species of Tropical Fruits. J Med Food 2018; 21(7): 734-43.
[http://dx.doi.org/10.1089/jmf.2017.0124] [PMID: 29481311]

[28]   Aarland RC, Bañuelos-Hernández AE, Fragoso-Serrano M, *et al.* Studies on phytochemical, antioxidant, anti-inflammatory, hypoglycaemic and antiproliferative activities of Echinacea purpurea and Echinacea angustifolia extracts. Pharm Biol 2017; 55(1): 649-56.
[http://dx.doi.org/10.1080/13880209.2016.1265989] [PMID: 27951745]

[29]   Coolborn AF, Bolatito B. Antibacterial and phytochemical evaluation of three medicinal plants. J Nat Prod 2010; 3: 27-34.

[30]   Chang CC, Yang MH, Wen HM, Chern JC. Estimation of total flavonoid content in propolis by two complementary colorimetric methods. Yao Wu Shi Pin Fen Xi 2002; 10: 178-82.

[31]   Kubola J, Siriamornpun S, Meeso N. Phytochemicals, Vitamin C, and sugar content of Thai wild fruit. Food Chem 2011; 126(3): 972-81.
[http://dx.doi.org/10.1016/j.foodchem.2010.11.104]

[32]   Whitam FF, Blaydes DF, Devlin RM. Experiments in Plant Physiology. New York, USA: Van Nostrand Reinhold C. 1971; p. 245.

[33]   Arzudia C, Martinez E, Ayala H, Martinez V. Sapotáceas del sur-occidente de Guatemala. Revista de Ciencia y Tecnología de la Universidad de San Carlos de Guatemala 1997; 1: 35-55.

[34]   Rodríguez-Carpena JG, Morcuende D, Andrade MJ, Kylli P, Estévez M. Avocado (Persea americana Mill.) phenolics, *in vitro* antioxidant and antimicrobial activities, and inhibition of lipid and protein oxidation in porcine patties. J Agric Food Chem 2011; 59(10): 5625-35.
[http://dx.doi.org/10.1021/jf1048832] [PMID: 21480593]

[35]   Arana-Argáez VE, Chan-Zapata I, Canul-Canche J, *et al.* Immunosuppressive effects of the methanolic extract of Chrysophyllum cainito leaves on macrophage functions. Afr J Tradit Complement Altern Med 2016; 14(1): 179-86.
[http://dx.doi.org/10.21010/ajtcam.v14i1.20] [PMID: 28480396]

[36]   Meira NA, Rocha LW, da Silva GF, *et al.* Chrysophyllum cainito leaves are effective against pre-clinical chronic pain models: Analysis of crude extract, fraction and isolated compounds in mice. J Ethnopharmacol 2016; 184: 30-41.
[http://dx.doi.org/10.1016/j.jep.2016.02.046] [PMID: 26945982]

[37]   N'guessan K, Amoikon KE, Tiebre MS, Kadja B, Zirihi GN. Effect of aqueous extract of Chrysophyllum cainito leaves on the glycaemia of diabetic rabbits. Afr J Pharm Pharmacol 2009; 3(10): 501-6.

[38]   Hegde K, Arathi AP, Mathew A. Evaluation of antidiabetic activity of hydro alcoholic extract of Chrysophyllum cainito fruits. Int J Pharm Sci Res 2016; 7(11): 4422-8.

[39]   Doan HV, Riyajan S, Iyara R, Chudapongse N. Antidiabetic activity, glucose uptake stimulation and α-glucosidase inhibitory effect of Chrysophyllum cainito L. stem bark extract. BMC Complement Altern Med 2018; 18(1): 267.
[http://dx.doi.org/10.1186/s12906-018-2328-0] [PMID: 30285723]

[40]   Déciga-Campos M, Ortiz-Andrade R, Sanchez-Recillas A, Flores-Guido JS, Ramírez Camacho MA. Antinociceptive and antihyperalgesic activity of a Traditional maya herbal preparation composed of Pouteria campechiana, Chrysophyllum cainito, Citrus limonum, and Annona muricata. Drug Dev Res 2017; 78(2): 91-7.
[http://dx.doi.org/10.1002/ddr.21378] [PMID: 28176363]

[41]   Tjølsen A, Berge OG, Hunskaar S, Rosland JH, Hole K. The formalin test: an evaluation of the method. Pain 1992; 51(1): 5-17.
[http://dx.doi.org/10.1016/0304-3959(92)90003-T] [PMID: 1454405]

[42]   Dowdall T, Robinson I, Meert TF. Comparison of five different rat models of peripheral nerve injury. Pharmacol Biochem Behav 2005; 80(1): 93-108.
[http://dx.doi.org/10.1016/j.pbb.2004.10.016] [PMID: 15652385]

[43]   Mao LM, Qi XW, Hao JH, Liu HF, Xu QH, Bu PL. *In vitro*, *ex vivo* and *in vivo* anti-hypertensive activity of Chrysophyllum cainito L. extract. Int J Clin Exp Med 2015; 8(10): 17912-21.
[PMID: 26770385]

[44]   Lin L, Lv S, Li B. Angiotensin-I-converting enzyme (ACE)-inhibitory and antihypertensive properties of squid skin gelatin hydrolysates. Food Chem 2012; 131: 225-30.
[http://dx.doi.org/10.1016/j.foodchem.2011.08.064]

[45]   Sánchez-Recillas A, Yáñez-Pérez V, Ibarra-Barajas M, *et al.* Pharmacological and toxicological study of a Traditional Mayan herbal preparation used as antihypertensive agent. European J Med Plants 2018; 24(3): 1-11.
[http://dx.doi.org/10.9734/EJMP/2018/42504]

[46]   da Rosa RL, de Almeida CL, Somensi LB, *et al.* Chrysophyllum cainito (Apple-star): a fruit with gastroprotective activity in experimental ulcer models Inflammopharmacol. Available from 2017; pp. 1-12. [Cited: 12th June 2019]

[47]   Mizui T, Doteuchi M. Effect of polyamines on acidified ethanol-induced gastric lesions in rats. Jpn J Pharmacol 1983; 33(5): 939-45.
[http://dx.doi.org/10.1254/jjp.33.939] [PMID: 6580476]

[48]   Eamlamnam K, Patumraj S, Visedopas N, Thong-Ngam D. Effects of Aloe vera and sucralfate on gastric microcirculatory changes, cytokine levels and gastric ulcer healing in rats. World J Gastroenterol 2006; 12(13): 2034-9.
[http://dx.doi.org/10.3748/wjg.v12.i13.2034] [PMID: 16610053]

[49]   Mowry R, Winkler CH. The coloration of acidic carbo hydrates of bacteria and fungi in tissue sections with special reference to capsules of Cryptococcus neoformans, Pneumococci and Staphilococci. Am J Pathol 1956; 32: 628-39.

[50]   Corne SJ, Morrissey SM, Woods RJA. Proceedings: A method for the quantitative estimation of gastric barrier mucus. J Physiol 1974; 242(2): 116P-7P.
[PMID: 4142046]

[51]   Rainsford KD, Whitehouse MW. Biochemical gastroprotection from acute ulceration induced by aspirin and related drugs. Biochem Pharmacol 1980; 29(9): 1281-9.

[http://dx.doi.org/10.1016/0006-2952(80)90286-5] [PMID: 7397011]

[52]   Beber AP, de Souza P, Boeing T, *et al.* Constituents of leaves from Bauhinia curvula Benth. exert gastroprotective activity in rodents: role of quercitrin and kaempferol. Inflammopharmacology 2018; 26(2): 539-50. [Cited: 13th June 2019].
[http://dx.doi.org/10.1007/s10787-017-0313-8] [PMID: 28176198]

[53]   Arrieta J, Benitez J, Flores E, Castillo C, Navarrete A. Purification of gastroprotective triterpenoids from the stem bark of Amphipterygium adstringens; role of prostaglandins, sulfhydryls, nitric oxide and capsaicin-sensitive neurons. Planta Med 2003; 69(10): 905-9.
[http://dx.doi.org/10.1055/s-2003-45098] [PMID: 14648392]

[54]   Matsuda H, Li Y, Yoshikawa M. Roles of capsaicin-sensitive sensory nerves, endogenous nitric oxide, sulfhydryls, and prostaglandins in gastroprotection by momordin Ic, an oleanolic acid oligoglycoside, on ethanol-induced gastric mucosal lesions in rats. Life Sci 1999; 65(2): PL27-32.
[http://dx.doi.org/10.1016/S0024-3205(99)00241-6] [PMID: 10416830]

[55]   Shay H, Komarov SA, Fels SS, Marenze D, Grunstein M, Siplet H. A simple method for the uniform production of gastric ulceration in the rat. Gastroenterology 1945; 5: 43-61.

[56]   Shailajan S, Gurjar D. Wound healing activity of Chrysophyllum cainito L. leaves: Evaluation in rats using excision wound model. J Young Pharm 2016; 8(2): 96-103.
[http://dx.doi.org/10.5530/jyp.2016.2.7]

SUBJECT INDEX

A

ABTS assays 199
Acid 47, 63, 78, 75, 99, 100, 101, 102, 132,
    135, 146, 155, 168, 170, 171, 175, 174,
    176, 177, 178, 194, 195, 197, 198
   acacic 170
   Angelic 132
   aristolochic 176
   ascorbic 146, 168, 174, 195
   chlorogenic 99, 100
   Cubebic 78
   deoxyribonucleic 63
   echinocystic 170
   ferulic 195
   gallic 171, 177, 194, 198
   hexacosanoic 171
   loganic 101, 102
   oleanolic 75, 135, 170, 172, 176, 178
   succinic 177
   uric 47
Actin cytoskeletons 18, 20
Activation 10, 16, 17, 18, 19, 20, 21, 22, 23,
    27, 28, 49, 110, 129, 130, 146, 148, 152,
    153
   of extracellular signal-regulated protein
     kinase 27
   mediated inflammatory 23
   metabolic 49
   serine/threonine kinase 28
Activity 20, 21, 46, 48, 49, 51, 63, 69, 70, 73,
    74, 81, 82, 84, 99, 103, 105, 106, 133,
    142, 143, 144, 148, 149, 153, 154, 155,
    156, 172, 173, 175, 176, 179, 200, 201,
    203, 205
   analgesic 175
   antiatherogenic 148
   antiatherosclerosis 48
   anti-atherosclerotic 155
   antibacterial 63
   anticholinesterase 144
   antidepressant 133
   anti-diabetic 69, 70, 73, 74, 103

   antiglycation 143
   anti-hyperglycemic 173
   anti-hypersensitivity 201
   antihypertensive 176, 203
   anti-hypertensive 81
   anti-inflammatory 46, 155, 175, 201
   antimutagenic 49
   antiproliferative 205
   hemostasis 156
   hepatoprotective 51
   hypertensive 179
   hypocholesterolemic 142
   hypoglycaemic 106
   hypolipidemic 149
   hypotensive 156
Adiponectin 10
Adipose tissue 4, 5, 22
   dysfunction 4, 5
   lipolysis 22
Agent 47, 63, 146, 148, 156, 180
   cardioprotective 146, 148
   non-toxic therapeutic 180
   strong anti-bacterial 63
Ajwa date 42, 51
Ajwain 177
Alcoholic extract 70, 74
Alcohols 40, 62, 79, 135
   arteannuic 79
Alkaline phosphatase 139, 142
Alkaloids 38, 41, 48, 50, 79, 169, 170, 171,
    189, 190, 192
   isoquinoline 171
Allium 83, 172, 173, 179
   cepa 82, 172, 179
   sativum 83, 173, 179
Alpha-adrenergic receptor antagonist 204
Alzheimer's disease 47, 48, 49
   curcumin 47
AMK-dependent mechanism 20
Amyloid angiopathy 68
Anchusa officinalis 69, 77
Ancient Chinese methods 67
Angiogenesis 141
Annona 173, 175, 199, 202

reductase 146
Glutathione peroxidase 143, 146, 152
  activities 143
  enzyme activities 143
Glycogenesis 67
Glycogenolysis 14
Glycogen 17, 18 19, 20
  synthase 17, 20
  synthesis 17, 18, 19
Glycolysis 14, 67, 76, 110, 154
Glycoprotein 27
Glycosides 41, 78, 79, 127, 169, 170, 205
  cyanogenic 205
Glycosylated hemoglobin levels 43, 139
Glycosylates hemoglobin 140
Glycyrrhetinic acid 127, 149, 150, 151
  acts on cardiac tissue 150
  cardioprotective activity of 150, 151
  in cardiovascular diseases 149
Glycyrrhetinic acid in diabetes 149
Grape-seed procyanidin extract (GSPE) 111
Growth 9, 17, 19, 28, 46, 63, 129, 131, 137
  cellular 28
  mycelial 63
  transforming 129
GTPase-activating protein 20
Gut 96, 103, 113
  lumen 113
  microbiota 103
  peptides 96

H

Haemoglobin 48 75
  glycosylated 48
Heart 64. 65, 85, 129
  attack 65, 85, 129
  stroke 64
Heartbeats, irregular 129
Heart failure 80, 129, 130
  congestive 80
Helicobacter pylori 63
Hemodynamic systems 127
Hepatic 13, 22, 25
  de novo lipogenesis 22
  glucose production (HGP) 13, 25
Hepatocyte 6, 40
  necrosis 40
  nuclear factor 6
Hepatoprotective action 47

Herbal medicine 41, 102
  therapeutic 102
  and diabetes mellitus 41
High 48, 64, 65, 68, 72, 79, 81, 85, 150, 152,
  167, 168, 176, 201
  blood pressure 64, 65, 68, 79, 81, 85, 167,
    168, 176
  -density lipoprotein (HDL) 48, 72, 150,
    152, 201
Homeostasis 11, 25, 98, 148
  lipid 148
  metabolic 25
Hormones 1, 9, 13, 28, 67, 115, 128, 131, 137
  anabolic peptide 1, 13, 28
  glucagonotropic 115
  pancreatic 67
Human renal cancer cells 46
Hypercholesterolemia 176, 179
Hyperglycemia 4, 7, 8, 12, 21, 23, 25, 38, 39,
  40, 66, 67, 69, 128, 129, 130, 141, 146
  chronic 4, 69
  fasting 5, 141
  reduced 146
Hyperinsulinemia 4, 12, 22, 23, 154, 168
  compensatory 4
  euglycemic 4
  hyperglycemic 4
Hyperlipidemia 47, 71, 154
Hypersensitivity 200
Hypertension 80, 144,1 48
  genetic 148
  intense 80
  monocrotaline-induced pulmonary 144
  reduced monocrotaline-induced 144
Hypertrophy-associated cardiac fibrosis 147
Hypoglycemic activity 41, 44, 47, 49, 50, 51,
  52, 74, 148, 173
  of *Gymnema sylvestre* 47
  of *Piper nigrum* 49
  of *Sesamum indicum* 50

I

Impaired 11, 12
  glucose tolerance (IGT) 11
  insulin action and hyperglycemia 12
Inflammation 4, 8, 12, 51, 127, 128, 154, 155,
  176, 179, 190, 199
  biological defense mechanism 51
Inflammatory 4, 46, 47, 201

effects 10, 17
Transcriptional factor 17, 51
  activity 17
  inhibitors 51
Transcriptional repressor 26, 27
  in liver cells 26
Transcription factors 6, 9, 12, 15, 17, 26
  activating 9
  phosphorylates 17
Transmission electron microscopy 150
Tumorigenesis 20
Tumour necrosis factor 12
Tyrosine autophosphorylation 15
Tyrosine kinase 12, 15, 16, 19, 20, 22, 28
  activity 15, 22
  antigen-related 20
  insulin receptor 19
  phosphorylation 12
  receptors 15, 28
Tyrosine phosphatases 16, 20, 153
  cytoplasmic protein 20
Tyrosine phosphorylation 15, 22, 23
  insulin-stimulated 22

U

Ulcer 203, 204
  indomethacin-induced 203
  indomethacin-induced gastric 204
Unfolded protein response (UPR) 10
Urine 25, 40, 66, 67, 141
  sugar levels 141
Ursolic acid 127, 135, 147, 148, 149, 194
  in cardiovascular diseases 148
  in diabetes 147
  oral treatment of 148

V

Vascular 46, 129, 168
  diseases 129, 168
  system 46
Vasodilatory activity of corosolic acid 155
Very-low-density lipoprotein (VLDL) 14

W

World Health Organisation (WHO) 2, 40, 41,
    61, 127, 128, 129, 156, 167

Wound healing 47, 141

Z

Zingiber officinale 85